Surgical Anatomy of the Internal Carotid Artery

Paolo Castelnuovo • Iacopo Dallan
Manfred Tschabitscher

Surgical Anatomy of the Internal Carotid Artery

An Atlas for Skull Base Surgeons

Springer

Authors
Paolo Castelnuovo
Department of Otorhinolaryngology
University of Insubria
Ospedale di Circolo e
Fondazione Macchi
Varese
Italy

Iacopo Dallan
Department of Otorhinolaryngology
University of Insubria
Ospedale di Circolo e
Fondazione Macchi
Varese
Italy

Manfred Tschabitscher
Medical University of Vienna
Vienna
Austria

ISBN 978-3-642-29663-5 ISBN 978-3-642-29664-2 (eBook)
DOI 10.1007/978-3-642-29664-2
Springer Heidelberg New York Dordrecht London

Library of Congress Control Number: 2012952507

Printed on acid-free paper

Springer is part of Springer Science+Business Media (www.springer.com)

To my friends Renato Galzio and in memoriam Axel Perneczky.
Manfred Tschabitscher

To Lorella and our children. Their presence and love make me go on studying and improving.
Paolo Castelnuovo

In loving memory of my father. I'm so grateful and proud to be your son!!
Iacopo Dallan

Foreword

> *All truths are easy to understand once they are discovered; the point is to discover them.*
>
> *Galileo Galilei* (*1564–1642*)

When running through the pages of the manuscript of this atlas for the first time, I could not find words to describe the stunning beauty of the images with their fascinating attention to detail, their unseen-before quality of anatomical preparation and dissection, the precision of both photographic as well as schematic documentation and explanations—and my first impression was: *What a piece of masterly art!*

Dissecting the internal carotid artery along its different segments in high quality, explaining the topographical relations in each of them, is one achievement the authors have met with excellence: to integrate and display views of different surgical corridors into their dissection opens "windows of opportunity" for skull base surgeons that have been explored over the last decade by a few—and shall I say daring?—expert surgeons only. This book makes available to all who are interested in skull base surgery the complexity of anatomy, yet at the same time the beauty of it: I consider this atlas a milestone in the history of endoscopic and other skull base surgery. The authors have to be congratulated for this masterpiece, which will become the gold standard for experts and beginners, for surgeons and anatomists, as well as for radiologists instantly:

> Can one desire too much of a good thing?
> William Shakespeare: As you like it

No!

Graz, Austria

Heinz Stammberger, M.D.
Department of Otorhinolaryngology
University of Graz

Preface

Sine anatomia non sciemus

Knowledge of human anatomy is one of the bases for the exercise of medicine. The considerable growth of core disciplines such as physiology, genetics, and immunology has led to major development of the teaching of these disciplines over the past 20 years, increasingly limiting the teaching of anatomy, which is sometimes considered a "too old" discipline. At the same time, during the last decade the growth and development of new surgical techniques (especially endoscopically assisted ones) and their everyday application has been phenomenal. This dichotomy is probably the most important reason for this book: Although we could be wrong, we strongly believe that there is a pressing need for a text atlas that provides essential (but not excessive) information pictorially accompanied by cadaveric correlation. In other words, an atlas that is simple, concise, and informative.

This book covers the relevant anatomy of the regions surrounding the internal carotid artery, which is the "queen structure" of the whole skull base. Arbitrarily, the book has been divided into three parts focusing on different segments of the internal carotid artery: the cervical, the skull base, and the intracranial. The text of each chapter is deliberately simple and clear, and the illustrations offer a three-dimensional multiperspective representation of the regions, with direct correlation to neuroradiological imaging.

Philosophically speaking, we are strongly convinced that there exists only *one anatomy*—but several ways of looking at it. So, all the effort has been directed toward offering a multiperspective visualization of the anatomic fields to create a three-dimensional, truly orienting vision of the spaces.

We wish to express our deep gratitude to all our coworkers for the support, help, and encouragement shown throughout the project.

We hope that this new anatomic atlas, deliberately dedicated to clinical and practical application, meets the modern requirement of simplification to the essential and will serve as a necessary step toward new surgical approaches. But above all, we hope that it will be a useful tool for all those who are involved in the fascinating field of skull base surgery.

Austria — Manfred Tschabitscher
Italy — Paolo Castelnuovo
Italy — Iacopo Dallan

Acknowledgement

Authors would like to thank Prof. Alberto Prats Galino and Matteo de Notaris for their kindness. Pictures 1.12, 1.28 (inferior-right), 1.32 (superior-right), 1.34 (inferior-left), 1.37 (inferior), 1.49 (right), 3.78 (inferior), 3.80, 3.84 have been taken in the Laboratory of Surgical Neuroanatomy (LSNA), Faculty of Medicine, University of Barcelona (Head Prof. Alberto Prats Galino).

Contents

Collaborators

- Paolo Battaglia
- Maurizio Bignami
- Mirco Cosottini
- Riccardo Lenzi
- Davide Locatelli
- Anna Mercuri
- Veronica Seccia
- Giustino Tomei
- Mario Turri-Zanoni

Cervical Segment 1

1.1 Anatomic Layout

The cervical segment of the internal carotid artery (ICA) starts in the neck at the common carotid artery (CCA) bifurcation and ends at the level of the carotid foramen. This segment is both extradural and extracranial. Conventionally, the cervical ICA can be divided into a proximal and distal part. The border between the two segments is not universally accepted. In this atlas, we assumed that the proximal segment extends from the carotid bifurcation to the point where the vessel is crossed by the posterior belly of the digastric muscle, and the distal segment is from this point to the entrance of the vessel into the carotid canal. These external landmarks are virtually useless when describing ICA anatomy from an anterior, endoscopic perspective.

1.1.1 Proximal Segment

At the level of the neck, the proximal part of the ICA usually presents a vertical course and a strict relationship with the internal jugular vein (IJV) and the vagus nerve. Usually, the carotid bifurcation is localized at the level of the upper border of the thyroid cartilage. Close to this, it is possible to visualize the *carotid sinus*, a localized area of dilation, and the *carotid body* (*glomus caroticum*). The last is appreciable on the posteromedial wall of the carotid bifurcation. Above the bifurcation, the ICAp (parapharyngeal portion of the ICA) ascends under the sternocleidomastoid muscle. This portion of the vessel presents, on its lateral surface, a critical relationship with the *hypoglossal nerve*, which courses along the inferior border of the posterior belly of the digastric muscle and goes toward the tongue. Above this level, the ICAp is crossed by the *occipital artery* (Janfaza and Fabian 2001a, b). More inferiorly, the *ansa hypoglossi* runs on the anterolateral surface of the CCA. The *vagus nerve* is placed deep between the CCA/ICA and the IJV, and it is enclosed in the carotid sheath while the *accessory nerve* runs beneath the most posterior aspect of the posterior belly of the digastric muscle, in 2/3 of the cases over the IJV and in 1/3 below, moving posteriorly and inferiorly toward the anterior border of the sternocleidomastoid muscle (Janfaza and Fabian 2001a, b). In more than 80 %, it passes through the sternocleidomastoid muscle (Janfaza and Fabian 2001a, b). Anteriorly to the ICA, the *superior laryngeal nerve* can be visualized. In more detail, the nerve can be identified in between the external carotid artery (ECA), stylohyoid muscle, and the superior thyroid artery, with which it usually maintains a close relationship. On its medial surface, the ICAp presents a close relationship with the superior constrictor muscle and to some extent to the tonsillar fossa.

1.1.2 Cranial Segment

Cranial to the posterior belly of the digastric muscle, the ICA is covered and separated from the ECA by the styloid apparatus. The ECA is

P. Castelnuovo et al., *Surgical Anatomy of the Internal Carotid Artery*,
DOI 10.1007/978-3-642-29664-2_1, © Springer-Verlag Berlin Heidelberg 2013

located anterolaterally to the ICA. With a lateral perspective, the stylohyoid muscle is the first muscle encountered; the stylopharyngeus muscle is the most medial. The styloglossus lies in between and anterior to the other two muscles. Below the inferior part of the styloid process, the glossopharyngeal nerve can be visualized. It lies medial to the styloid process and lateral and in close proximity to the stylopharyngeus muscle. The nerve courses in a posterior-to-anterior direction, first posterior to the stylopharyngeus muscle and then lateral and anterior to it. At the end, it runs medially, innervating the pharyngeal wall muscles. Usually, the glossopharyngeal nerve is accompanied by the pharyngeal branch(es) from the vagus nerve. The glossopharyngeal nerve can be identified in a triangle given by the styloglossus/stylopharyngeus, the ECA, and the facial artery (Cavalcanti et al. 2010). At this level, the ICA is "covered" by a thick fascia, *stylopharyngeal aponeurosis*, connecting the posteromedial surface of the styloid process to the pharyngeal recess (Rhoton 2000). This fascia separates the *carotid space* (previously named the *poststyloid compartment*) from the prestyloid compartment, and belongs to the styloid diaphragm. More exactly, it represents its medial aspect. Anatomically speaking, the styloid diaphragm is given by the posterior belly of the digastric muscle, stylohyoid, stylopharyngeus, and stylopharygeal aponeurosis.

Posteriorly, the ICA presents a close relationship with the *longus capitis muscle* (in its lateral aspect), the superior sympathetic chain and ganglion, the vagus nerve, and to some extent the IJV. At this level (more or less C1), the "jugular" and hypoglossal nerves pass between the ICA and the IJV (Janfaza and Fabian 2001a, b). The superior cervical ganglion lies on the longus capitis muscle, medial to the vagus nerve and within a duplication of the prevertebral fascia, at the C2–3 level. After its exit from the jugular foramen (JF), the IJV initially lies on the rectus capitis lateralis muscle, crosses the transverse process of C1, and then presents an anterior and lateral position with respect to the transverse processes of the other vertebrae. Going inferiorly, it becomes lateral to the ICA/CCA and lies on the surface of the levator scapulae and middle and anterior scalene muscles. Superiorly and laterally, it is separated from the parotid gland by the stylopharyngeus muscle and the styloid process. The *vagus nerve* remains behind and somewhat between the vessels during its pathway. The *accessory nerve* runs inferiorly as the most posterior of the three nerves, crossing the IJV (in 2/3 of the cases, above the IJV). It presents a strict relationship with the transverse process of C1. The *hypoglossal nerve*, once it exits from its own foramen, comes in close relationship with the IX, X, and XI cranial nerves. It lies medial to the IJV and ICA and passes laterally and inferiorly, together with the sympathetic trunk, between the IJV and ICA. At the level of the transverse process of C1, it turns anteriorly on the lateral surface of the ICA, and then it curves around the occipital artery and runs first to the lateral and then to the anterior surface of the ECA. Inferiorly, it lies lateral to ICA and ECA and deep to the styloid process.

1.1.3 Jugular Foramen Region

Anatomically speaking, the JF does not correspond to a single hole but is a canal given by the basioccipital bone (posteromedially) and the petrous bone (anterolaterally) (Rhoton 2003; Roche et al. 2008). Within the JF, three compartments can be described: a large posterolateral venous channel (*sigmoid*); a small anteromedial venous compartment (*petrosal*), which receives the drainage of the inferior petrosal sinus (IPS); and an intermediary neural compartment (*intrajugular*), located between the venous ones (Katsuta et al. 1997; Rhoton 2003).

The *anterior or petrosal compartment* is given by a small venous channel that receives the IPS.

The relationship with the IPS is highly variable. This sinus drains into the anterior aspect of the jugular bulb in more than 90 % of cases (Roche et al. 2008); in less than 10 % of cases, it drains directly into the IJV. Sometimes, a poorly developed IPS has connection with the plexus of the hypoglossal canal (also named the anterior condylar vein), the petroclival vein, or the posterior condylar emissary vein. This last vein puts the vertebral venous plexus into communication with the jugular bulb (Roche et al. 2008).

The *medial intrajugular compartment* includes neural structures, venous channels, and arterial vessels. The glossopharyngeal nerve is separated from the vagus and accessory nerve by means of a dural fold (*dural septum*) and a venous channel. If the dural fold is ossificated it is called Hayek's bridge. The *glossopharyngeal nerve,* when it exits through the JF, forms a superior and inferior ganglion. The inferior ganglion is placed in a small fossa, the *fossula petrosa*, placed between the carotid canal and the jugular foramen. Then, the nerve courses along the posteromedial aspect of the ICA; at the level of the skull base, it gives the *Jacobson's nerve*, which enters its own canaliculus (*canaliculus tympanicus*) to reach the middle ear (Lang 1995; Osawa et al. 2008). Then, the nerve, after giving some anastomotic branches for cranial nerve X, runs on the lateral surface of the ICA and buries itself within the vagina carotica, coursing anteriorly and inferiorly to the vessel. At the level of the inferior ganglion, there are some twigs that anastomose with similar ones from the vagus nerve and from the sympathetic chain to form the *ramus sinus carotici of Hering*.

The *vagus nerve* enters the dura through the *vagal meatus* (Rhoton 2003), and it is immediately joined by the accessory nerve. Immediately lateral to the intrajugular process of the temporal bone, the superior ganglion lies. At this level, the vagus nerve branches off the Arnold nerve (auricular branch), which enters a mastoid canaliculus and goes toward the third part of the facial nerve. When the vagus nerve emerges from the superior ganglion, it passes posteriorly to the carotid sheath together with the accessory nerve. The inferior ganglion is located anterior to the transverse process of C1–C2. At this level, a small pharyngeal branch arises, which connects with the pharyngeal branch of cranial nerve IX. Below this, the superior laryngeal nerve arises.

The *accessory nerve* lies immediately lateral to the vagus nerve and presents a close relationship with it. It divides into 2 rami at the JF. The internal one (accessory ramus of the vagus nerve) joins the vagus nerve just below the JF, while the external one acts as the accessory nerve for trapezius and sternocleidomastoid muscle. Both nerves (accessory and vagus) are posterior to the glossopharyngeal nerve. Below the JF, usually they are on the posteromedial wall of the IJV. Obviously, the nerve position can be different with respect to the IJV. In about 60 %, the nerve is anterior to the IJV; in the remaining cases, it is behind the IJV. Rarely, it can run through the connecting vein between the IPS and the IJV and then course dorsal to the styloid process.

The *posterior compartment* is occupied by a wide venous channel that drains the sigmoid sinus. It is mainly given by the superior jugular bulb, which is housed in the jugular fossa. Usually the posterior meningeal artery enters this space.

Anatomically speaking, the hypoglossal nerve does not belong to the JF, but given its close relationship, it is included in a description of the JF region. The exit point of the hypoglossal nerve is medial and below the JF. The nerve exits from the anterior condylar foramen and lies posterior to IX, X and XI cranial nerves and on the medial surface of the IJV. Then, it passes laterally between the IJV and the ICA (through the carotid sheath) (Janfaza et al. 2001). So, from an anatomic viewpoint, the hypoglossal nerve does not transverse the JF but joins the "jugular" nerves just below the skull. At the level of the transverse process of C1, it turns frontward, lying on the lateral surface of the ICA.

1.2 Anatomic Pictures

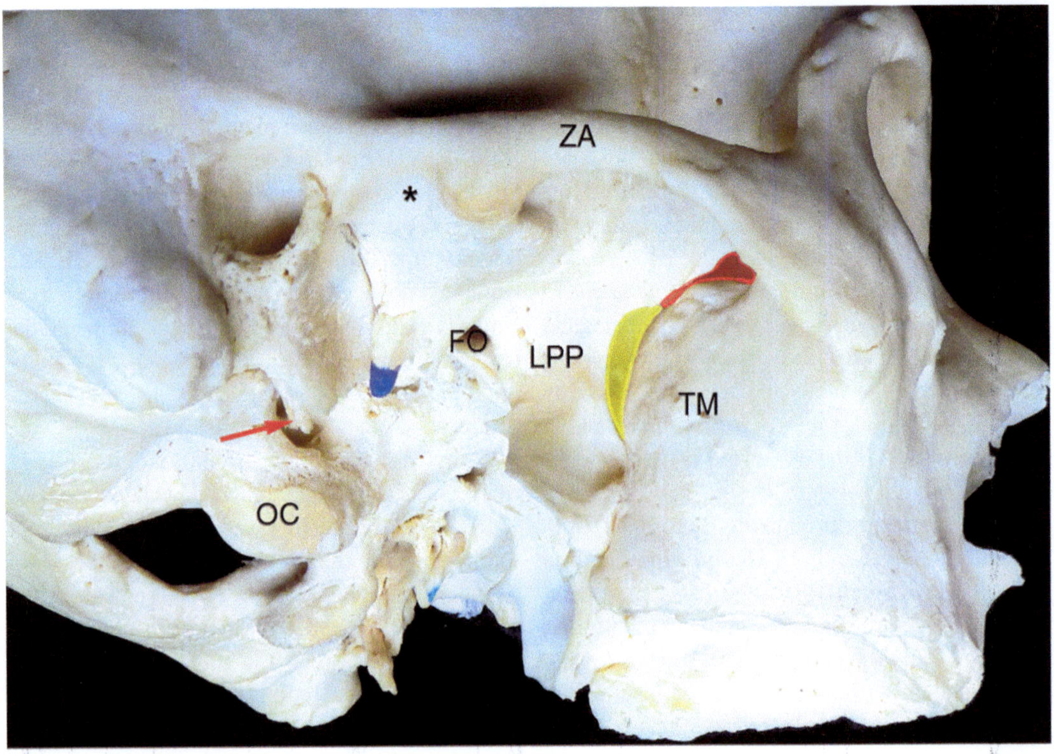

Fig. 1.1 Infratemporal fossa-osteology

FO **foramen ovale,** ***LPP*** **lateral pterygoid plate,** ***OC*** **occipital condyle,** ***TM*** **tuberosity of the maxilla,** ***ZA*** **zygomatic arch,** ***black asterisk*** **glenoid fossa,** ***blue*** **spine of the sphenoid,** ***yellow*** **pterygopalatine fissure,** ***red*** **inferior orbital fissure,** ***red arrow*** **styloid process**

The pterygomaxillary fissure is a narrow V shaped fissure between the LPP and the superior portion of the tuberosity of the maxilla. The upper part of the pterygomaxillary fissure joins the inferior orbital fissure. The pterygo-palatine fossa communicates with the infratemporal fossa (ITF) by means of the pterygomaxillary fissure laterally. Behind the inferior orbital fissure lies the ITF, which is mainly located below the greater wing of the sphenoid.

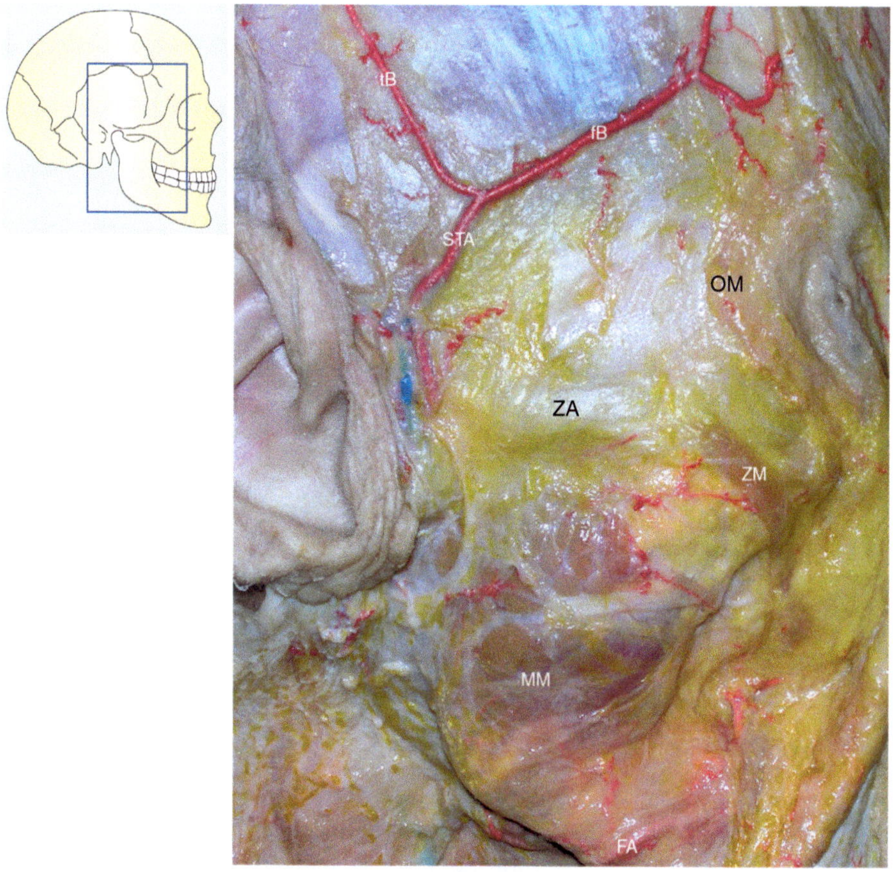

Fig. 1.2 Lateral vision of the temporozygomatic region

***FA* facial artery, *fB* frontal branch, *MM* masseter muscle, *OM* orbicularis oculi muscle, *STA* superficial temporal artery, *tB* temporal branch, *ZA* zygomatic arch, *ZM* zygomatic muscle**

The parotid-masseteric fascia covers the masseteric muscle and surrounds the parotid gland. It attaches superiorly to the zygomatic arch and extends deep to the posterior border of the ramus of the mandible, fusing with the fascia of the posterior belly of the digastric muscle, to give the stylomandibular ligament (Janfaza and Fabian 2001b).

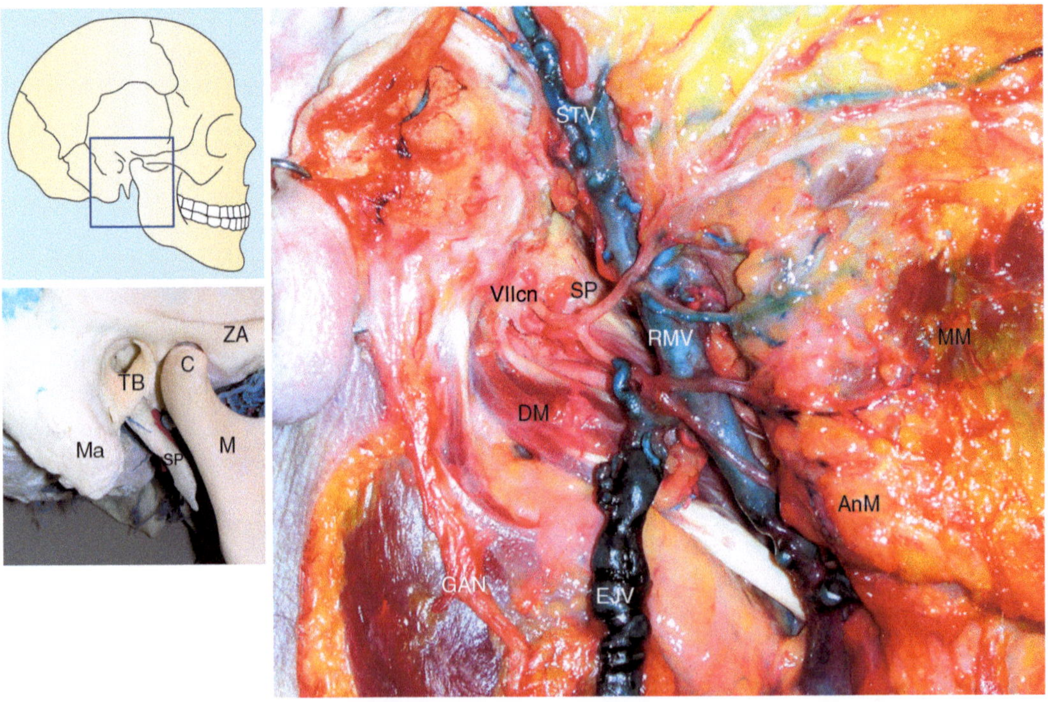

Fig. 1.3 Lateral vision of the parotid-cervical region. The facial nerve has been dissected and the parotid gland removed

AnM **angle of the mandible,** ***C*** **condyle,** ***EJV*** **external jugular vein,** ***GAN*** **greater auricular nerve,** ***M*** **mandible,** ***Ma*** **mastoid,** ***MM*** **masseter muscle,** ***RMV*** **retromandibular vein,** ***SP*** **styloid process,** ***STV*** **superficial temporal vein,** ***TB*** **tympanic bone,** ***ZA*** **zygomatic arch,** ***VIIcn*** **facial nerve**

The maxillary vein joins the superficial temporal vein in the parotid gland, forming the RMV. The facial nerve lies lateral to the RMV.

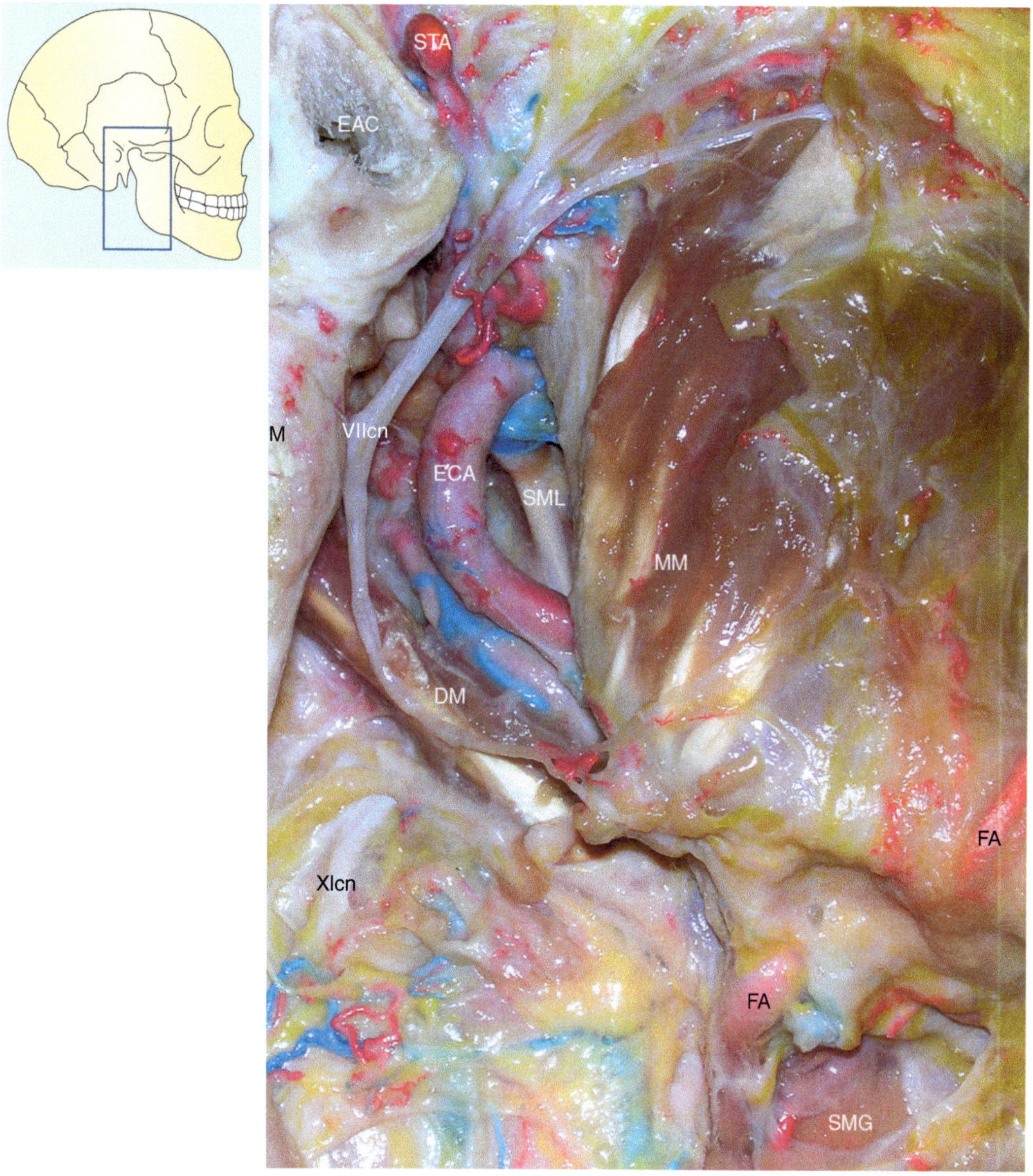

Fig. 1.4 Parotid fossa. The parotid gland has been removed and the deeper areas exposed

***DM* digastric muscle (posterior belly), *EAC* external acoustic canal, *ECA* external carotid artery, *FA* facial artery, *M* mastoid, *MM* masseter muscle, *SMG* submandibular gland, *SML* spheno-mandibular ligament, *STA* superficial temporal artery, *VIIcn* facial nerve, *XI* accessory nerve**

The parotid-masseteric fascia covers the masseteric muscle and splits to involve the parotid gland. Deeply and posteriorly, it fuses with the fascia of the digastric muscle to give the stylo-mandibular ligament.

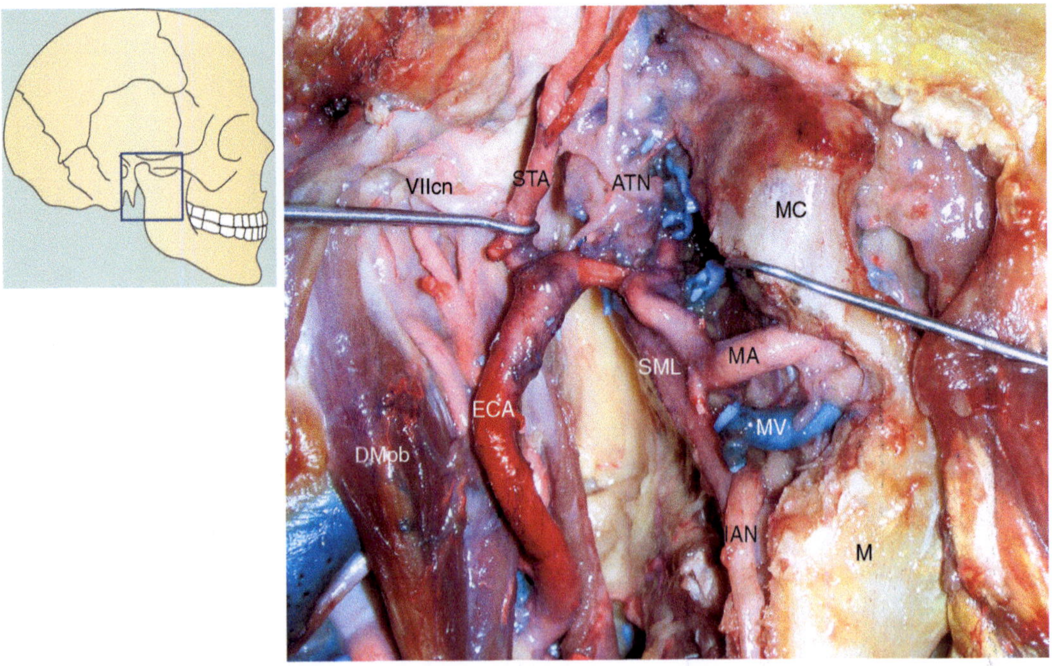

Fig. 1.5 Parotid region. The inferior part of the neck of the mandibular condyle has been partially removed

ATN **auriculotemporal nerve,** ***DMpb*** **posterior belly of the digastric muscle,** ***ECA*** **external carotid artery,** ***IAN*** **inferior alveolar nerve,** ***M*** **mandible,** ***MA*** **maxillary artery,** ***MC*** **mandibular condyle,** ***MV*** **maxillary vein,** ***SML*** **sphenomandibular ligament,** ***STA*** **superficial temporal artery,** ***VIIcn*** **facial nerve**

The MA enters the infratemporal fossa, passing between the mandibular condyle and the SML. At this level, it usually lies below the ATN and above the MV. Usually, it passes lateral to the nerves, and only in less than 5 % of cases it is deep to all the branches of V3. Only the first part of the MA is accompanied by the MV, the second and third parts are accompanied by a venous plexus. The MV(s) unite with the superficial temporal vein to form the retromandibular vein. The ATN emerges from the upper border of the parotid gland behind the temporomandibular joint and then runs over the root of the zygomatic arch posterior to the STA.

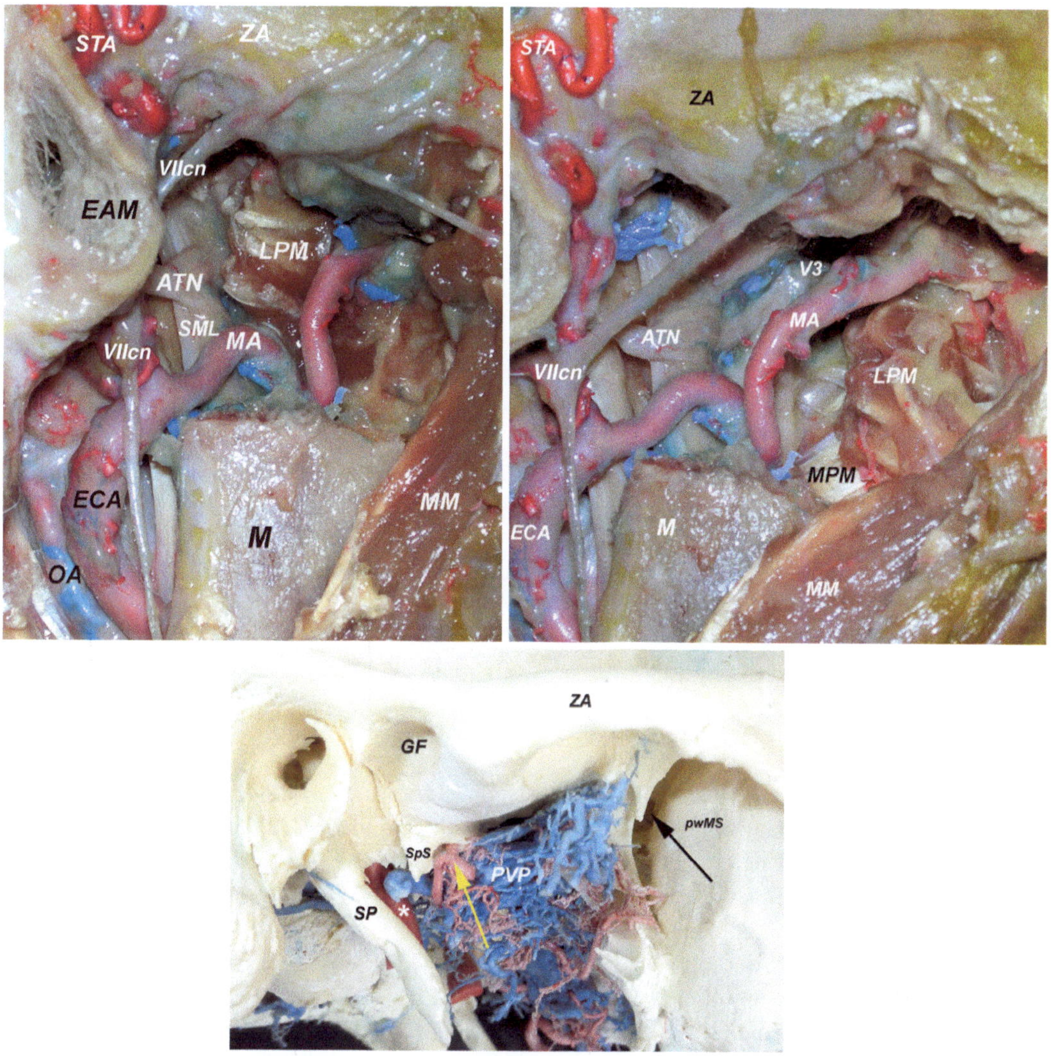

Fig. 1.6 Infratemporal fossa exposure. The condyle and the neck of the mandible have been removed

ATN **auriculotemporal nerve,** ***EAM*** **external acoustic meatus,** ***ECA*** **external carotid artery,** ***GF*** **glenoid fossa,** ***LPM*** **lateral pterygoid muscle,** ***M*** **mandible,** ***MA*** **maxillary artery,** ***MM*** **masseter muscle,** ***MPM*** **medial pterygoid muscle,** ***OA*** **occipital artery,** ***pwMS*** **posterior wall of the maxillary sinus,** ***PVP*** **pterygoid venous plexus,** ***SML*** **sphenomandibular ligament,** ***SP*** **styloid process,** ***SpS*** **spine of the sphenoid,** ***STA*** **superficial temporal artery,** ***ZA*** **zygomatic arch,** ***V3*** **third branch of the trigeminal nerve,** ***VIIcn*** **facial nerve,** ***black arrow*** **pterygopalatine fossa,** ***yellow arrow*** **middle meningeal artery,** ***white asterisk*** **parapharyngeal portion of the internal carotid artery**

The infratemporal fossa communicates medially with pterygopalatine fossa and posteromedially with the parapharyngeal space. The MA is 1 of the 2 terminal branches of the ECA; the other is the STA. During its course within the infratemporal fossa, its relationship with the LPM is highly variable. The PVP lies between temporalis, lateral, and medial pterygoid muscles (Janfaza and Montgomery 2001). PVP can comunicate directly with the cavernous sinus through Foramen of Vesalius (when it is present). The pterygoid fascia encases both pterygoid muscles and attaches to the stylomandibular ligament. The sphenomandibular ligament is a fascial condensation between the spine of the sphenoid and the lingula of the mandible (Janfaza and Fabian 2001).

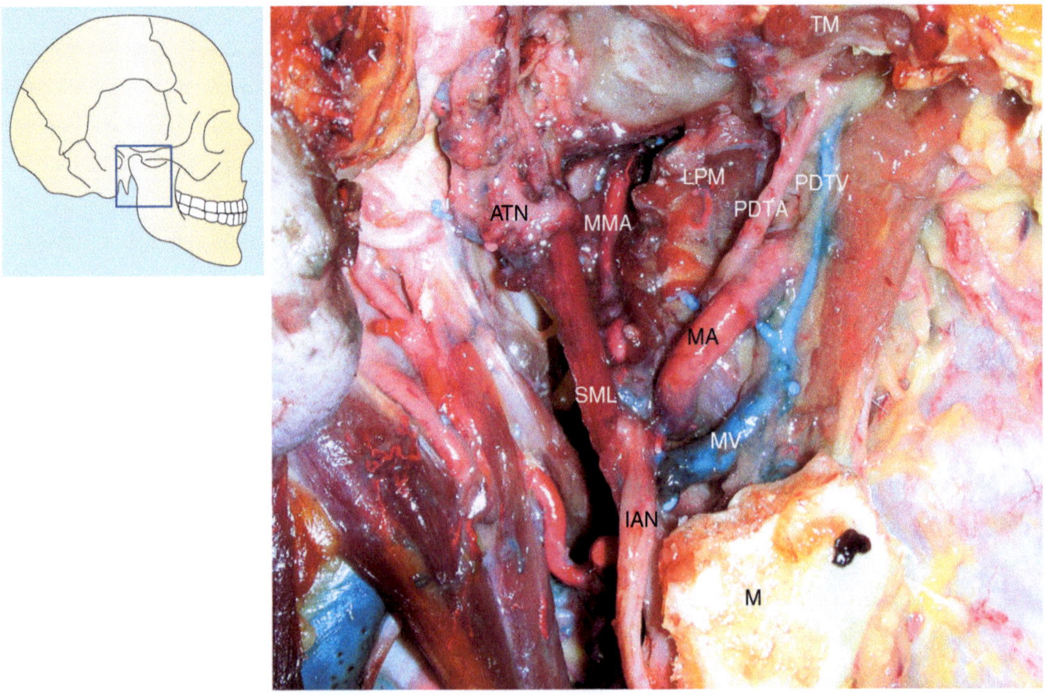

Fig. 1.7 Parotid and retrocondylar region

ATN **auriculotemporal nerve,** ***IAN*** **inferior alveolar nerve,** ***LPM*** **lateral pterygoid muscle,** ***M*** **mandible,** ***MA*** **maxillary artery,** ***MMA*** **middle meningeal artery,** ***MV*** **maxillary vein,** ***PDTA*** **posterior deep temporal artery,** ***PDTV*** **posterior deep temporal vein,** ***SML*** **sphenomandibular ligament,** ***TM*** **temporal muscle**

Usually, the MMA is posterior to the lateral pterygoid muscle. The ATN passes laterally, around the MMA and between the neck of the mandible and the SML. Similarly, the IAN passes inferiorly between the neck of the mandible and the SML. This last one is a thin fibrous connection between the spine of the sphenoid and the lingula of the mandible (Janfaza et al. 2001). Sometimes, there is an accessory middle meningeal artery that can share a common trunk with the MMA. It accompanies the mandibular nerve and enters the cranial cavity through the foramen ovale.

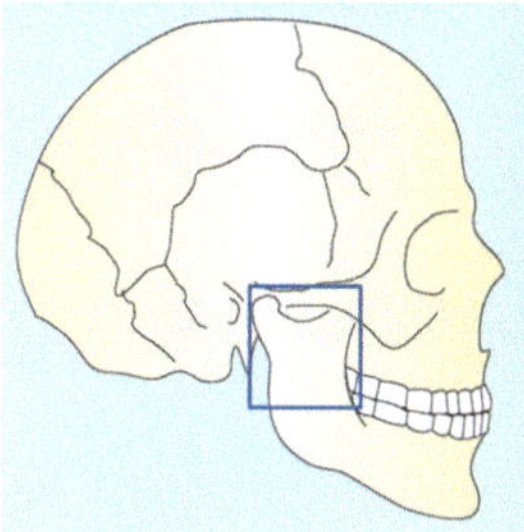

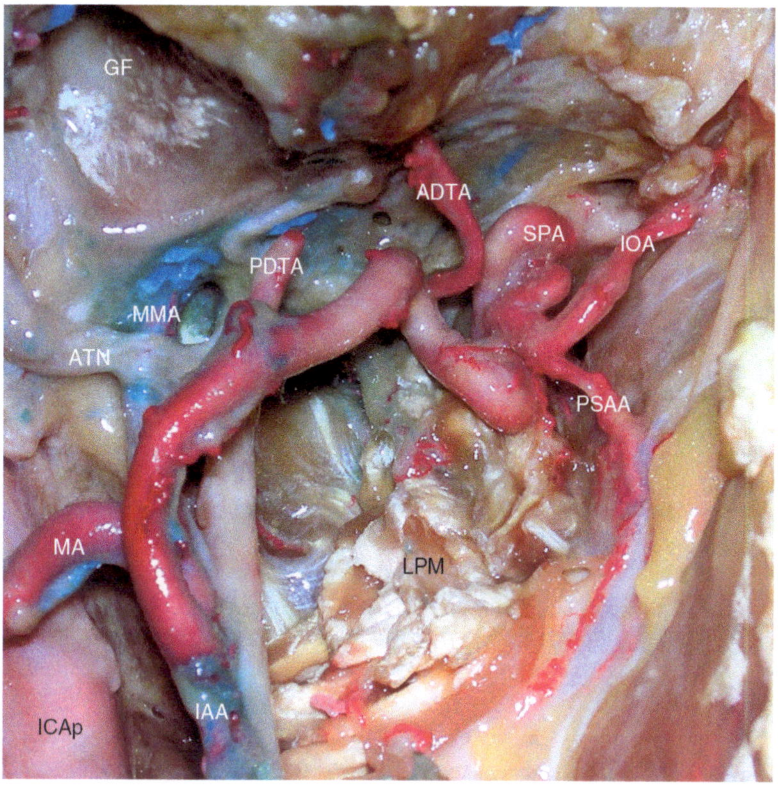

Fig. 1.8 Infratemporal fossa exposure, focus on the maxillary artery

ADTA **anterior deep temporal artery,** ***ATN*** **auriculotemporal nerve,** ***GF*** **glenoid fossa,** ***IAA*** **inferior alveolar artery,** ***ICAp*** **parapharyngeal portion of the internal carotid artery,** ***IOA*** **infraorbital artery,** ***LPM*** **lateral pterygoid muscle,** ***MA*** **maxillary artery,** ***MMA*** **middle meningeal artery,** ***PDTA*** **posterior deep temporal artery,** ***PSAA*** **posterosuperior alveolar artery,** ***SPA*** **sphenopalatine artery**

The first small branches of the MA are the deep auricular and anterior tympanic arteries. The IAA usually arises from the MA between the sphenomandibular ligament and the neck of the mandible. The DTAs travel superiorly between the temporalis muscle and pericranium. Usually, the PSAA present a common trunk with the IOA. It runs over the tuberosity of the maxilla in close relationship with the posterior superior alveolar nerve. The IOA courses within the infraorbital groove, with the infraorbital nerve. Usually, the PDTA and the MMA are separated by the lateral pterygoid muscle.

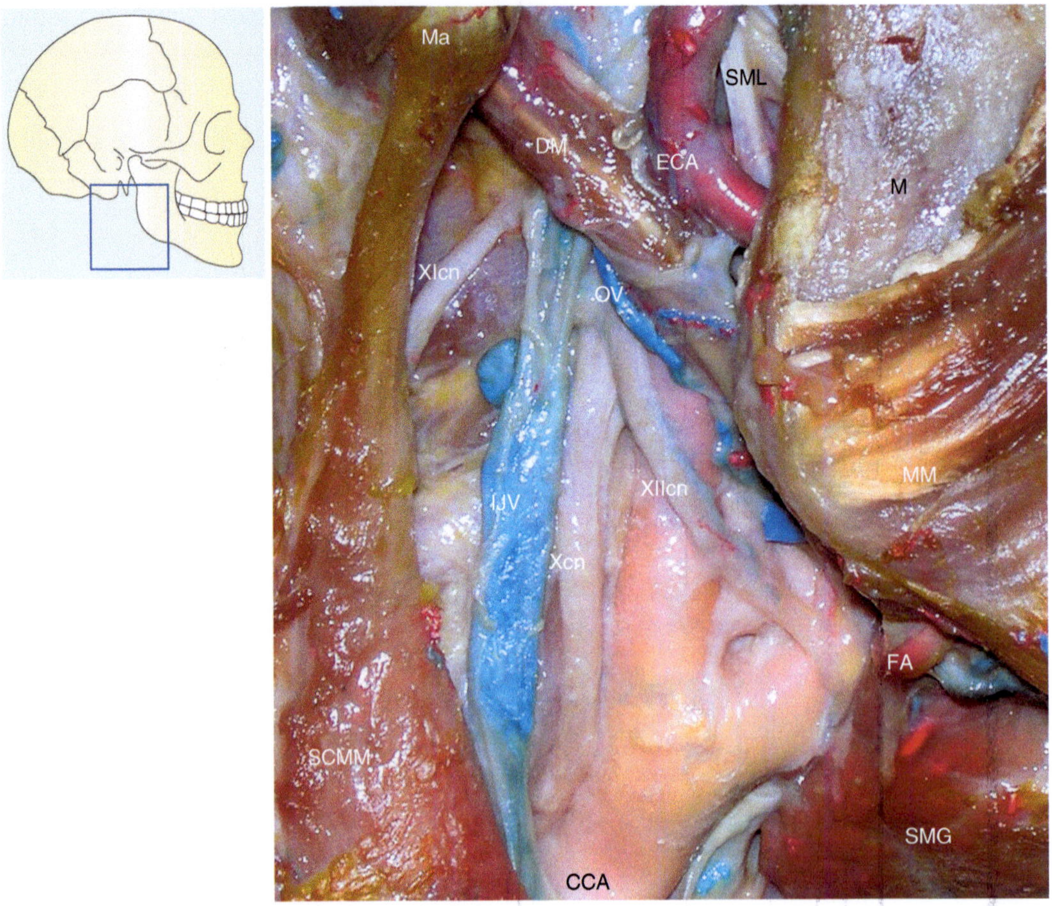

Fig. 1.9 Upper laterocervical and parotid regions

CCA **common carotid artery,** ***DM*** **digastric muscle,** ***ECA*** **external carotid artery,** ***FA*** **facial artery,** ***IJV*** **internal jugular vein,** ***M*** **mandible,** ***Ma*** **mastoid (tip),** ***MM*** **masseter muscle,** ***OV*** **occipital vein,** ***SCMM*** **sternocleidomastoid muscle,** ***SMG*** **submandibular gland,** ***SML*** **sphenomandibular ligament,** ***Xcn*** **vagus nerve,** ***XIcn*** **accessory nerve,** ***XIIcn*** **hypoglossal nerve**

The internal carotid artery origins at the level of the carotid bifurcation. Two segments can be described. The proximal segment extends from the bifurcation to the point where the artery is crossed by the posterior belly of the digastric muscle (Beretta et al. 2006). The distal segment is from this point to the carotid canal at the skull base.

The hypoglossal nerve courses along the inferior aspect of the posterior belly of the digastric muscle and crosses both internal and external carotid artery.

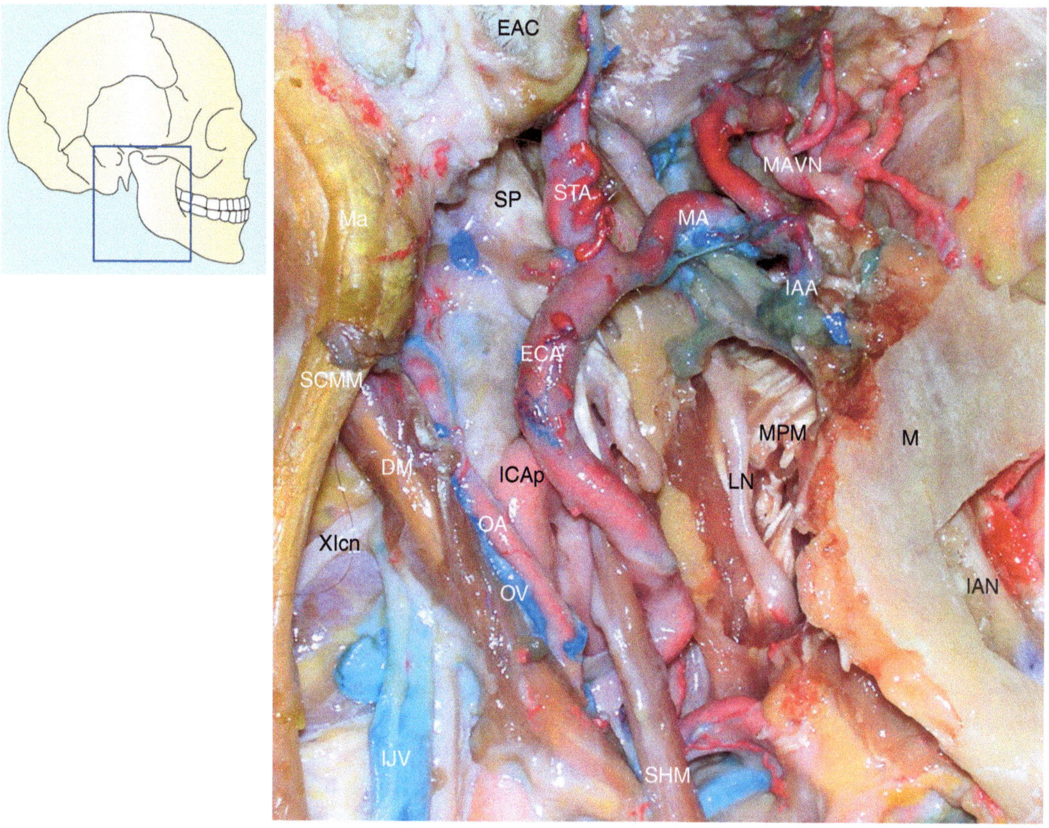

Fig. 1.10 Infratemporal, parapharyngeal, and upper laterocervical regions. The mandible has been partially cut, pushed forward and inferiorly, and the inferior alveolar nerve dissected in its own canal

DM **digastric muscle,** ***EAC*** **external acoustic canal,** ***ECA*** **external carotid artery,** ***IAA*** **inferior alveolar artery,** ***IAN*** **inferior alveolar nerve,** ***ICAp*** **parapharyngeal portion of the internal carotid artery,** ***IJV*** **internal jugular vein,** ***LN*** **lingual nerve,** ***M*** **mandible,** ***Ma*** **mastoid,** ***MA*** **maxillary artery,** ***MAVN*** **maxillary artery vascular network,** ***MPM*** **medial pterygoid muscle,** ***OA*** **occipital artery,** ***OV*** **occipital vein,** ***SCMM*** **sternocleidomastoid muscle,** ***SHM*** **stylohyoid muscle,** ***SP*** **styloid process,** ***STA*** **superficial temporal artery,** ***XIcn*** **accessory nerve**

The styloid apparatus separates the internal carotid artery from the external carotid artery. The stylohyoid muscle is the most lateral element of the styloid apparatus, while the stylopharyngeus the most medial.

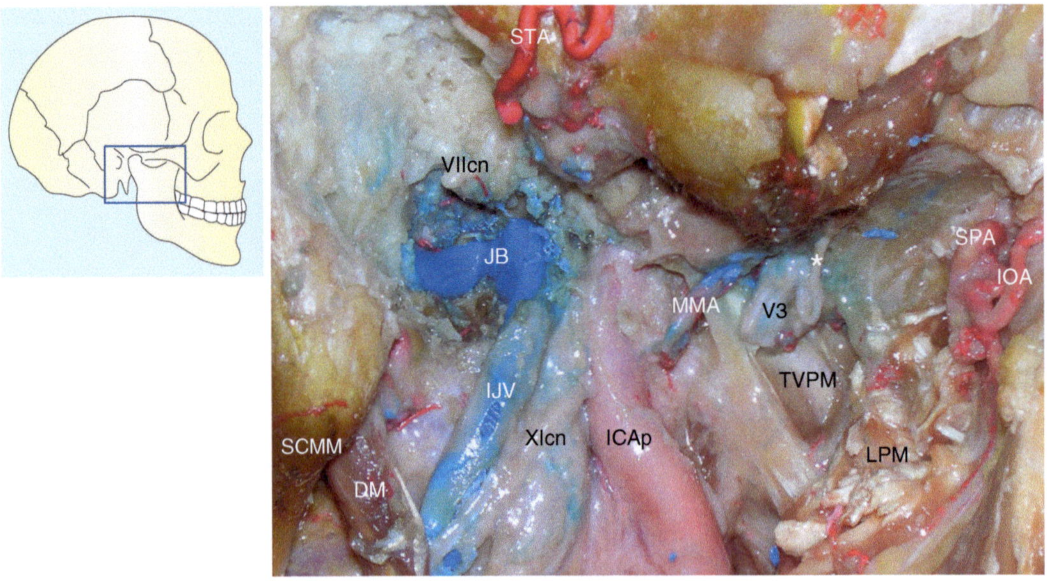

Fig. 1.11 Infratemporal fossa and jugular foramen exposure

DM **digastric muscle,** ***ICAp*** **parapharyngeal portion of the internal carotid artery,** ***IJV*** **internal jugular vein,** ***IOA*** **infraorbital artery,** ***LPM*** **lateral pterygoid muscle,** ***MMA*** **middle meningeal artery,** ***SCMM*** **sternocleidomastoid muscle,** ***SPA*** **sphenopalatine artery,** ***STA*** **superficial temporal artery,** ***TVPM*** **tensor veli palatini muscle,** ***V3*** **third branch of the trigeminal nerve,** ***VIIcn*** **facial nerve,** ***XIcn*** **accessory nerve,** ***white asterisk*** **branch for the middle cranial fossa dura**

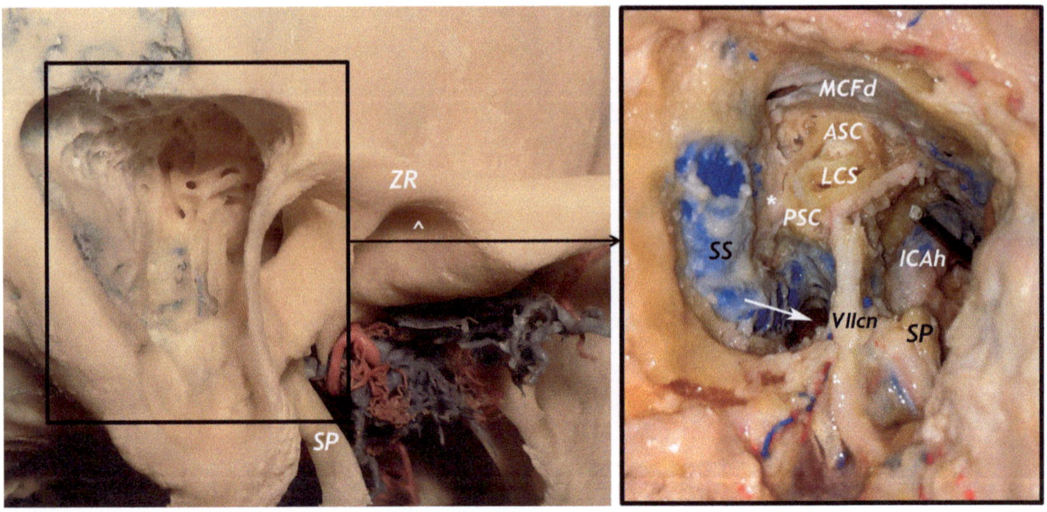

Fig. 1.12 Jugular foramen region: transpetrous exposure

ASC **anterior semicircular canal,** ***ICAh*** **horizontal portion of the internal carotid artery,** ***LSC*** **lateral semicircular canal,** ***MCFd*** **dura of the middle cranial fossa,** ***PSC*** **posterior semicircular canal,** ***SP*** **styloid process,** ***SS*** **sigmoid sinus,** ***ZR*** **zygomatic root,** ***VIIcn*** **facial nerve,** ***white arrow*** **jugular tubercle,** ***white asterisk*** **endolymphatic sac,** ***white arrowhead*** **glenoid fossa**

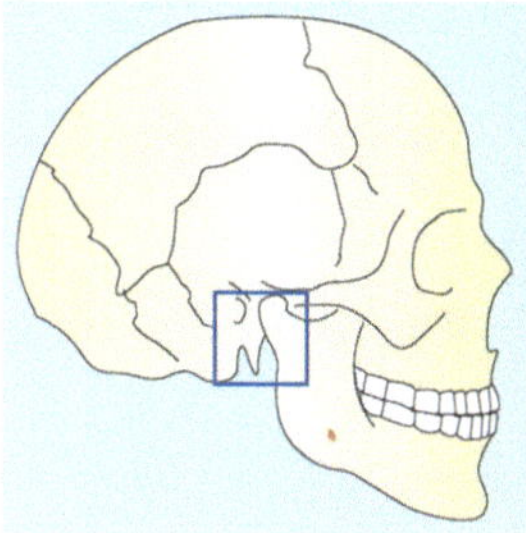

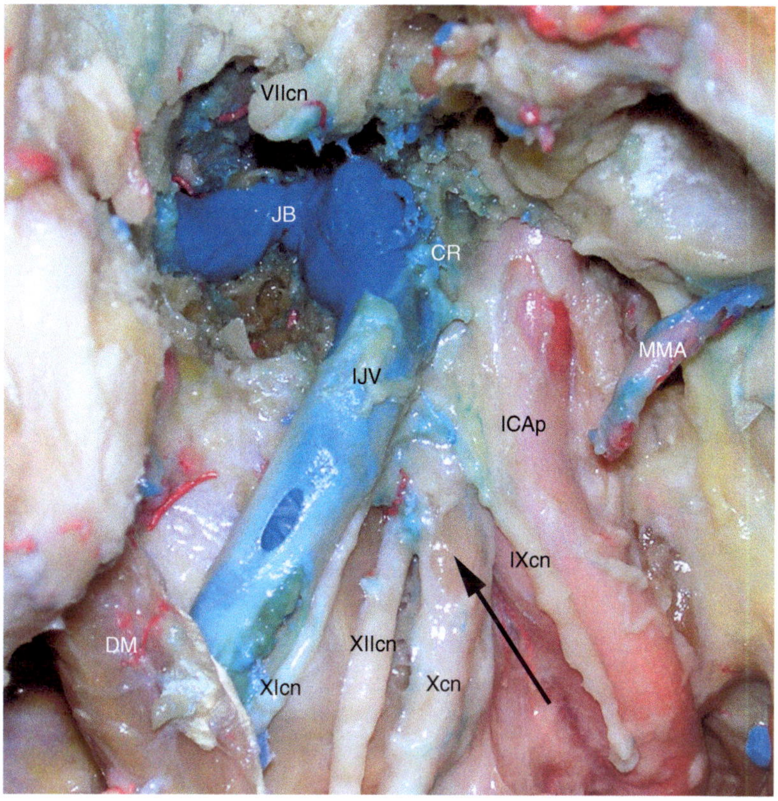

Fig. 1.13 Jugular foramen region

CR **carotid ridge,** ***DM*** **digastric muscle (posterior belly),** ***ICAp*** **parapharyngeal portion of the internal carotid artery,** ***IJV*** **internal jugular vein,** ***JB*** **jugular bulb,** ***MMA*** **middle meningeal artery,** ***VIIcn*** **facial nerve,** ***IX*** **glossopharyngeal nerve,** ***X*** **vagus nerve,** ***XI*** **accessory nerve,** ***XII*** **hypoglossal nerve,** ***black arrow*** **inferior ganglion of vagus nerve**

The jugular bulb lies beneath the floor of the middle ear cavity (Roche et al. 2008). It can be of variable shape and size. All the lower cranial nerves (*LCNs*) exit the foramen anteromedially to the jugular bulb, separated from it by connective tissue. The superior ganglion of the vagus nerve is within the jugular foramen (*JF*). At the level of the intraforaminal course, there is a strict connection between the LCNs. The vagus nerve exits the JF vertically, behind IXcn and ICAp (Roche et al. 2008) and gives its inferior ganglion on the outer skull base surface. The accessory nerve lies immediately lateral to the vagus nerve.

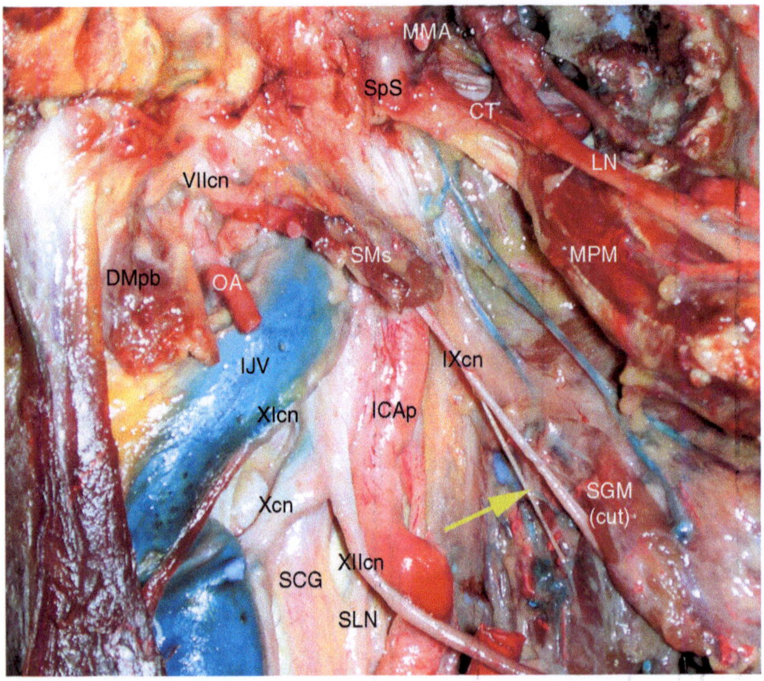

Fig. 1.14 Upper parapharyngeal region below the jugular foramen. Note that the styloid muscles covering the parapharyngeal vessels are partially removed

CT **chorda tympani,** ***DMpb*** **posterior belly of the digastric muscle,** ***ICAp*** **parapharyngeal portion of the internal carotid artery,** ***IJV*** **internal jugular vein,** ***LN*** **lingual nerve,** ***MMA*** **middle meningeal artery,** ***MPM*** **medial pterygoid muscle,** ***OA*** **occipital artery,** ***SCG*** **superior cervical ganglion (sympathetic),** ***SGM*** **styloglossus muscle,** ***SLN*** **superior laryngeal nerve,** ***SMs*** **styloid muscles,** ***SpS*** **spine of the sphenoid,** ***VIIcn*** **facial nerve,** ***IXcn*** **glossopharyngeal nerve,** ***Xcn*** **vagus nerve,** ***XIcn*** **accessory nerve,** ***XIIcn*** **hypoglossal nerve,** ***yellow arrow*** **pharyngeal branch of IX cranial nerve**

The lower cranial nerves and the IJV present an intimate relationship with the transverse process of C1. In its upper segment, the IJV lies behind the ICAp on the levator scapulae (Janfaza and Fabian 2001b). The stylopharyngeus muscle and the styloid process separate the IJV from the parotid gland. Usually, the pharyngeal branch of cranial nerve IX runs anteriorly between the internal and external carotid arteries inferior to the main trunk of cranial nerve IX (Janfaza and Fabian 2001b).

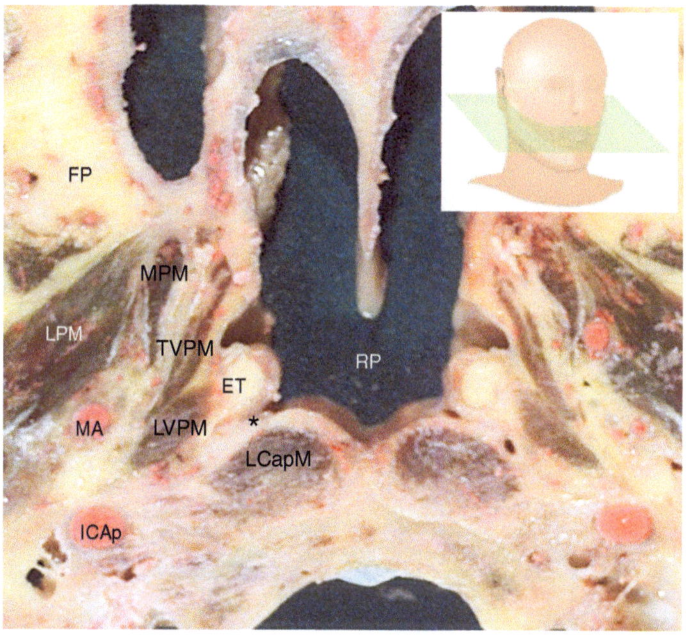

Fig. 1.15 Axial view of the parapharyngeal region

ET **eustachian tube,** ***FP*** **fat pad,** ***ICAp*** **parapharyngeal portion of the internal carotid artery,** ***LCapM*** **longus capitis muscle,** ***LPM*** **lateral pterygoid muscle,** ***LVPM*** **levator veli palatini muscle,** ***MA*** **maxillary artery,** ***MPM*** **medial pterygoid muscle,** ***RP*** **rhinopharynx,** ***TVPM*** **tensor veli palatini muscle,** ***black asterisk*** **Rosenmuller's fossa**

The upper parapharyngeal region is demonstrated. In particular, the position of the muscles is evident. The prestyloid compartment is now identified as the true parapharyngeal space, while the poststyloid compartment is now named the carotid space (Stambuk and Patel 2008). The prestyloid space is separated from the poststyloid regions by means of a fascial layer connecting the styloid process to the pharyngeal wall. The true parapharyngeal space contains the tensor veli palatine muscle and the tensor-styloid fascia, which reflects from the TVPM and reaches the pharyngeal wall (Janfaza et al. 2001).

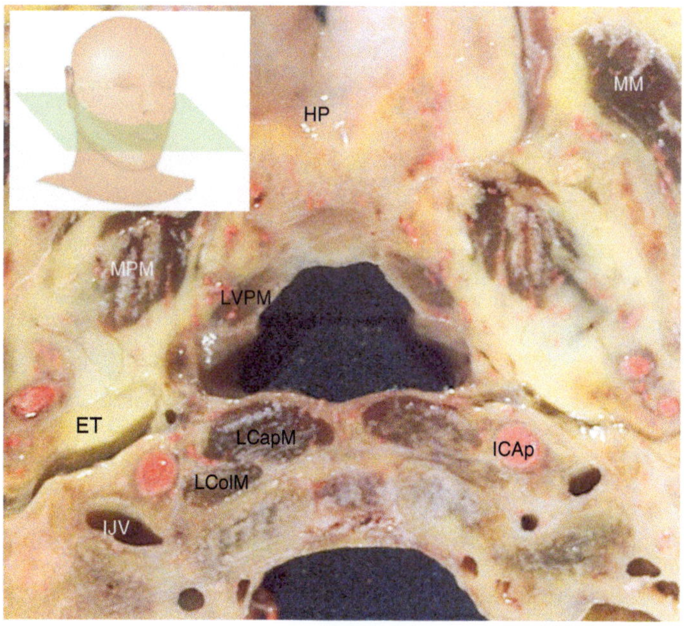

Fig. 1.16 Axial view of the parapharyngeal region (more caudally in respect to the previous image)

ET **eustachian tube,** ***HP*** **hard palate,** ***ICAp*** **parapharyngeal portion of the internal carotid artery,** ***IJV*** **internal jugular vein,** ***LCapM*** **longus capitis muscle,** ***LColM*** **longus colli muscle,** ***LVPM*** **levator veli palatini muscle,** ***MM*** **masseter muscle,** ***MPM*** **medial pterygoid muscle**

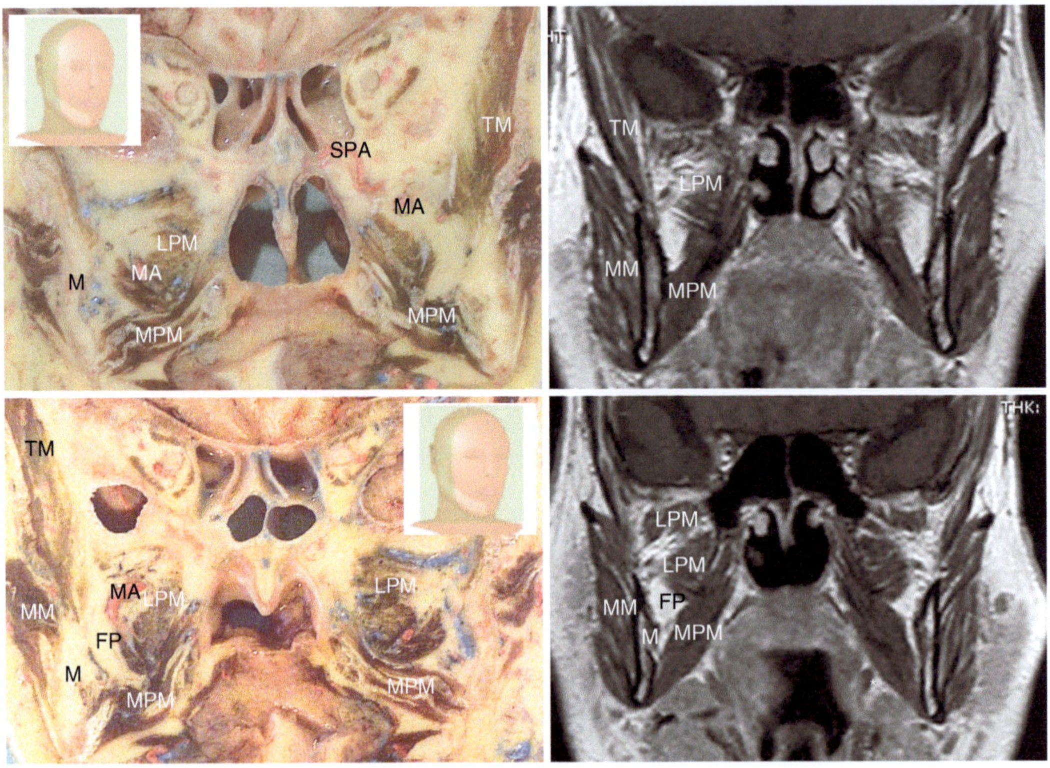

Fig. 1.17 Coronal views of the infratemporal fossa

FP **fat pad,** ***LPM*** **lateral pterygoid muscle,** ***M*** **mandible,** ***MA*** **maxillary artery,** ***MM*** **masseter muscle,** ***MPM*** **medial pterygoid muscle,** ***SPA*** **sphenopalatine artery,** ***TM*** **temporal muscle**

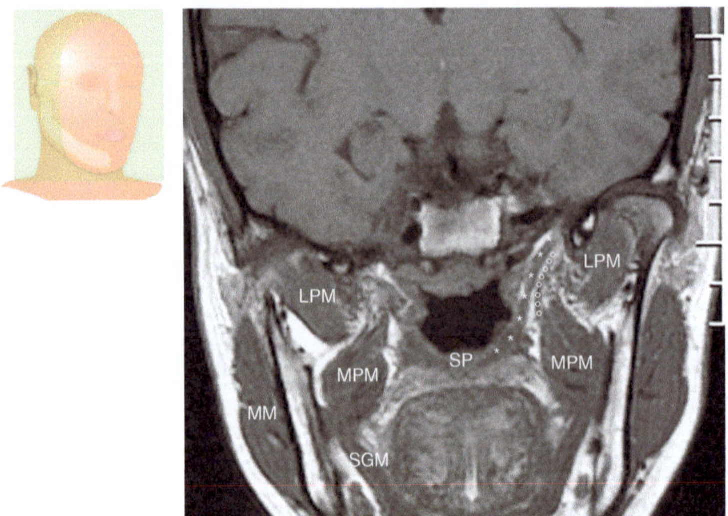

Fig. 1.18 Coronal view of the infratemporal fossa

LPM **lateral pterygoid muscle,** ***MM*** **masseter muscle,** ***MPM*** **medial pterygoid muscle,** ***SGM*** **styloglossus muscle,** ***SP*** **soft palate,** ***white asterisks*** **levator veli palatini muscle,** ***white circles*** **tensor veli palatini muscle**

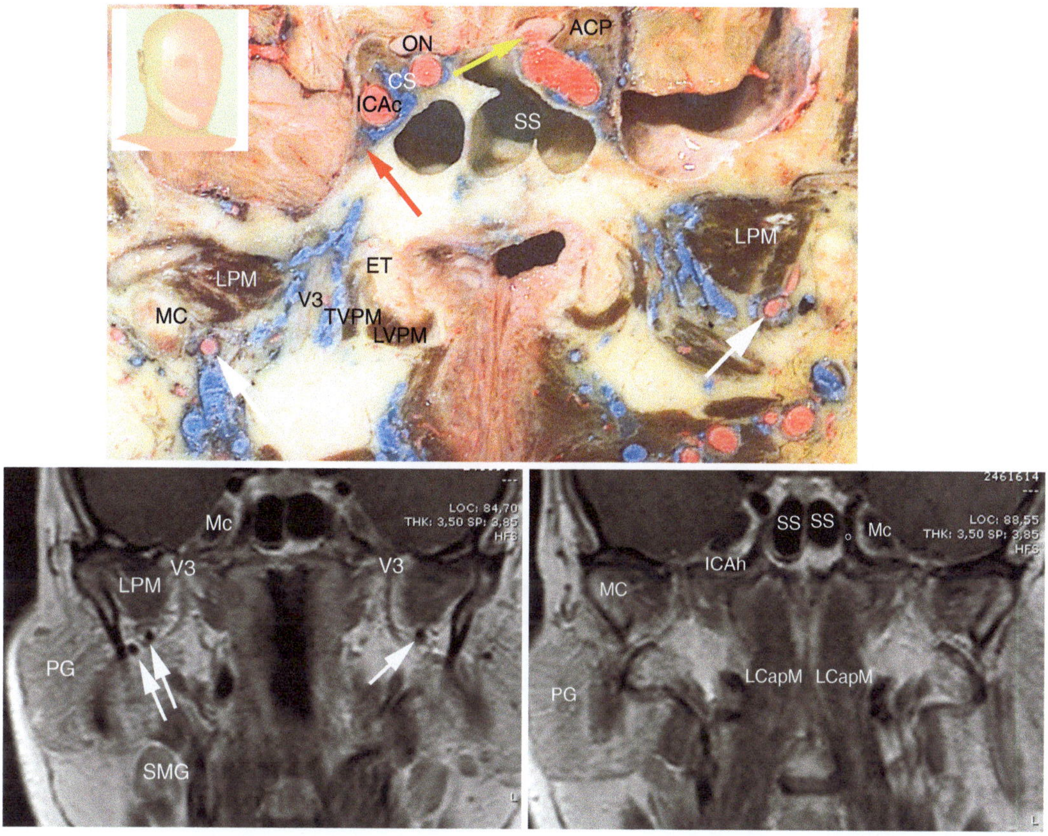

Fig. 1.19 Coronal views of the infratemporal fossa and parapharyngeal region

ACP **anterior clinoid process,** ***CS*** **cavernous sinus,** ***ET*** **eustachian tube,** ***ICAc*** **cavernous portion of the internal carotid artery,** ***ICAh*** **horizontal portion of the internal carotid artery,** ***LCapM*** **longus capitis muscle,** ***LPM*** **lateral pterygoid muscle,** ***LVPM*** **levator veli palatini muscle,** ***MC*** **mandibular condyle,** ***Mc*** **Meckel's cave,** ***ON*** **optic nerve,** ***PG*** **parotid gland,** ***SMG*** **submandibular gland,** ***SS*** **sphenoid sinus,** ***TVPM*** **tensor veli palatini muscle,** ***V3*** **third branch of the trigeminal nerve,** ***yellow arrow*** **ophthalmic artery,** ***red arrow*** **second branch of the trigeminal nerve,** ***white arrows*** **maxillary artery,** ***white circle*** **cavernous (vertical) portion of the internal carotid artery**

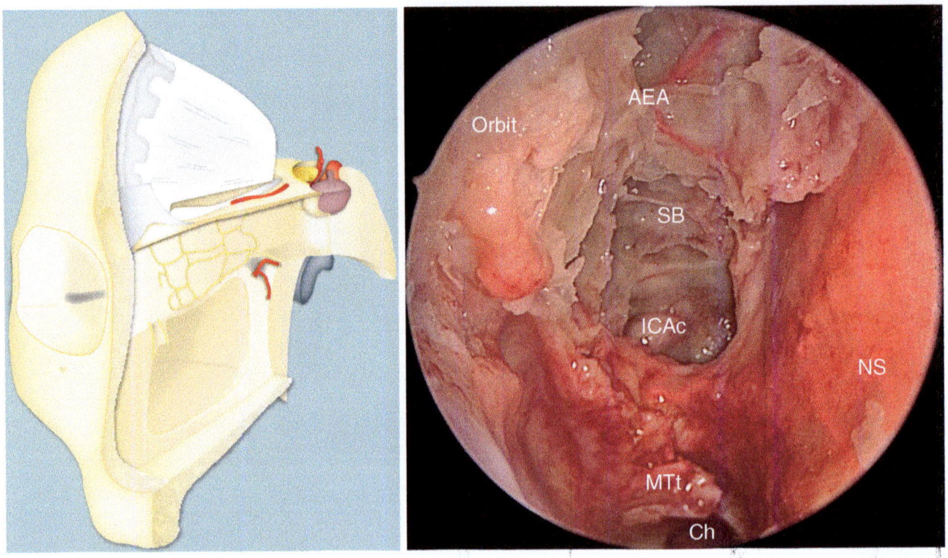

Fig. 1.20 Panoramic endoscopic vision of the sphenoethmoidal spaces and 3D reconstruction of the pterygomaxillo-orbital region

AEA **anterior ethmoidal artery,** ***Ch*** **choana,** ***ICAc*** **cavernous portion of the internal carotid artery,** ***MTt*** **tail of the middle turbinate,** ***NS*** **nasal septum,** ***SB*** **skull base**

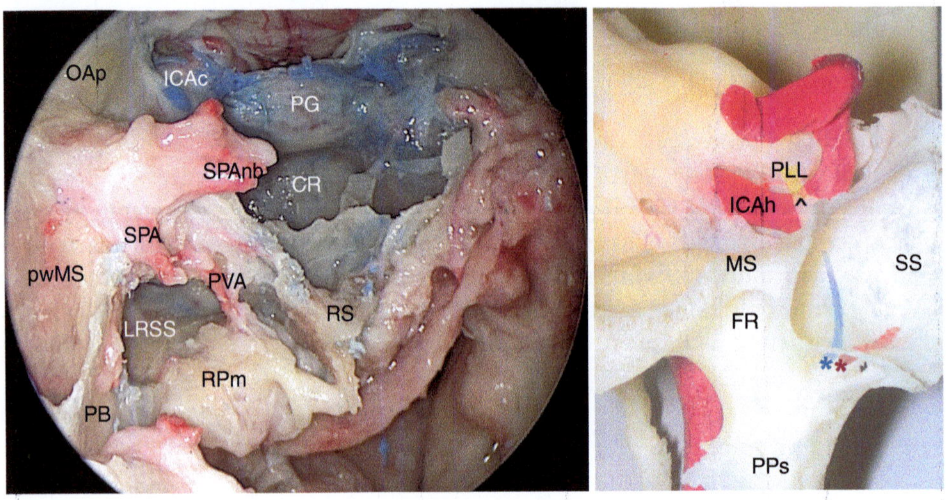

Fig. 1.21 Close endoscopic vision of the sphenopalatine region and related osteology

CR **clival recess,** ***FR*** **foramen rodundum,** ***ICAc*** **cavernous portion of the internal carotid artery,** ***ICAh*** **horizontal portion of the internal carotid artery,** ***MS*** **maxillary strut,** ***OAp*** **orbital apex,** ***PB*** **palatine bone,** ***PG*** **pituitary gland,** ***PLL*** **petrolingual ligament (*****yellow*****),** ***PPs*** **pterygoid plates,** ***PVA*** **palatovaginal artery,** ***pwMS*** **posterior wall of the maxillary sinus,** ***RPm*** **rhinopharyngeal mucosa,** ***RS*** **rostrum sphenoidale,** ***SPA*** **sphenopalatine artery,** ***SPAnb*** **nasal branch of the sphenopalatine artery,** ***SS*** **sphenoid sinus,** ***black arrowhead*** **lingula of the sphenoid,** ***blue-sky asterisk*** **and** ***line*** **vidian canal,** ***violet asterisk*** **and** ***line*** **palatovaginal canal**

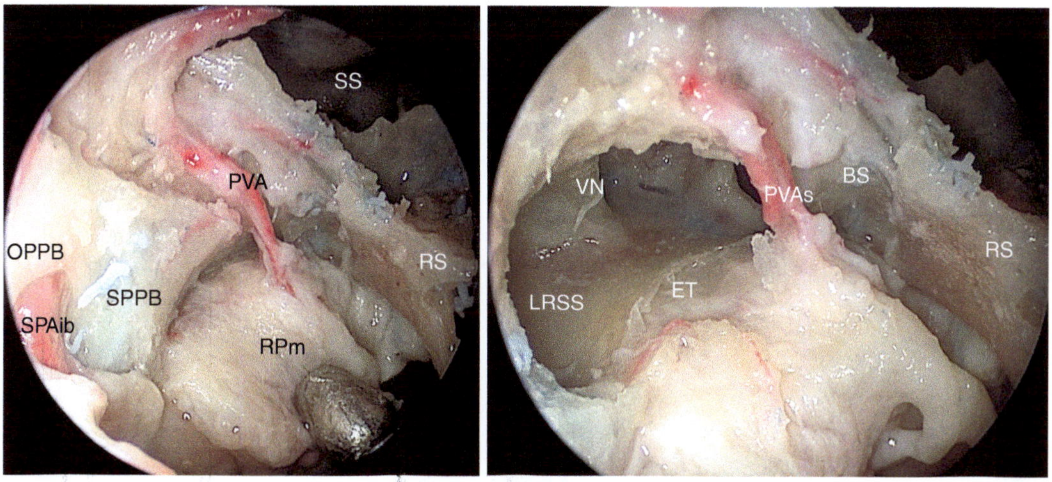

Fig. 1.22 Close vision of the pterygoid and basisphenoid region. The position of the palatovaginal artery is evident

BS **basisphenoid,** ***ET*** **eustachian tube,** ***LRSS*** **lateral recess of the sphenoid sinus,** ***OPPB*** **orbital process of the palatine bone,** ***PVA(s)*** **palatovaginal artery(ies),** ***RPm*** **rhinopharyngeal mucosa,** ***SPAib*** **inferior branch of the sphenopalatine artery,** ***SPPB*** **sphenoidal process of the palatine bone,** ***SS*** **sphenoid sinus,** ***RS*** **rostrum sphenoidale,** ***VN*** **vidian nerve**

The PVA (also called the pharyngeal artery) lies within the palatovaginal canal accompanied by the pharyngeal nerve (from the pterygopalatine ganglion). The palatovaginal (or pharyngeal) canal is given superiorly by a groove in the basisphenoid and inferiorly by the sphenoidal process of the palatine bone.

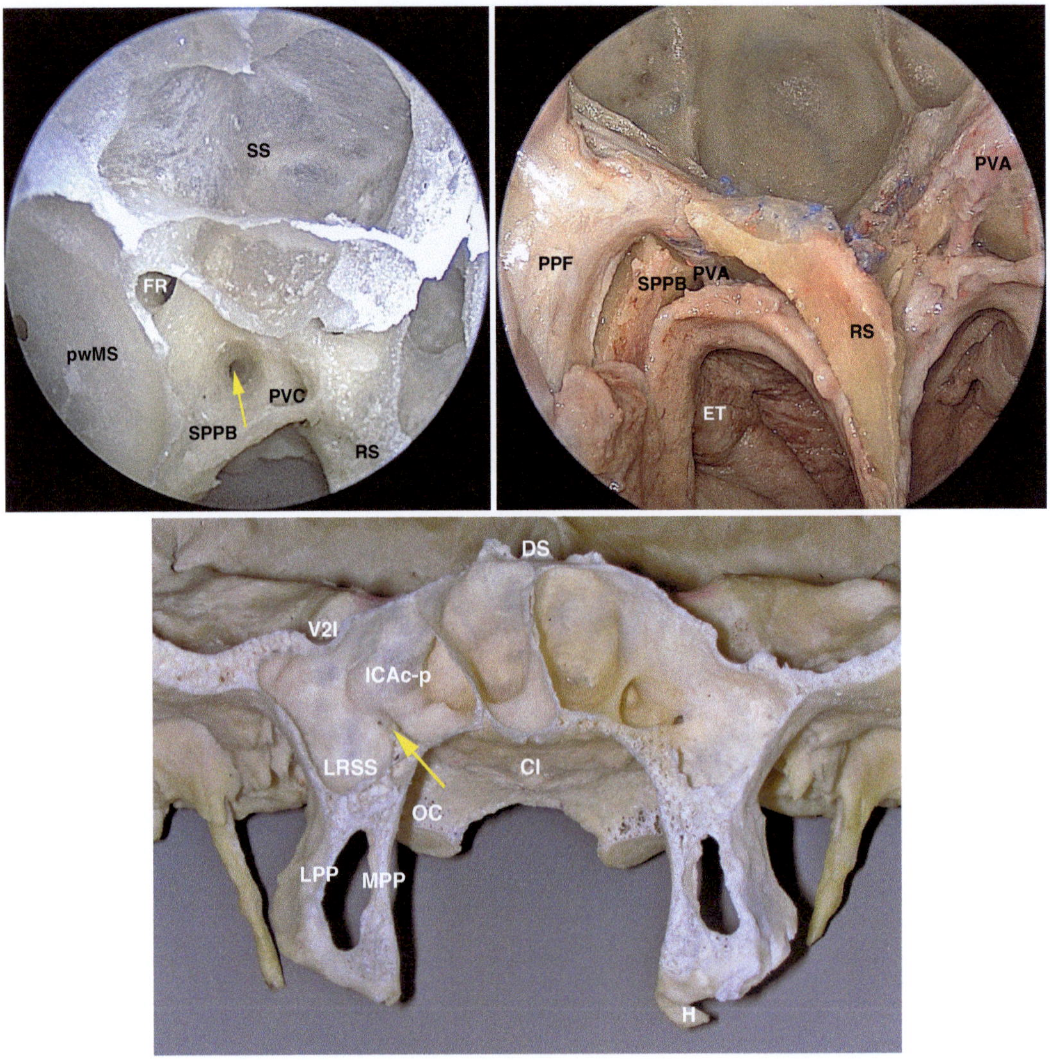

Fig. 1.23 Pterygoid and basisphenoid region

Cl **clivus,** ***DS*** **dorsum sellae,** ***ET*** **eustachian tube,** ***FR*** **foramen rotundum,** ***H*** **hamulus,** ***ICAc-p*** **protuberance of the cavernous portion of the internal carotid artery,** ***LPP*** **lateral pterygoid plate,** ***LRSS*** **lateral recess of the sphenoid sinus,** ***MPP*** **medial pterygoid plate,** ***OC*** **occipital condyle,** ***PPF*** **pterygopalatine fossa,** ***PVA*** **palatovaginal artery,** ***PVC*** **palatovaginal canal,** ***pwMS*** **posterior wall of the maxillary sinus,** ***RS*** **rostrum sphenoidale,** ***SPPB*** **sphenoidal process of the palatine bone,** ***SS*** **sphenoidal sinus,** ***V2I*** **incisure of V2,** ***yellow arrow*** **vidian canal**

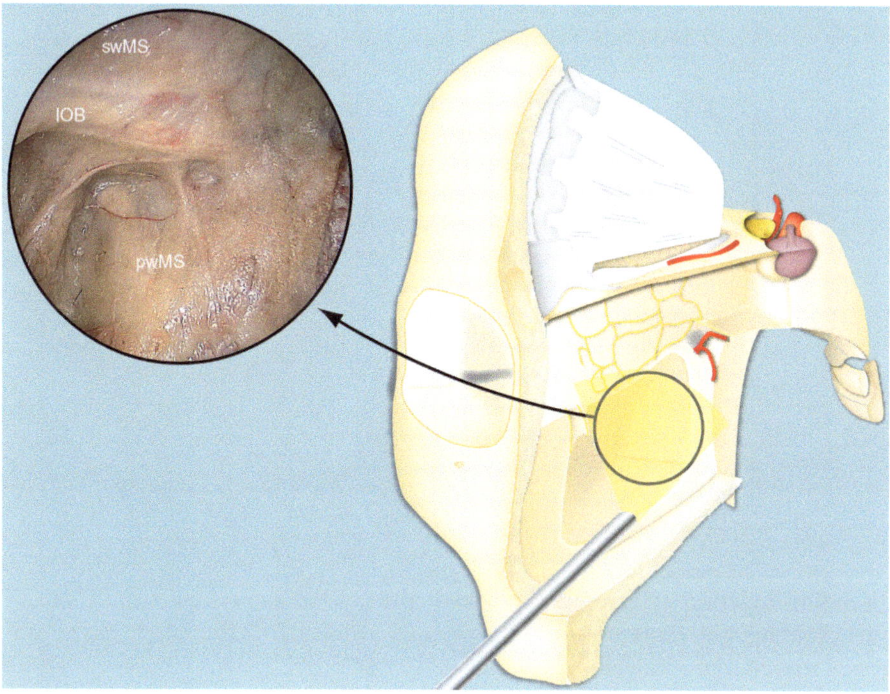

Fig. 1.24 Maxillary window

***IOB* infraorbital bundle, *pwMS* posterior wall of the maxillary sinus, *swMS* superior wall of the maxillary sinus**

Through the maxillary window, usually associated with a transpterygoid approach, it is possible to gain access to the infratemporal fossa and upper parapharyngeal space.

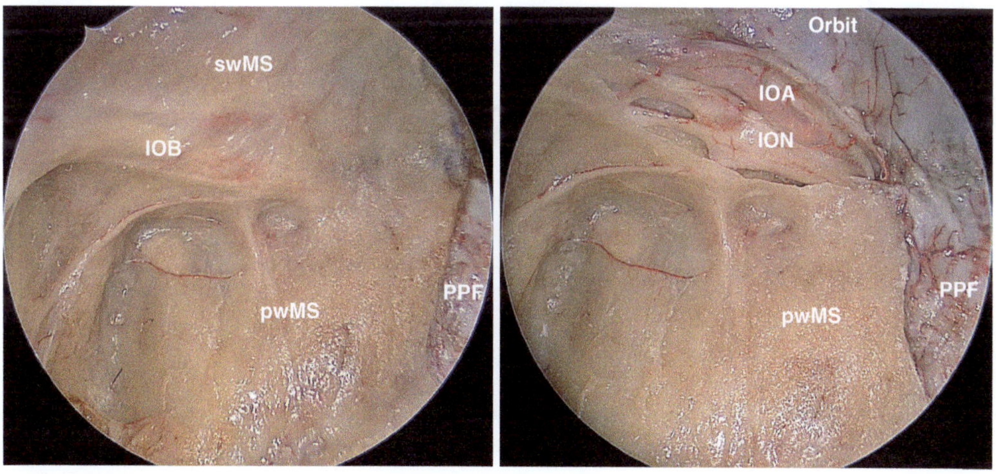

Fig. 1.25 Endoscopic view of the maxillary window

***IOA* infraorbital artery, *IOB* infraorbital bundle, *ION* infraorbital nerve, *pwMS* posterior wall of the maxillary sinus, *swMS* superior wall of the maxillary sinus, *PPF* pterygopalatine fossa**

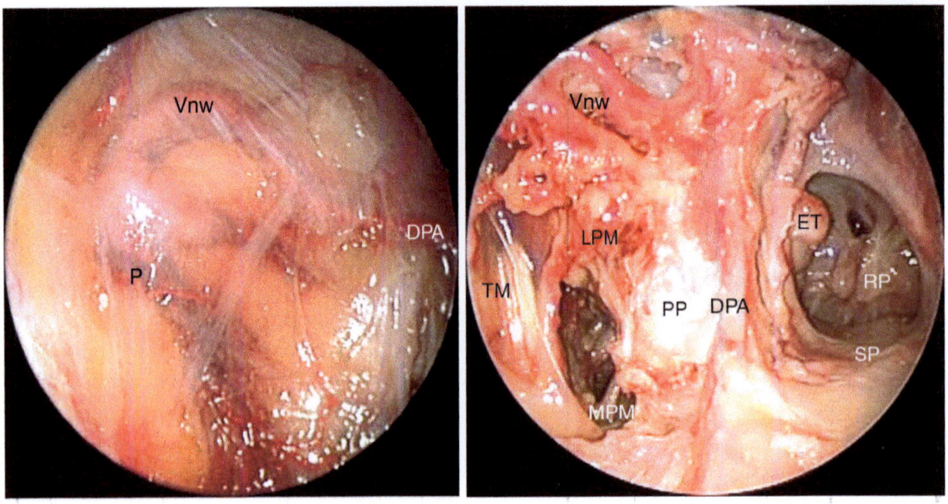

Fig. 1.26 Endoscopic view of the maxillary window

DPA **descending palatine artery,** ***ET*** **eustachian tube,** ***LPM*** **lateral pterygoid muscle,** ***MPM*** **medial pterygoid muscle,** ***P*** **periostium,** ***PP*** **pterygoid process,** ***RP*** **rhinopharynx,** ***SP*** **soft palate,** ***TM*** **temporal muscle,** ***Vnw*** **vascular network**

The fat pad filling the space between the medial pterygoid, lateral pterygoid, and temporal muscle is in direct continuation with the Bichat's fat pad.

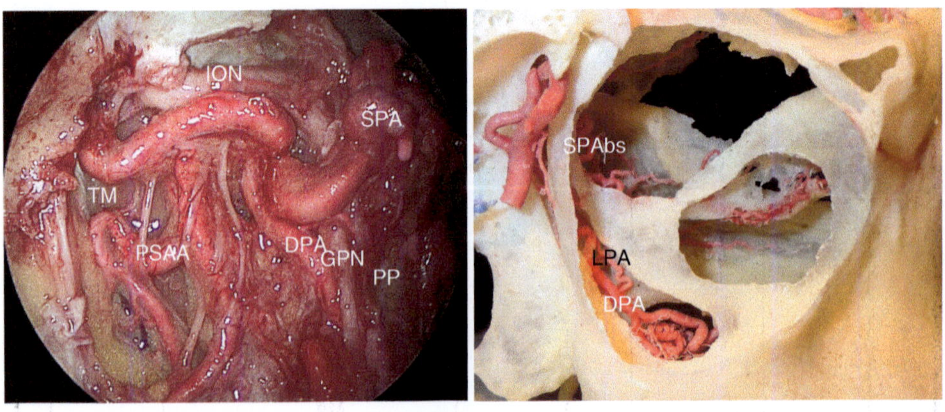

Fig. 1.27 Endoscopic view of the vascular plane below the periostium and focus on the "palatine vessels" (external view)

DPA **descending palatine artery,** ***GPN*** **greater palatine nerve,** ***ION*** **infraorbital nerve,** ***LPA*** **lesser palatine artery,** ***PP*** **pterygoid plate,** ***PSAA*** **posterosuperior alveolar artery,** ***SPA*** **sphenopalatine artery,** ***SPAbs*** **sphenopalatine branches,** ***TM*** **temporal muscle**

The PSAA often presents a common trunk with the infraorbital artery (*IOA*). The IOA runs forward in the infraorbital groove and canal accompanying the ION. The DPA descends with the GPN and becomes the greater palatine artery after exiting from the greater palatine foramen. The LPA is a branch of the DPA and exits the nasal cavity through the lesser palatine foramen and feeds mainly the soft palate.

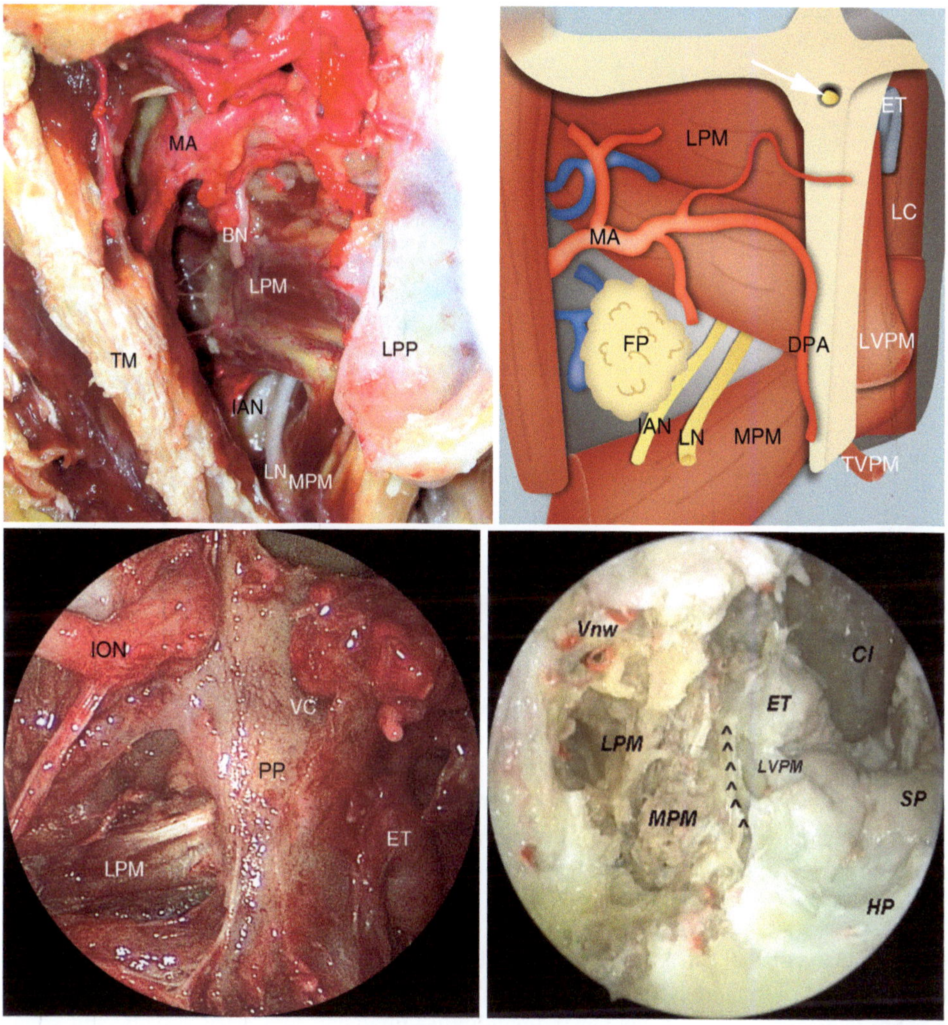

Fig. 1.28 Anterior views of the infratemporal fossa. The muscular wall given by the lateral pterygoid muscle, with the overlying vascular network, is evident. Between the lateral and the medial pterygoid muscle, the lingual and the inferior alveolar nerves are visible

BN **buccal nerve,** ***Cl*** **clivus,** ***DPA*** **descending palatine artery,** ***ET*** **eustachian tube,** ***FP*** **fat pad,** ***HP*** **hard palate,** ***IAN*** **inferior alveolar artery,** ***ION*** **infraorbital nerve,** ***LC*** **longus capitis,** ***LN*** **lingual nerve,** ***LPM*** **lateral pterygoid muscle,** ***LPP*** **lateral pterygoid plate,** ***LVPM*** **levator veli palatini muscle,** ***MA*** **maxillary artery,** ***MPM*** **medial pterygoid muscle,** ***PP*** **pterygoid plate,** ***SP*** **soft palate,** ***TM*** **temporal muscle,** ***TVPM*** **tensor veli palatini muscle,** ***VC*** **vidian canal,** ***Vnw*** **vascular network,** ***white arrow*** **vidian nerve,** ***black arrowheads*** **tensor veli palatini muscle**

LPM connects the lateral surface of the pterygoid plate and the surrounding skull base (infratemporal crest of the greater wing of the sphenoid) to the anterior surface of the neck of the mandible and the articular capsule. The muscular "wall" given by the LPM covers the deeper structures and should be cut and removed to gain wide access to the infratemporal fossa and upper paraphargeal space (Dallan et al. 2010). The buccal nerve passes between the two heads of the LPM and runs toward the medial aspect of the temporal muscle. Then, it passes close to the ramus of the mandible to lie on the lateral surface of the buccinator muscle in the cheek and innervate the mucosa of the cheek. The buccal nerve can be accompanied by the buccal artery. The FP between the LMP, MPM, and TM is a prolongation of the buccal fat pad, which lies on the lateral surface of the buccinator muscle. The position of the MA in respect to the LPM is highly variable.

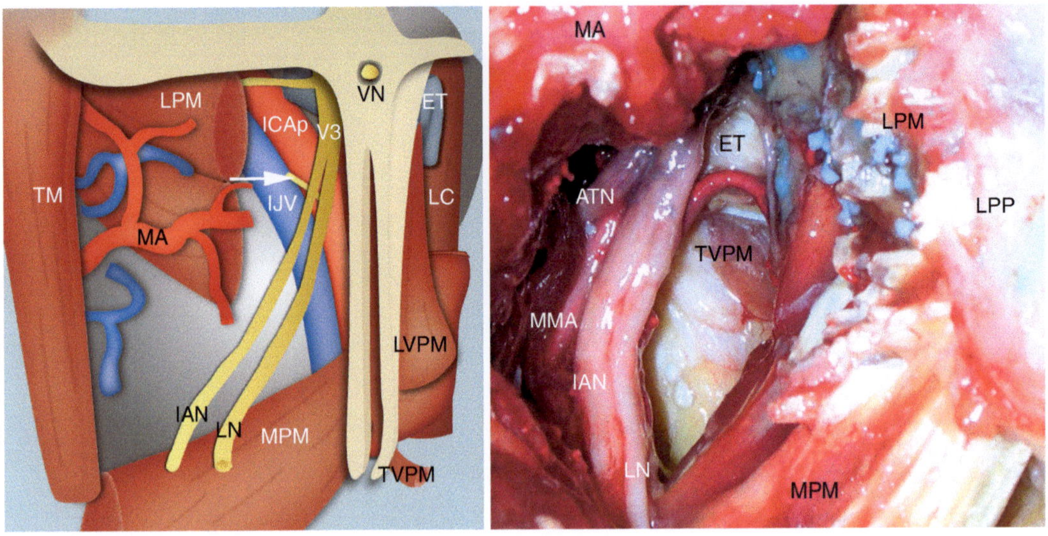

Fig. 1.29 Anterior view of the infratemporal fossa. The lateral pterygoid muscle has been cut, and V3 and the Eustachian Tube are exposed. Through this muscular window access to the upper parapharyngeal space can be gained

ATN **auricolotemporal nerve,** ***ET*** **eustachian tube,** ***IAN*** **inferior alveolar nerve,** ***ICAp*** **parapharyngeal portion of the internal carotid artery,** ***IJV*** **internal jugular vein,** ***LC*** **longus capitis,** ***LN*** **lingual nerve,** ***LPM*** **lateral pterygoid muscle,** ***LPP*** **lateral pterygoid plate,** ***LVPM*** **levator veli palatini muscle,** ***MA*** **maxillary artery,** ***MMA*** **middle meningeal artery,** ***MPM*** **medial pterygoid muscle,** ***TM*** **temporal muscle,** ***TVPM*** **tensor veli palatini muscle,** ***VN*** **vidian nerve,** ***V3*** **third branch of the trigeminal nerve,** ***white arrow*** **chorda tympani**

MPM connects the medial surface of the lateral pterygoid plate and the tuberosity of the maxilla with the medial surface of the ramus and angle of the mandible. On its lateral surface, LN and IAN lie. A relationship is also present with the sphenomandibular ligament, maxillary vessels, and sometimes with a parotid process. The medial surface of the MPM presents a relationship with the TVPM, styloglossus, stylopharyngeus, and superior constrictor muscles.

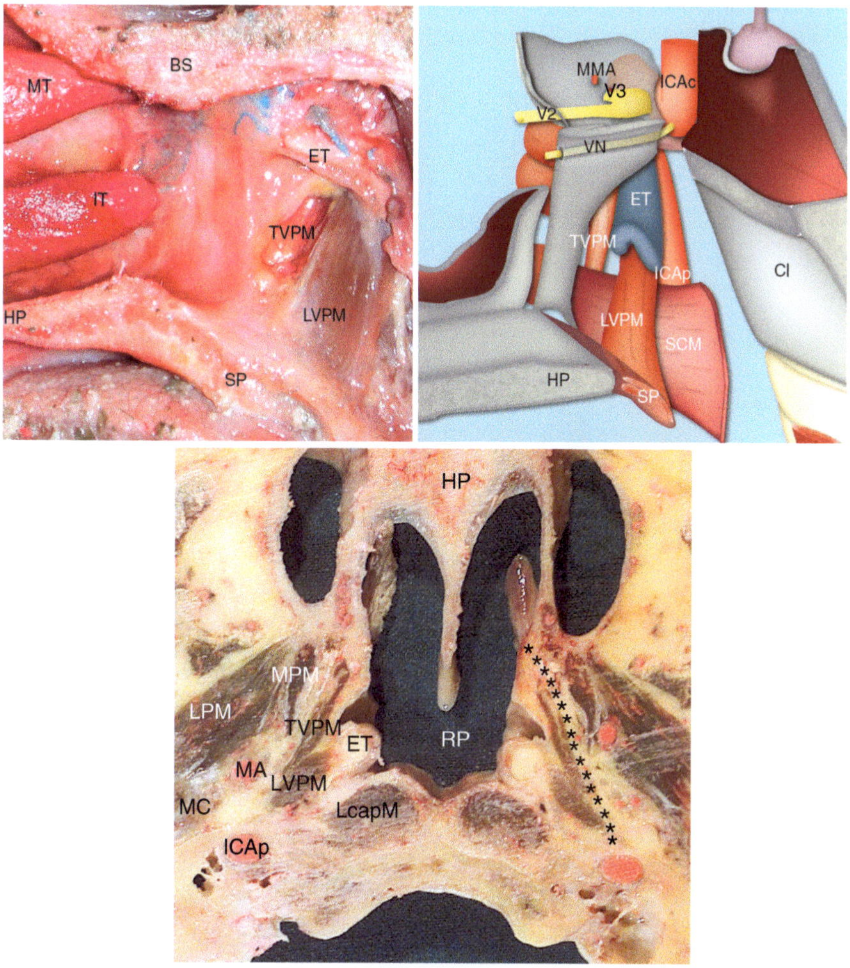

Fig. 1.30 Rhinopharyngeal region, medial to lateral and axial views

***BS* basisphenoid, *Cl* clivus, *ET* eustachian tube, *HP* hard palate, *ICAc* cavernous portion of the internal carotid artery, *ICAp* parapharyngeal portion of the internal carotid artery, *IT* inferior turbinate, *LCapM* longus capitis muscle, *LVPM* levator veli palatini muscle, *MA* maxillary artery, *MC* mandibular condyle, *MMA* middle meningeal artery, *MPM* medial pterygoid muscle, *MPP* medial pterygoid plate, *MT* middle turbinate, *RP* rhinopharynx, *SCM* superior constrictor muscle, *SP* soft palate, *TVPM* tensor veli palatini muscle, *VN* vidian nerve, *V2* second branch of the trigeminal nerve, *V3* third branch of the trigeminal nerve, *black asterisks* medial corridor to ICAp**

Cranially, the TVPM attaches to the lateral side of the ET, spine of the sphenoid bone, and scaphoid fossa. It runs inferiorly between the medial pterygoid muscle and plate, and then it turns medially at the level of the hamulus of the medial pterygoid plate to join, in the soft palate, the muscle from the opposite side (it also attaches to the posterior margin of the hard palate). The cranial origin of LVPM is at the level of the petrous bone anterior to the carotid canal, but mainly from the inferior surface of the cartilaginous portion of the ET. The muscle runs inferiorly parallel to the ET, medial to the SCM to join, in the soft palate, the muscle from the opposite side.

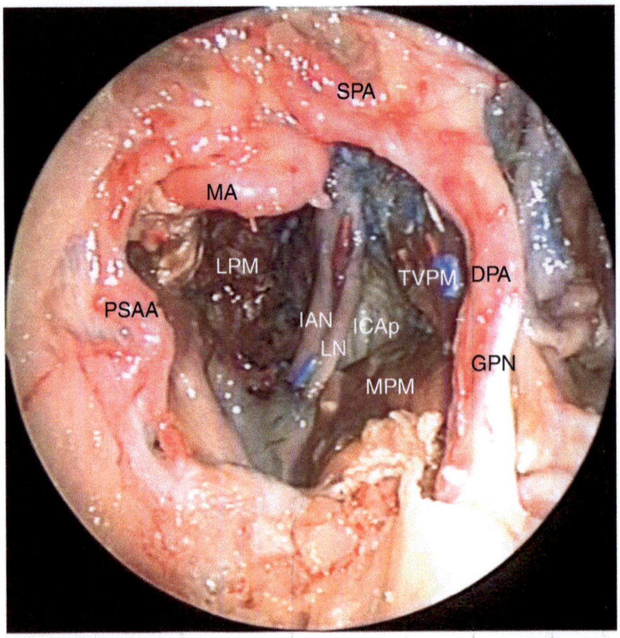

Fig. 1.31 Panoramic endoscopic vision of the infratemporal fossa. The lateral pterygoid muscle and the fat pad have been removed, and a panoramic vision on the infratemporal fossa is achieved. The inferior alveolar and the lingual nerves are visible on the lateral surface of the medial pterygoid muscle

DPA **descending palatine artery,** ***GPN*** **greater palatine nerve,** ***IAN*** **inferior alveolar nerve,** ***ICAp*** **parapharyngeal portion of internal carotid artery,** ***LN*** **lingual nerve,** ***LPM*** **lateral pterygoid muscle,** ***MA*** **maxillary artery,** ***MPM*** **medial pterygoid muscle,** ***PSAA*** **posterosuperior alveolar artery,** ***SPA*** **sphenopalatine artery,** ***TVPM*** **tensor veli palatini muscle**

DPA descends with the GPN and becomes the greater palatine artery after exiting from the greater palatine foramen. The PSAA frequently origins as a common trunk with the infraorbital artery; it runs over the tuberosity of the maxilla and accompains the posterior superior alveolar nerve.

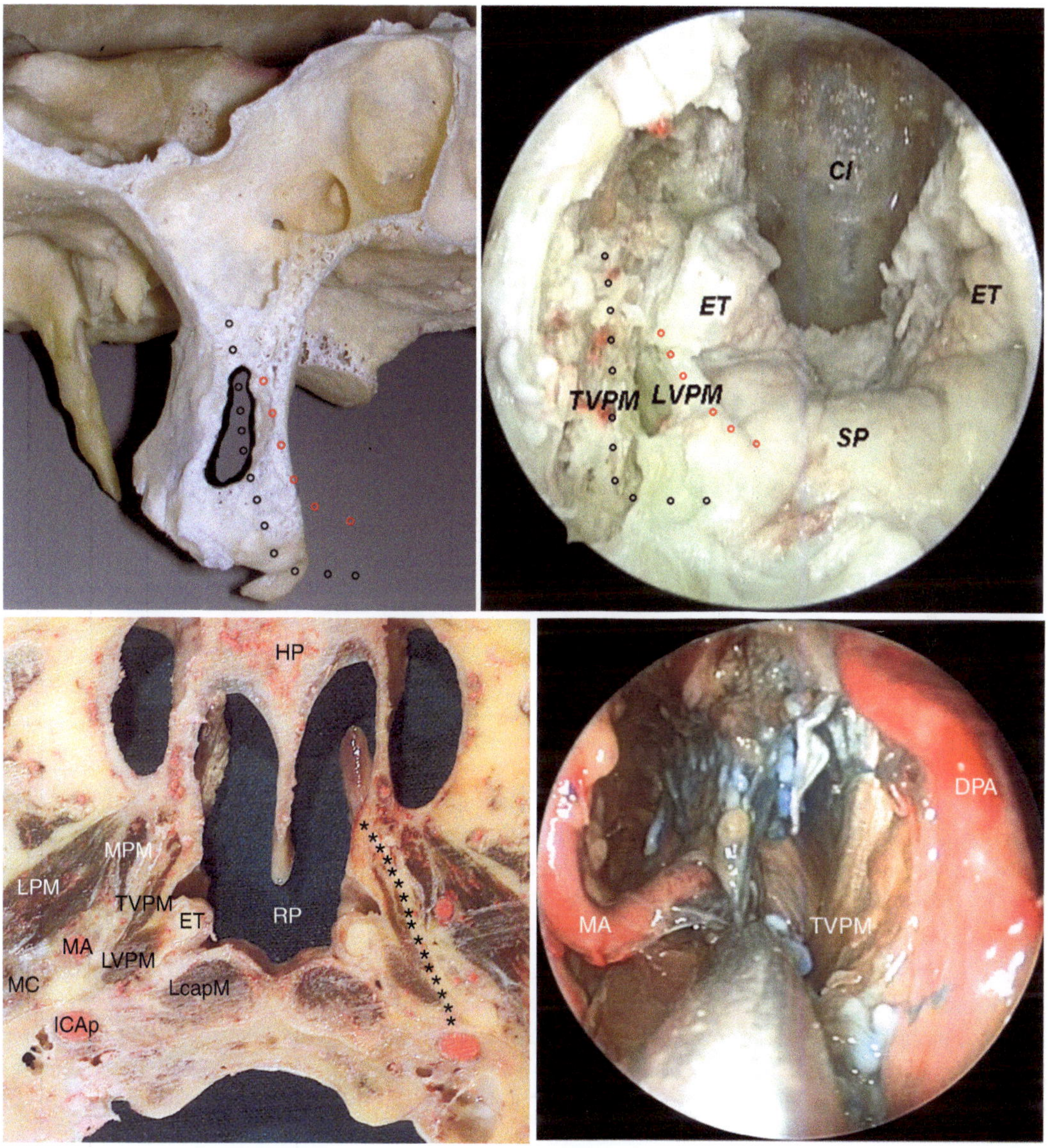

Fig. 1.32 Vision of the "medial wall" given by the muscular plane

Cl **clivus,** ***DPA*** **descending palatine artery,** ***ET*** **eustachian tube,** ***HP*** **hard palate,** ***ICAp*** **parapharyngeal portion of the internal carotid artery,** ***LCapM*** **longus capitis muscle,** ***LPM*** **lateral pterygoid muscle,** ***LVPM*** **levator veli palatini muscle,** ***MA*** **maxillary artery,** ***MC*** **mandibular condyle,** ***MPM*** **medial pterygoid muscle,** ***RP*** **rhinopharynx,** ***SP*** **soft palate,** ***TVPM*** **tensor veli palatini muscle,** ***black asterisks*** **medial corridor to ICAp,** ***black circles*** **tensor veli palatini muscle,** ***red circles*** **levator veli palatini muscle**

The TVPM belongs to the prestyloid compartment (Janfaza et al. 2001). Actually, the prestyloid compartment is considered the true parapharyngeal space (Stambuk and Patel 2008). Posterior to the TVPM lies the carotid space. Fibers from the LVPM follow eustachian tube orientation to insert at the soft palate. By passing laterally, in relation to the TVPM, it is possible to reach the ICAp and, immediatly lateral to it, the internal jugular vein and lower cranial nerves (Dallan et al. 2010)

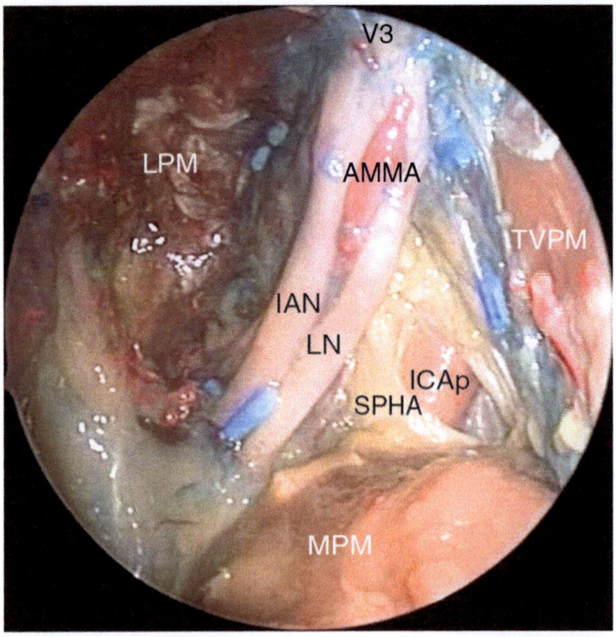

Fig. 1.33 Endoscopic view of the infratemporal fossa. The lingual and inferior alveolar nerves, two of the three branches of the posterior trunk of the third branch of the trigeminal nerve, are clearly visible, lying on the lateral surface of medial pterygoid muscle

***AMMA* accessory middle meningeal artery, *IAN* inferior alveolar nerve, *ICAp* parapharyngeal portion of the internal carotid artery, *LN* lingual nerve, *LPM* lateral pterygoid muscle, *MPM* medial pterygoid muscle, *SPHA* stylopharyngeal aponeurosis, *TVPM* tensor veli palatini muscle, *V3* third branch of the trigeminal nerve**

The LN emerges from the inferior border of the LPM and curves downward and forward in the pterygomandibular space. Passing inferiorly, it lies close to the lingual alveolar plate of the mandibular third molar. Sometimes, a small lingual comitant artery can be present that follows the LN. More consistent is the inferior alveolar artery, which follows the IAN, giving off a branch (mylohyoid branch) at the level of the mandibular foramen.

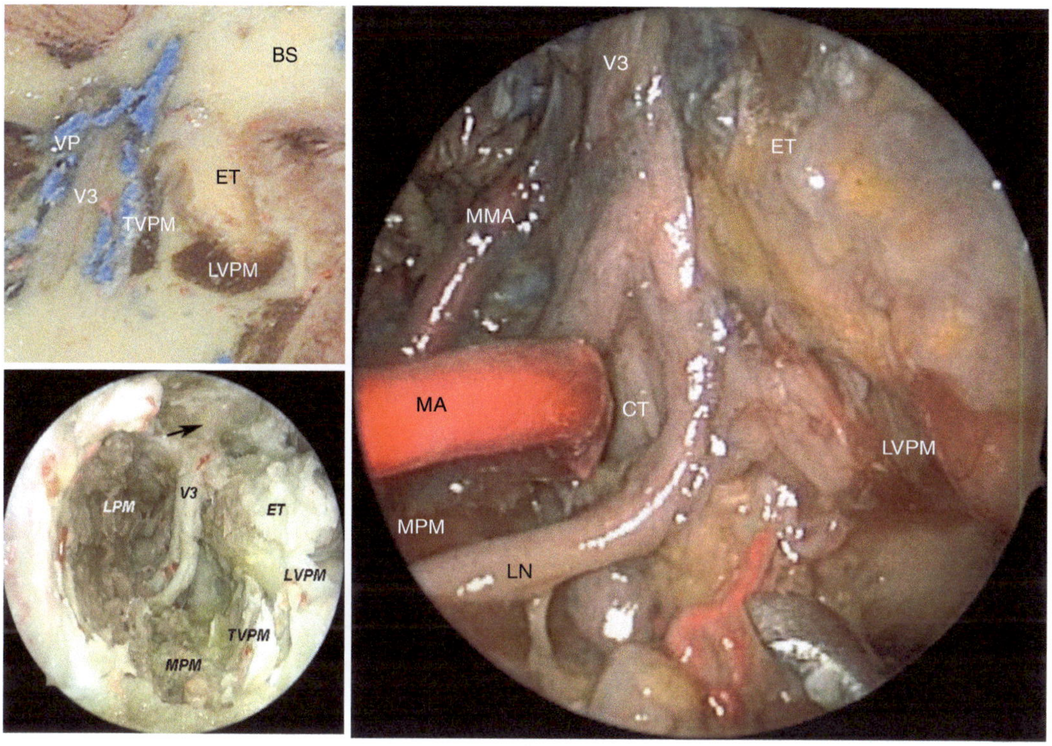

Fig. 1.34 Endoscopic view of the infratemporal fossa. Focus on the close relationship between the eustachian tube and the mandibular nerve (V3). V3 belongs to the pre-styloid compartment

BS **basisphenoid,** ***CT*** **chorda tympani,** ***ET*** **eustachian tube,** ***LN*** **lingual nerve,** ***LPM*** **lateral pterygoid muscle,** ***LVPM*** **levator veli palatini muscle,** ***MA*** **maxillary artery,** ***MMA*** **middle meningeal artery,** ***MPM*** **medial pterygoid muscle,** ***TVPM*** **tensor veli palatini muscle,** ***VP*** **venous plexus around** ***V3*****,** ***V3*** **third branch of trigeminal nerve,** ***black arrow*** **the canal of** ***V3*** **within the skull base**

V3 is an important landmark to locate the poststyloid compartment, being just anterior to this space (Falcon et al. 2011). No foramina of the skull base is included within the borders of the parapharyngeal space (Stambuk and Patel 2008). On the anterolateral surface of the ET, it is possible to identify the tubal incisure. This is a groove in the medial lamella of the ET that accommodates the LVPM. Around V3 a wide venous plexus is well evident.

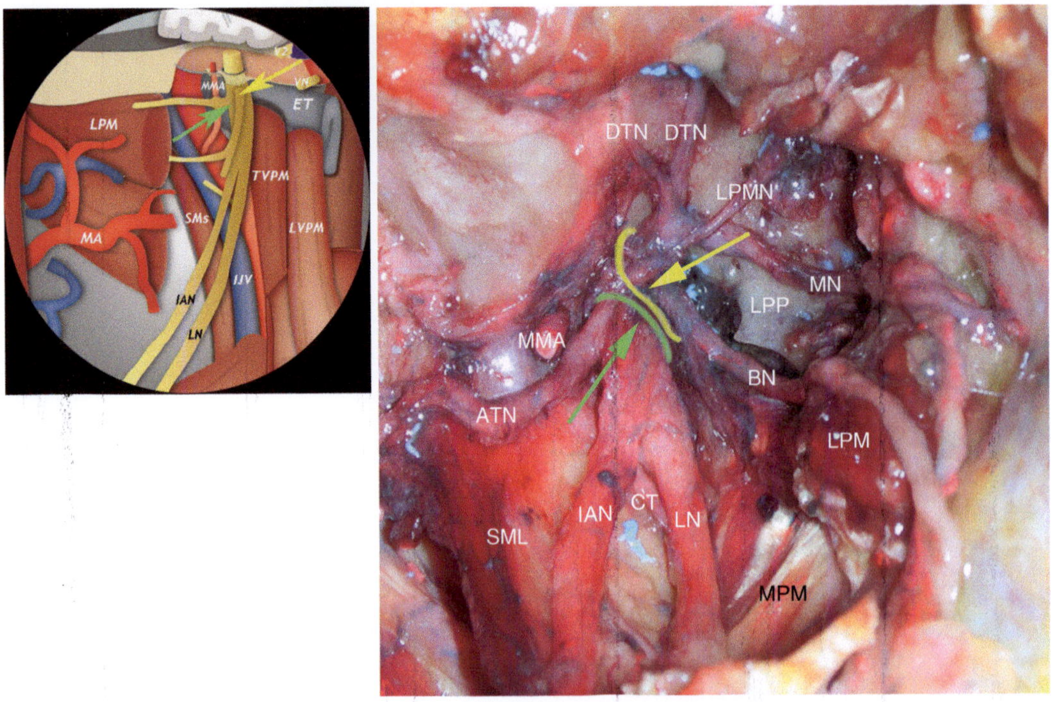

Fig. 1.35 View from below of the main branches of V3. The infratemporal fossa has been subtotally cleaned

***ATN* auricolotemporal nerve, *BN* buccal nerve, *CT* chorda tympani, *DTN* deep temporal nerve, *ET* eustachian tube, *IAN* inferior alveolar nerve, *LN* lingual nerve, *LPM* lateral pterygoid muscle, *LPMN* lateral pterygoid muscle nerve, *LPP* lateral pterygoid plate, *LVPM* levator veli palatini muscle, *MA* maxillary artery, *MMA* middle meningeal artery, *MN* masseteric nerve, *MPM* medial pterygoid muscle, *SML* sphenomandibular ligament, *SMs* styloid muscles, *TVPM* tensor veli palatini muscle, *VN* vidian nerve, *V2* second branch of the trigeminal nerve, *green arrow* posterior trunk, *yellow arrow* anterior trunk**

V3 divides at a short distance from the skull base. Before splitting into an anterior and posterior trunk, it offers some branches/nerves: meningeal, medial pterygoid, tensor tympani, and tensor veli palatine nerves. In close proximity to V3, on its dorso-medial surface, lies the otic ganglion. It is in close relationship with the lateral surface of the ET and just below the skull base. The CT comes out from the petrotympanic fissure and passes over the spine of the sphenoid bone to join the posterior aspect of the LN. The CT is usually accompanied by the anterior tympanic artery (branch of the maxillary artery). Within the infratemporal fossa, anastomotic nerve(s) between the IAN and the LN can be present.

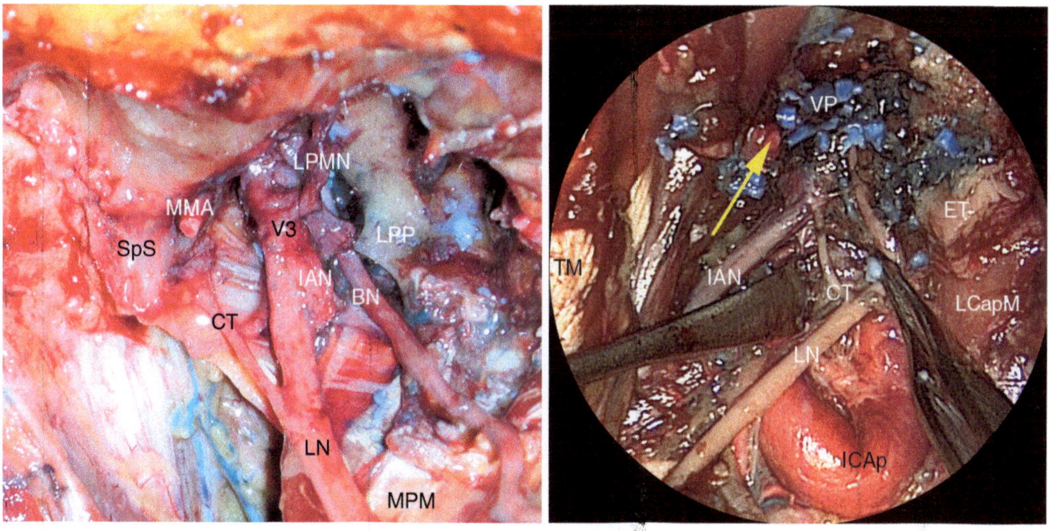

Fig. 1.36 External and endoscopic anterior view of the close relationship between chorda tympanic and the lingual nerve

BN **buccal nerve,** ***CT*** **chorda tympani,** ***ET*** **eustachian tube,** ***IAN*** **inferior alveolar nerve,** ***ICAp*** **parapharyngeal portion of the internal carotid artery,** ***LCapM*** **longus capitis muscle,** ***LN*** **lingual nerve,** ***LPMN*** **lateral pterygoid muscle nerve,** ***LPP*** **lateral pterygoid plate,** ***MMA*** **middle meningeal artery,** ***MPM*** **medial pterygoid muscle,** ***SpS*** **spine of the sphenoid,** ***TM*** **temporal muscle,** ***VP*** **venous plexus around** ***V3*****,** ***V3*** **third branch of the trigeminal nerve,** ***yellow arrow*** **maxillary artery (cut)**

The meningeal nerve enters the cranial cavity through the foramen spinosum, with the MMA. LN runs inferiorly on the lateral surface of the medial pterygoid muscle, passing between this muscle and the body of the mandible.

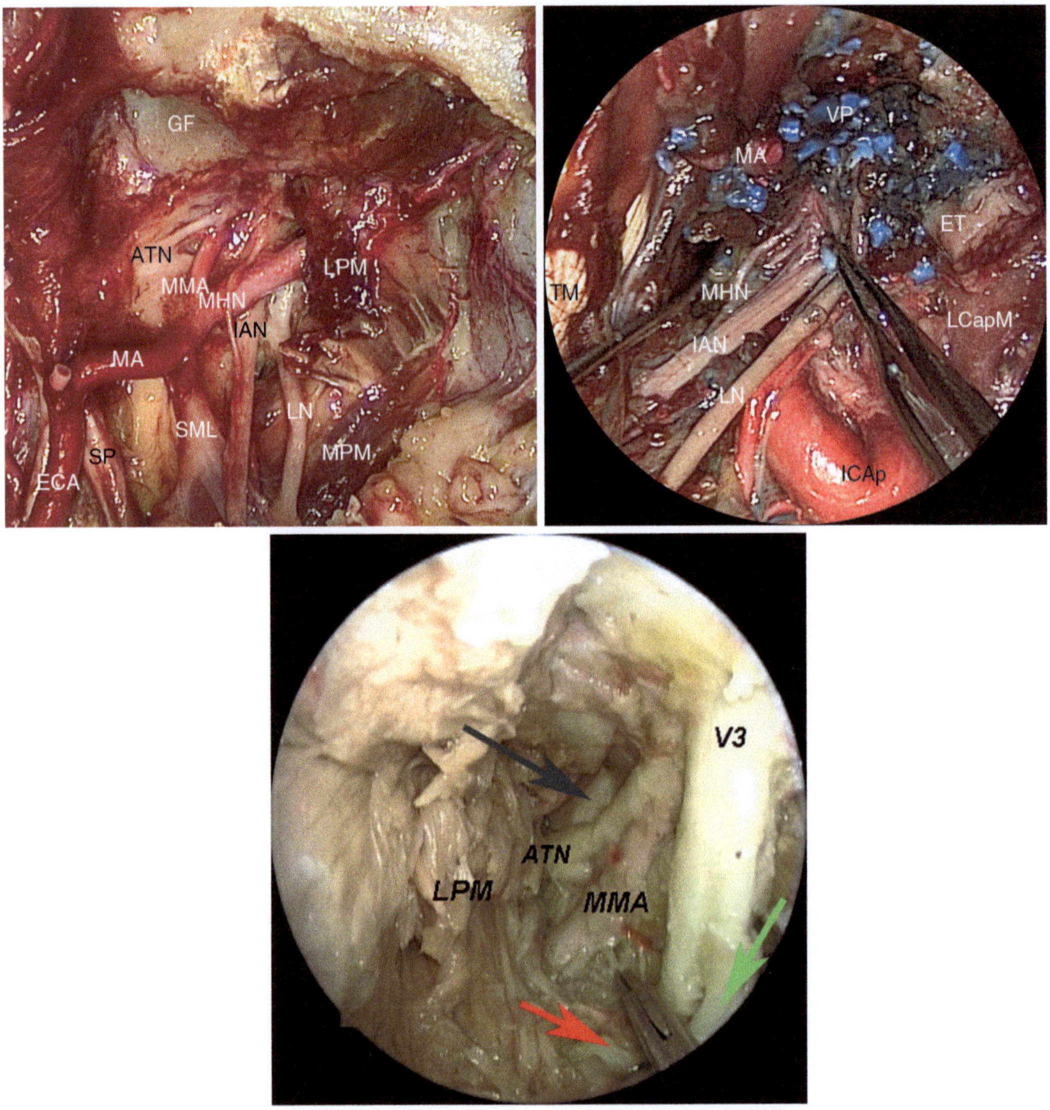

Fig. 1.37 External (lateral) and endoscopic anterior view of the main branches of the posterior trunk of V3

ATN **auricolotemporal nerve,** ***ECA*** **external carotid artery,** ***ET*** **eustachian tube,** ***GF*** **glenoid fossa,** ***IAN*** **inferior alveolar nerve,** ***ICAp*** **parapharyngeal portion of the internal carotid artery,** ***LCapM*** **longus capitis muscle,** ***LN*** **lingual nerve,** ***LPM*** **lateral pterygoid muscle,** ***MA*** **maxillary artery,** ***MHN*** **mylohyoid nerve,** ***MMA*** **middle meningeal artery,** ***MPM*** **medial pterygoid muscle,** ***SML*** **sphenomandibular ligament,** ***SP*** **styloid process,** ***TM*** **temporal muscle,** ***VP*** **venous plexus around V3, V3 third branch of the trigeminal nerve,** ***blue arrow*** **sphenomandibular ligament,** ***green arrow*** **lingual nerve,** ***red arrow*** **inferior alveolar nerve**

The MHN can be branched off at different heights, just below the foramen ovale or before the mandibular foramen (Janfaza and Fabian 2001a). The ATN splits around the MMA in about 75 % of the cases. It passes between the neck of the mandible and the SML and courses posteriorly to the temporomandibular joint. The spine of the sphenoid is a little bit posterior and lateral to the foramen spinosum. The SML connects the spine of the sphenoid to the lingula of the mandibular foramen (on the medial aspect of the mandible).

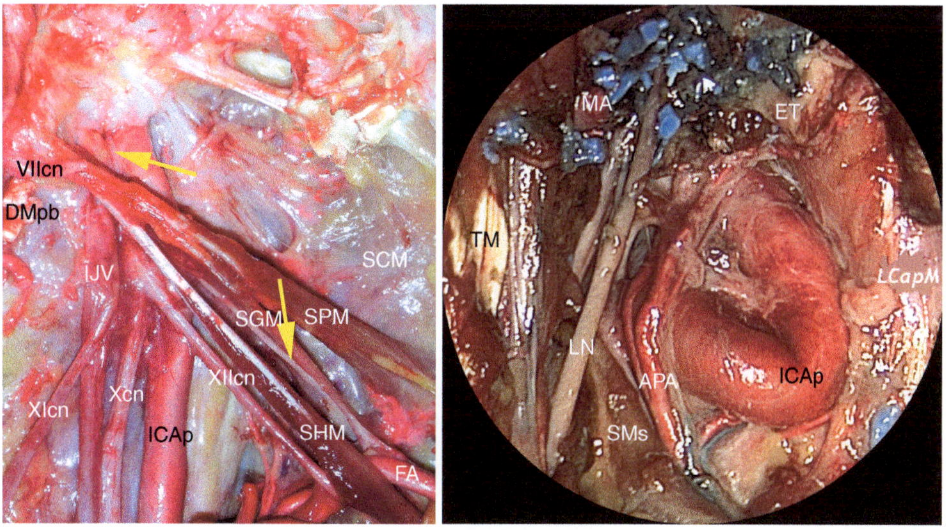

Fig. 1.38 Endoscopic and external view of the upper parapharyngeal space. Note the extreme loop of the parapharyngeal portion of the internal carotid artery

***APA* ascending pharyngeal artery, *DMpb* posterior belly of the digastric muscle, *ET* eustachian tube, *FA* facial artery, *ICAp* parapharyngeal portion of the internal carotid artery, *IJV* internal jugular vein, *LCapM* longus capitis muscle, *LN* lingual nerve, *MA* maxillary artery (cut), *SCM* superior constrictor muscle, *SGM* styloglossus muscle, *SHM* stylohyoid muscle, *SMs* styloid muscles, *SPM* stylopharyngeus muscle, *TM* temporal muscle, *VIIcn* facial nerve, *Xcn* vagus nerve, *XIcn* accessory nerve, *XIIcn* hypoglossal nerve, *yellow arrows* glossopharyngeal nerve**

Note the role of the styloid muscles that "cover" the ICAp. Unfortunately, the presence of looping and kinking of the ICAp makes segment(s) of this vessel anterior to the styloid "apparatus." The styloid diaphragm is given by the posterior belly of the digastric muscle, the stylohyoid and stylopharyngeus muscles, and the stylopharyngeal aponeurosis (Falcon et al. 2011; Rhoton 2000).

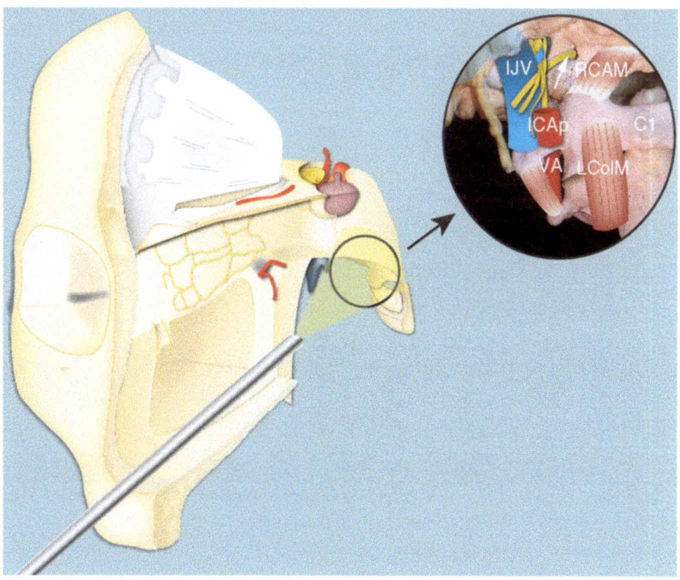

Fig. 1.39 Three-dimensional reconstruction of the endoscopic approach to craniovertebral junction and jugular foramen area

***C1* atlas, *ICAp* parapharyngeal portion of the internal carotid artery, *IJV* internal jugular vein, *LColM* longus colli muscle, *RCAM* rectus capitis anterior muscle, *VA* vertebral artery, *white arrow* hypoglossal nerve**

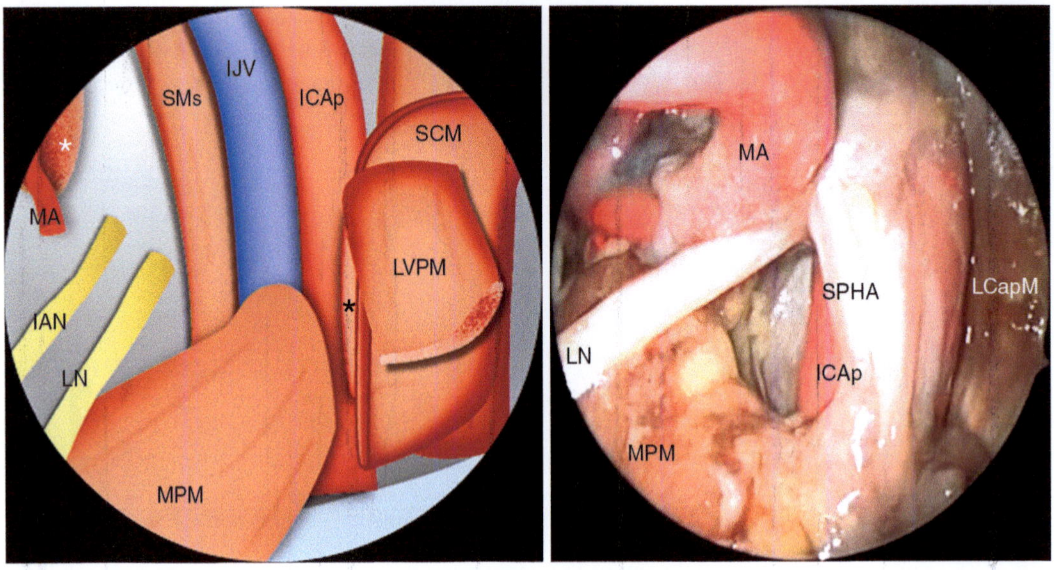

Fig. 1.40 Endoscopic view and reconstruction of the medial corridor to the parapharyngeal vessels

***IAN* inferior alveolar nerve, *ICAp* parapharyngeal portion of the internal carotid artery, *LCapM* longus capitis muscle, *LN* lingual nerve, *LVPM* levator veli palatini muscle, *MA* maxillary artery, *MPM* medial pterygoid muscle, *SPHA* stylopharyngeal aponeurosis, *SCM* superior constrictor muscle, *SMs* styloid muscles, *black asterisk* ascending pharyngeal artery, *white asterisk* lateral pterygoid muscle**

Theoretically, the role of the SCM in indicating the ICAp could be critical. Unfortunately, in real conditions it is hard to identify this structure in endoscopic approach. Anatomically speaking, the SCM does not reach the skull base laterally, but it is attached to the cranial base by means of the pharyngobasilar fascia. This fascia originates from the pharyngeal tubercle, courses laterally toward the petrous bone, turns anteromedially just in front of the carotid foramen, and attaches along the cartilaginous portion of the eustachian tube and the medial pterygoid plate (Janfaza et al. 2001).

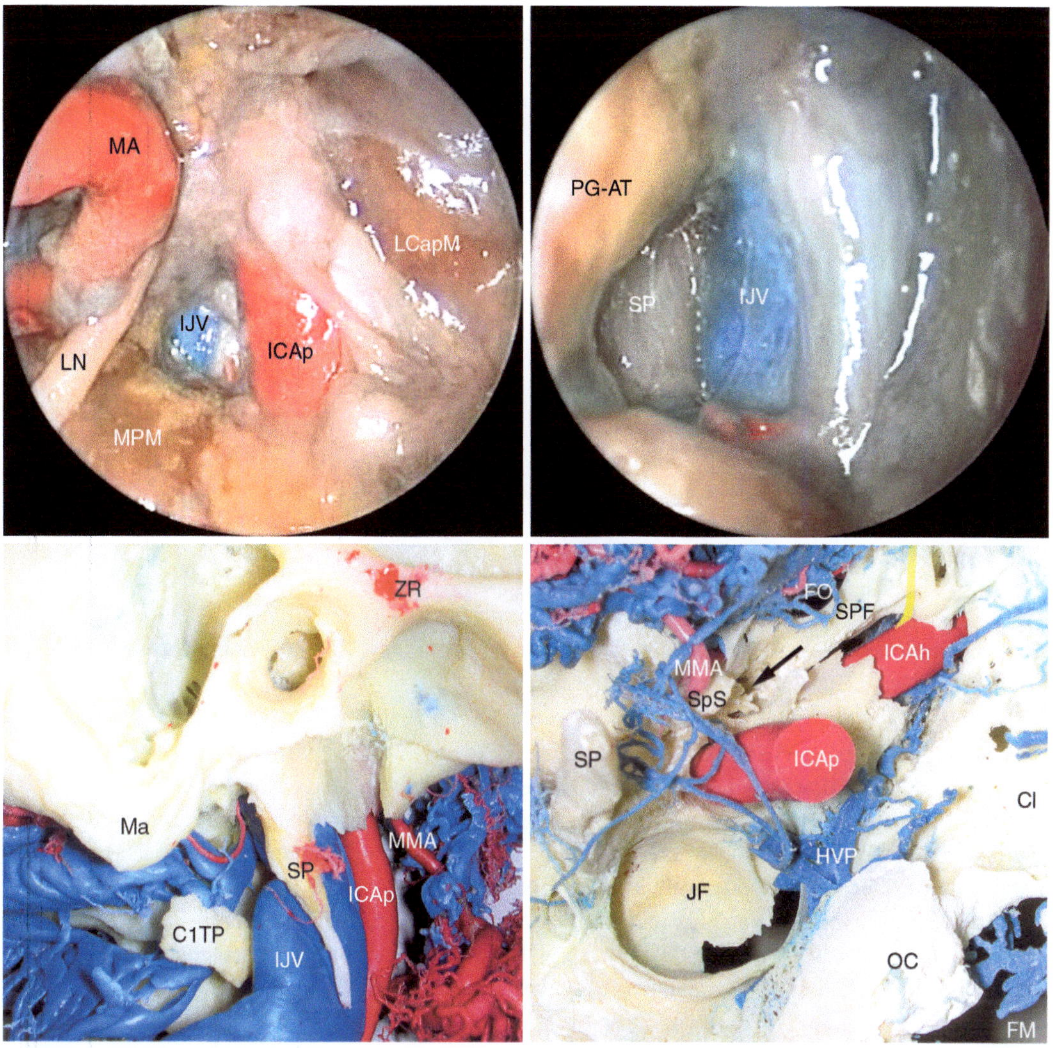

Fig. 1.41 Jugular foramen and styloid process

C1TP **transverse process of C1,** ***Cl*** **clivus,** ***FM*** **foramen magnum,** ***FO*** **foramen ovale,** ***HPV*** **hypoglossal venous plexus,** ***ICAh*** **horizontal segment of the internal carotid artery,** ***ICAp*** **parapharyngeal segment of the internal carotid artery,** ***IJV*** **internal jugular vein,** ***JF*** **jugular foramen,** ***LCapM*** **longus capitis muscle,** ***LN*** **lingual nerve,** ***Ma*** **mastoid (tip),** ***MMA*** **middle meningeal artery,** ***MPM*** **medial pterygoid muscle,** ***OC*** **occipital condyle,** ***PG-AT*** **parotid gland-adipose tissue,** ***SP*** **styloid process,** ***SPF*** **sphenopetrosal fissure,** ***SpS*** **spine of the sphenoid,** ***ZR*** **zygomatic root,** ***black arrow*** **opening of the musculo-tubal canal,** ***yellow line*** **vidian nerve**

The styloid process is laterally located with respect to the IJV. The stylopharyngeal aponeurosis (*SPHA*) extends from the SP and the stylopharyngeus muscle to the lateral pharyngeal recess (Falcon et al. 2011). The SPHA separates the prestyloid from the poststyloid compartment in its most medial aspect and encases major neurovascular structures (Rhoton 2000).

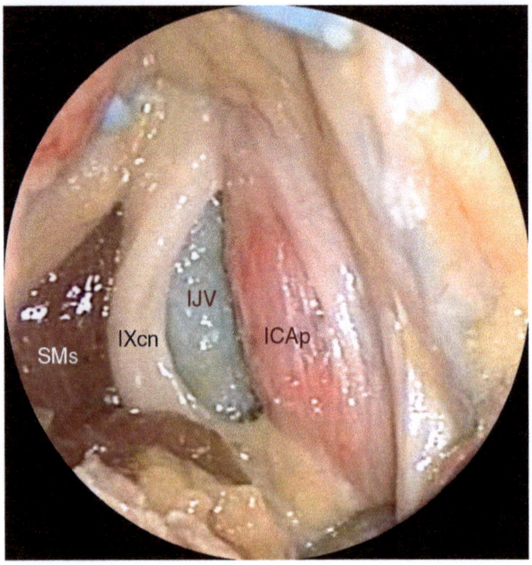

Fig. 1.42 Endoscopic view of the jugular foramen area

***ICAp* parapharyngeal portion of the internal carotid artery, *IJV* internal jugular vein, *SMs* styloid muscles, *IXcn* glossopharyngeal nerve**

The glossopharyngeal nerve is located between the ICAp and IJV, enclosed within the stylopharyngeal aponeurosis. It runs downward on the lateral aspect of the stylopharyngeus muscle. The vagus nerve emerges from the superior ganglion and passes posteriorly to the carotid sheath, between the ICAp and the IJV. It is posterior to the ICAp and can be visualized only by displacing the vessel. The accessory and hypoglossal nerves are posteriorly located with respect to the vagus nerve. The accessory nerve is located in between the ICAp and IJV, enclosed by the stylopharyngeal fascia. It runs immediately posterior to the vagus nerve, while the relationship with the IJV is variable. In fact, the nerve runs posteriorly to the IJV in 33 % of cases and anteriorly in 66 % of cases (Cavalcanti et al. 2010).

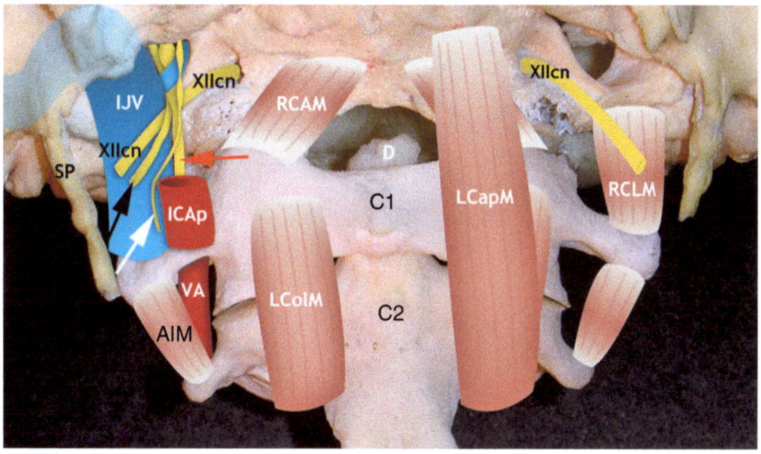

Fig. 1.43 Jugular foramen region

AIM **anterior intertransversarius muscle,** ***C1*** **atlas,** ***C2*** **axis,** ***D*** **dens,** ***ICAp*** **parapharyngeal portion of the internal carotid artery,** ***IJV*** **internal jugular vein,** ***LCapM*** **longus capitis muscle,** ***LColM*** **longus colli muscle,** ***RCAM*** **rectus capitis anterior muscle,** ***RCLM*** **rectus capitis lateralis muscle,** ***SP*** **styloid process,** ***VA*** **vertebral artery,** ***XIIcn*** **hypoglossal nerve,** ***black arrow*** **accessory nerve,** ***white arrow*** **glossopharyngeal nerve,** ***red arrow*** **vagus nerve**

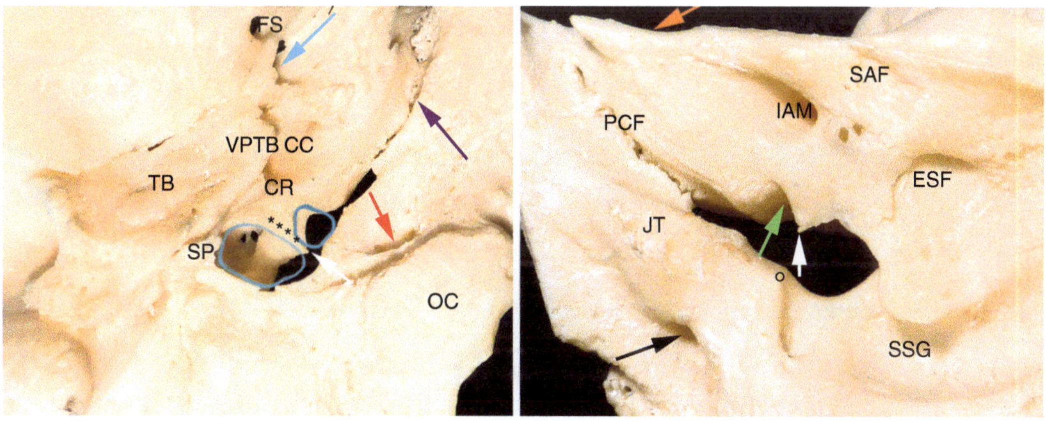

Fig. 1.44 Osteology of the jugular foramen area, exocranial and endocranial views

CC **carotid canal,** ***CR*** **carotid ridge,** ***ESF*** **endolymphatic sac fossa,** ***FS*** **foramen spinosum,** ***IAM*** **internal acoustic meatus,** ***JT*** **jugular tubercle,** ***OC*** **occipital condyle,** ***PCF*** **petroclival fissure,** ***SAF*** **subarcuate fossa,** ***SP*** **styloid process,** ***SSG*** **sigmoid sinus groove,** ***TB*** **tympanic bone,** ***VPTB*** **vaginal process of the tympanic bone,** ***white arrow*** **intrajugular process of the temporal bone,** ***red arrow*** **external orifice of the hypoglossal canal,** ***violet arrow*** **petroclival fissure,** ***blue-sky arrow*** **tubal isthmus,** ***black arrow*** **endocranial orifice of the hypoglossal canal,** ***orange arrow*** **trigeminal impression,** ***green arrow*** **pyramidal fossa,** ***black asterisks*** **intrajugular ridge,** ***black circle*** **intrajugular process of the occipital bone**

Within the JF area 2 venous compartement can be identified: a large postero-lateral_SIGMOID_venous channel and a small antero-medial_PETROSAL_venous channel which can receive the drainage of the inferior petrosal sinus (IPS). Anyway, the relationship with the IPS is highly variable. An intermediary neural compartment is located between the venous ones and houses lower cranial nerves (IX, X, XI).

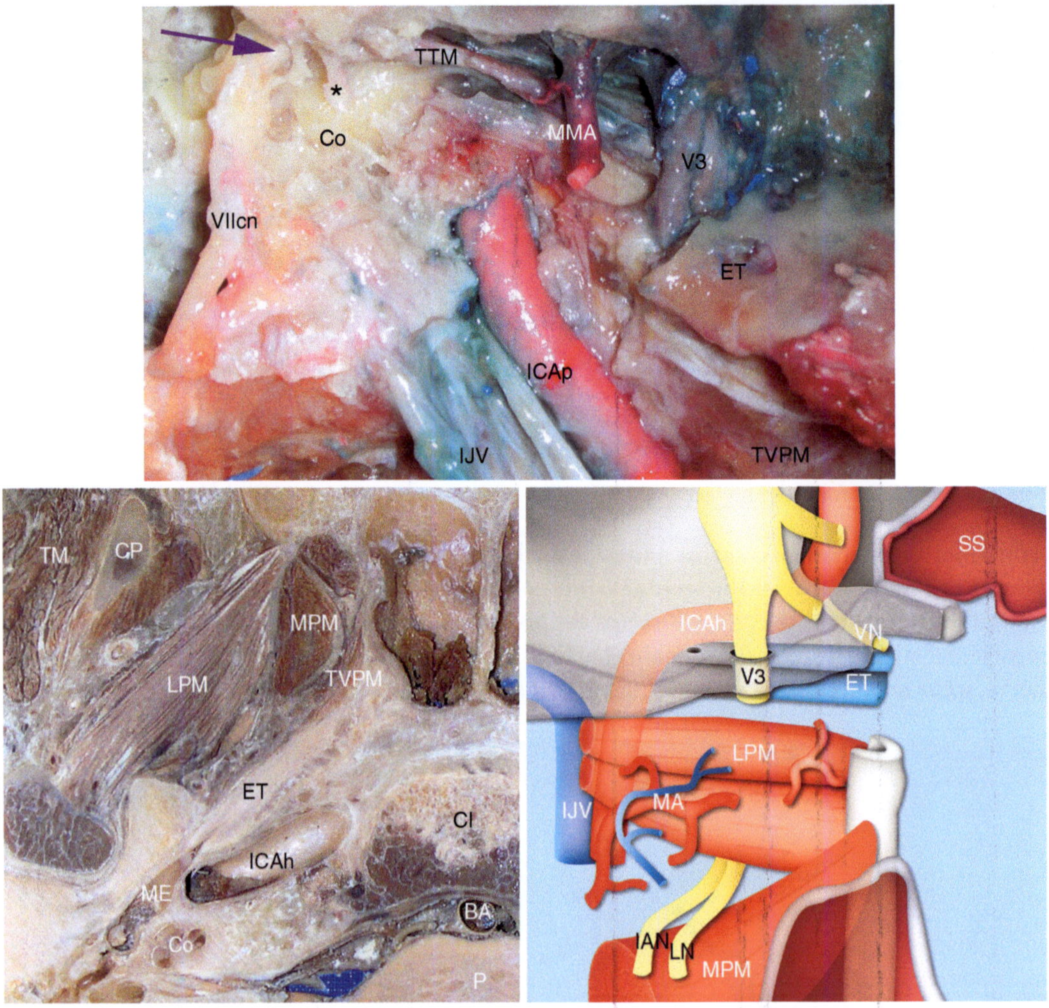

Fig. 1.45 Relationship between the carotid canal and the eustachian tube

BA **basilar artery,** ***Cl*** **clivus,** ***Co*** **cochlea,** ***CP*** **coronoid process,** ***ET*** **eustachian tube,** ***IAN*** **inferior alveolar nerve,** ***ICAp*** **parapharyngeal portion of the internal carotid artery,** ***ICAh*** **horizontal portion of the internal carotid artery,** ***IJV*** **internal jugular vein,** ***LN*** **lingual nerve,** ***LPM*** **lateral pterygoid muscle,** ***MA*** **maxillary artery,** ***ME*** **middle ear,** ***MMA*** **middle meningeal artery,** ***MPM*** **medial pterygoid muscle,** ***P*** **pons,** ***SS*** **sphenoid sinus,** ***TM*** **temporal muscle,** ***TTM*** **tensor tympani muscle,** ***TVPM*** **tensor veli palatini muscle,** ***VN*** **vidian nerve,** ***V3*** **third branch of the trigeminal nerve,** ***VIIcn*** **facial nerve,** ***violet arrow*** **tympanic segment of the facial nerve,** ***black asterisk*** **malleus**

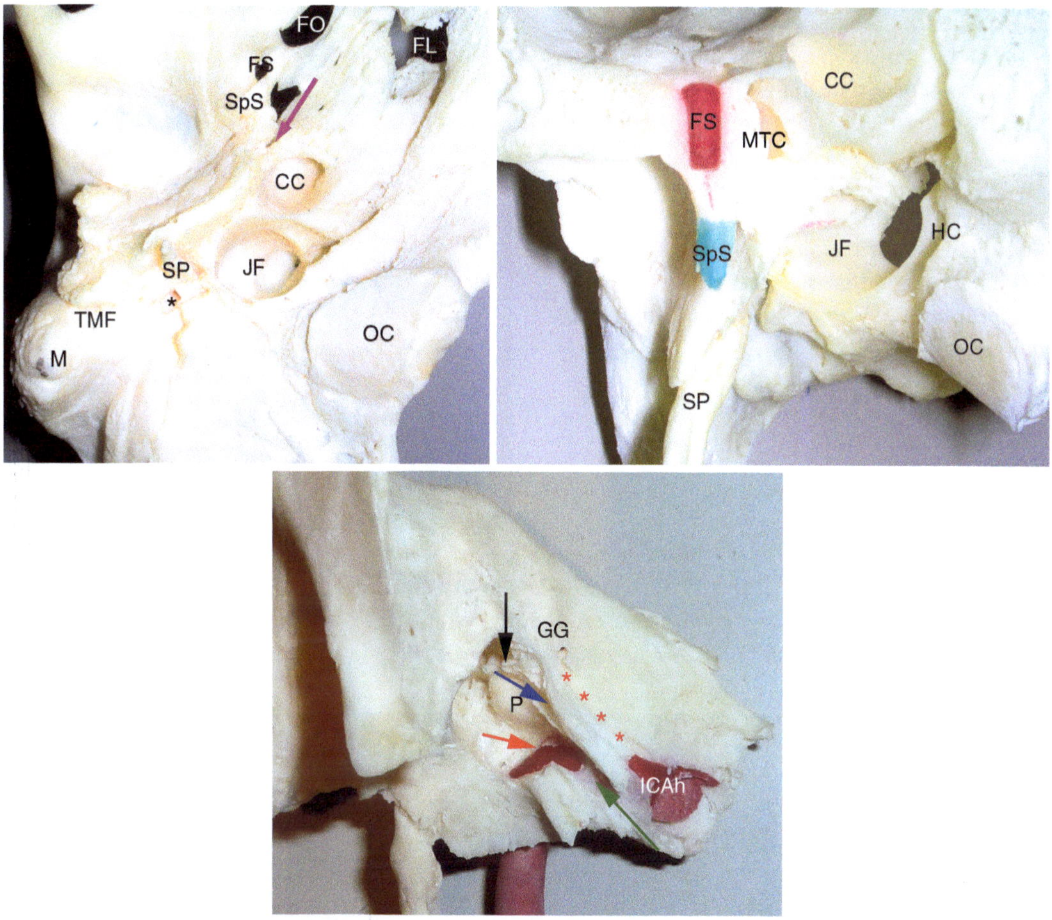

Fig. 1.46 Bony eustachian tube and carotid canal relationship

CC **carotid canal,** ***FL*** **foramen lacerum,** ***FO*** **foramen ovale,** ***FS*** **foramen spinosum,** ***GG*** **geniculate ganglion area,** ***HC*** **hypoglossal canal,** ***JF*** **jugular foramen,** ***ICAh*** **horizontal portion of the internal carotid artery,** ***M*** **mastoid (tip),** ***MTC*** **musculo-tubal canal,** ***OC*** **occipital condyle,** ***P*** **promontory,** ***SP*** **styloid process,** ***SpS*** **spine of the sphenoid,** ***TMF*** **tympanomastoid fissure,** ***red arrow*** **posterior bend of the ICAh,** ***green arrow*** **bony portion of the ET (musculo-tubal canal),** ***blue arrow*** **canal of the tensor tympani muscle,** ***violet arrow*** **opening of the musculo-tubal canal,** ***black arrow*** **cochleariform process,** ***black asterisk*** **stylomastoid foramen,** ***red asterisks*** **groove of the greater petrosal nerve**

The cartilaginous portion of the tube passes posteromedially along the border between the petrous bone and the greater wing of the sphenoid bone to attach the bony eustachian tube immediately anterior to the carotid canal (Janfaza et al. 2001). The isthmus lies immediately behind the SpS.

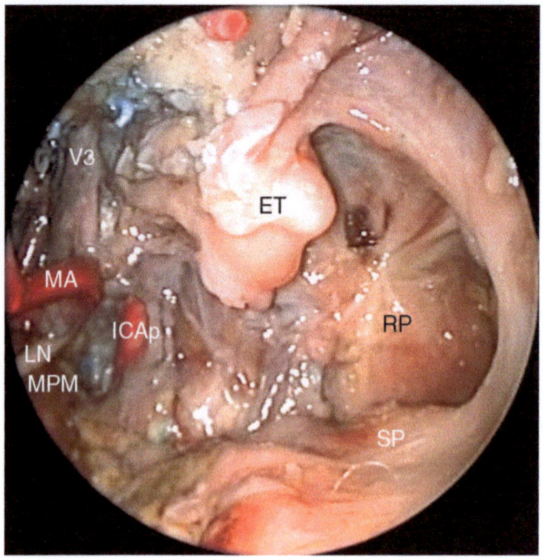

Fig. 1.47 Endoscopic view of the infratemporal fossa and upper parapharyngeal space. The role of the eustachian tube in pointing the carotid canal is underlined

ET **eustachian tube,** ***ICAp*** **parapharyngeal portion of the internal carotid artery,** ***LN*** **lingual nerve,** ***MA*** **maxillary artery,** ***MPM*** **medial pterygoid muscle,** ***RP*** **rhinopharynx,** ***SP*** **soft palate,** ***V3*** **third branch of the trigeminal nerve**

The cartilaginous portion of the ET is 2 cm long. It inserts at the back of the medial pterygoid plate immediately above the pharyngobasilar fascia (Janfaza et al. 2001).

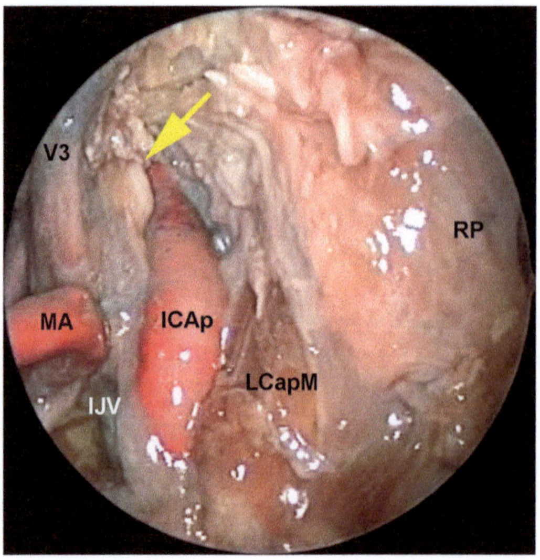

Fig. 1.48 Endoscopic view of the upper parapharyngeal space. The cartilaginous portion of the eustachian tube has been removed. The upper part of the parapharyngeal portion of the internal carotid artery entering the carotid canal is visible

ICAp **parapharyngeal portion of the internal carotid artery,** ***IJV*** **internal jugular vein,** ***LCapM*** **longus capitis muscle,** ***MA*** **maxillary artery,** ***RP*** **rhinopharynx,** ***V3*** **third branch of the trigeminal nerve,** ***yellow arrow*** **indicates bony tube (immediately anterior to the carotid canal)**

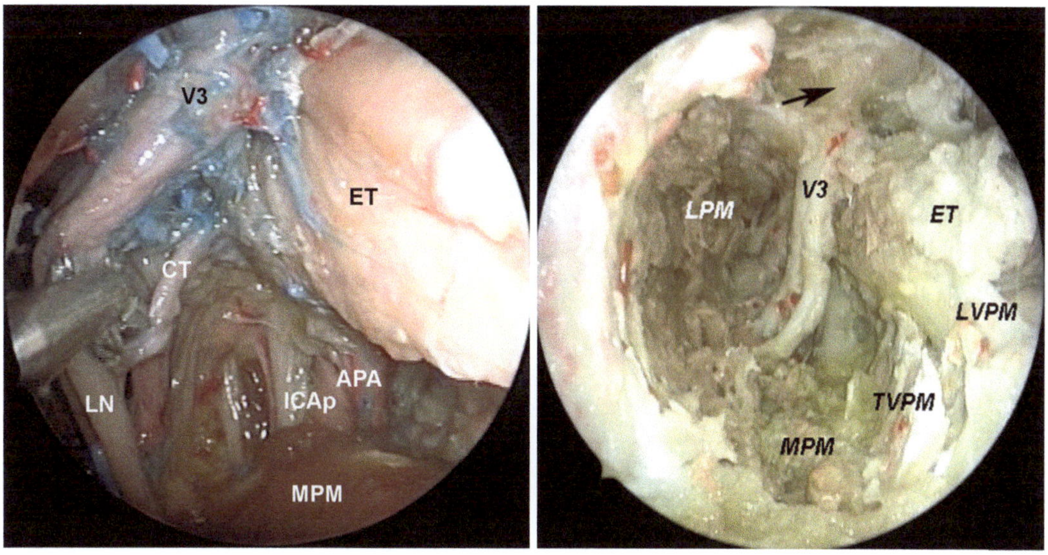

Fig. 1.49 Relationship between the eustachian tube and V3. The connection between the chorda tympani and the lingual nerve is visible

APA **ascending pharyngeal artery,** ***CT*** **chorda tympani,** ***ET*** **Eustachian tube,** ***ICAp*** **parapharyngeal portion of the internal carotid artery,** ***LN*** **lingual nerve,** ***LPM*** **lateral pterygoid muscle,** ***LVPM*** **levator veli palatini muscle,** ***MPM*** **medial pterygoid muscle,** ***TVPM*** **tensor veli palatini muscle,** ***V3*** **third branch of the trigeminal nerve,** ***black arrow*** **canal of** ***V3*** **within the skull base**

The cartilaginous part of the ET inserted in the posterior border of the medial pterygoid plate. It is attached posteriorly to foramen lacerum and clivus, and superiorly to the sphenopetrosal fissure region. V3 lies anteriorly to cartilaginous portion of ET, and presents an intimate relationship with the ET. The nerve, at the skull base, is surrounded by a wide venous plexus. V3 is an important landmark to locate the post-styloid compartment, as it is anterior to this space (Falcon et al. 2011).

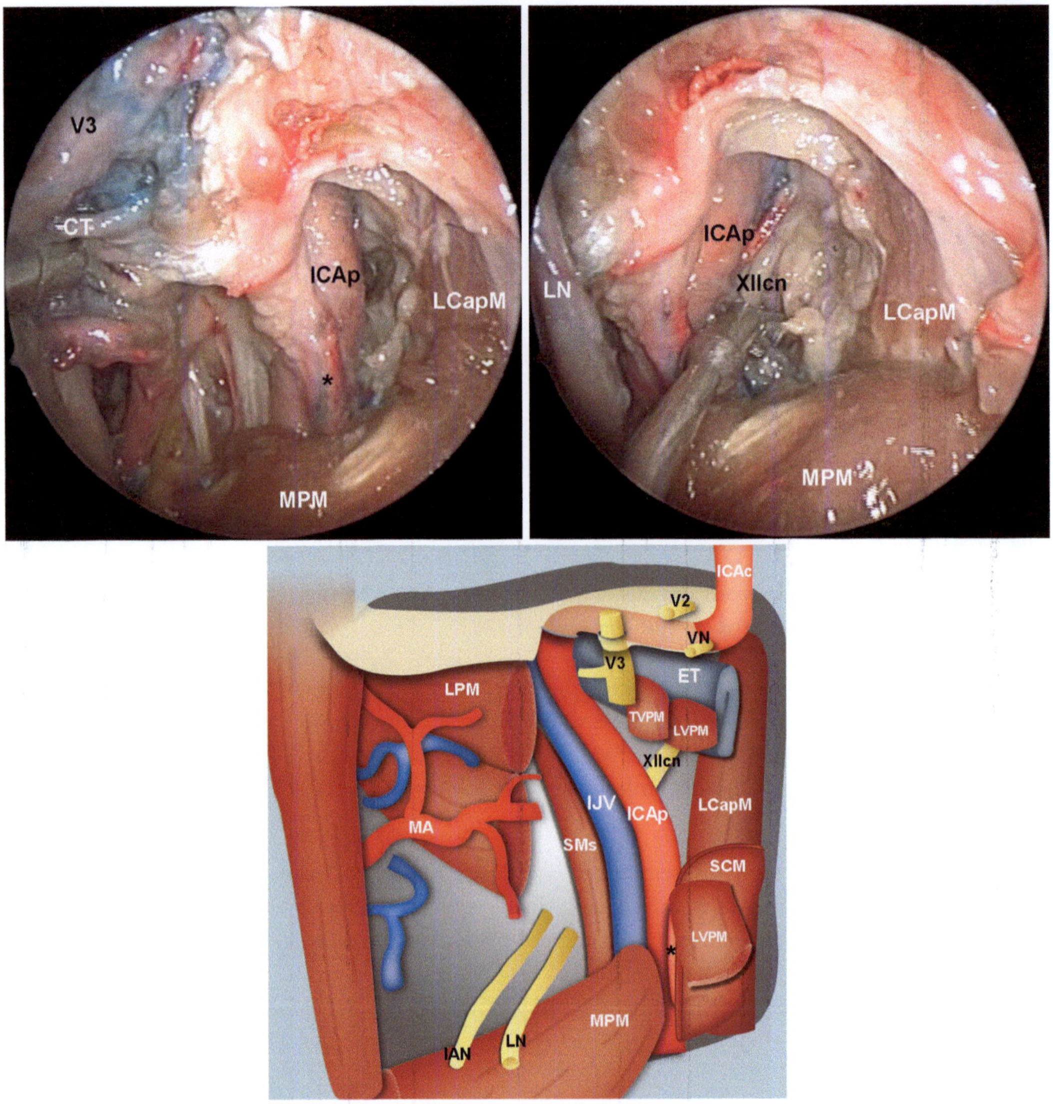

Fig. 1.50 Endoscopic view of parapharyngeal and laterovertebral regions

CT **chorda tympani,** ***ET*** **eustachian tube,** ***IAN*** **inferior alveolar nerve,** ***ICAc*** **cavernous portion of the internal carotid artery,** ***ICAp*** **parapharyngeal portion of the internal carotid artery,** ***IJV*** **internal jugular vein,** ***LCapM*** **longus capitis muscle,** ***LN*** **lingual nerve,** ***LPM*** **lateral pterygoid muscle,** ***LVPM*** **levator veli palatini muscle,** ***MA*** **maxillary artery,** ***MPM*** **medial pterygoid muscle,** ***SCM*** **superior constrictor muscle,** ***SMs*** **styloid muscles,** ***TVPM*** **tensor veli palatini muscle,** ***VN*** **vidian nerve,** ***XIIcn*** **hypoglossal nerve,** ***V2*** **second branch of the trigeminal nerve,** ***V3*** **third branch of the trigeminal nerve,** ***black asterisk*** **ascending pharyngeal artery**

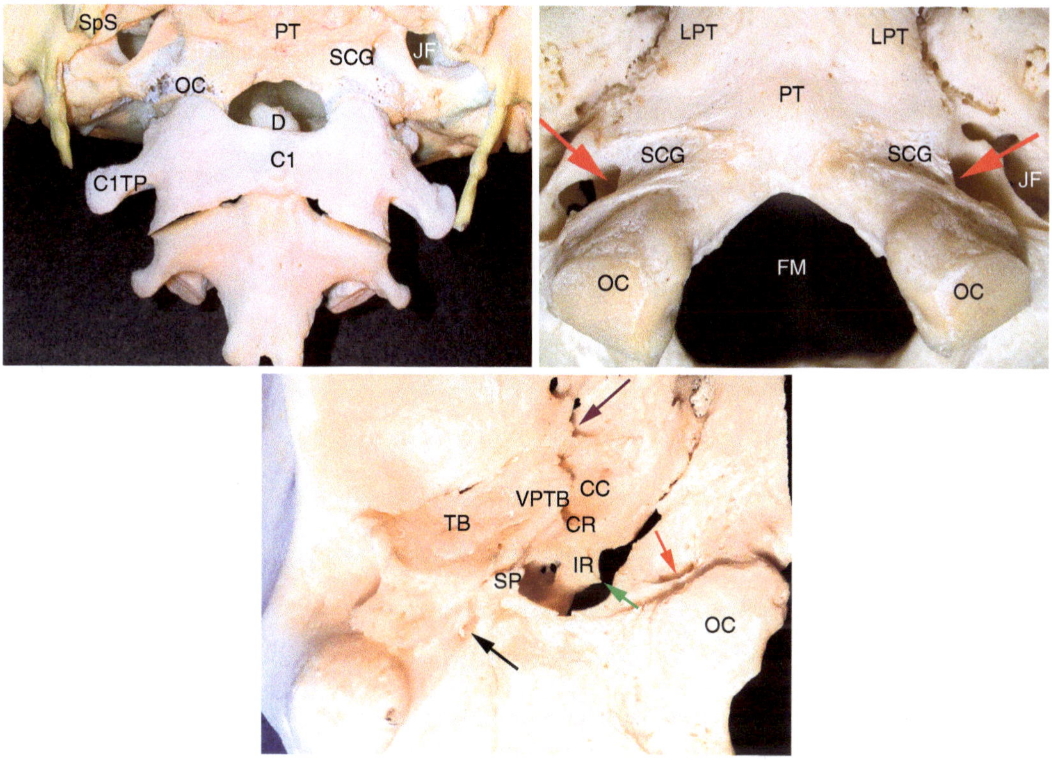

Fig. 1.51 Anterior view of the lower clivus and foramen magnum region and inferior view of jugular foramen area

CC **carotid canal,** ***CR*** **carotid ridge,** ***C1*** **atlas,** ***C1TP*** **transverse process of the atlas,** ***D*** **dens,** ***FM*** **foramen magnum,** ***IR*** **intrajugular ridge,** ***JF*** **jugular foramen,** ***LPT*** **lateral pharyngeal tubercle,** ***OC*** **occipital condyle,** ***PT*** **pharyngeal tubercle,** ***SCG*** **supracondylar groove,** ***SP*** **styloid process,** ***SpS*** **spine of the sphenoid,** ***TB*** **tympanic bone,** ***VPTB*** **vaginal process of the tympanic bone,** ***black arrow*** **stylomastoid foramen,** ***red arrow*** **hypoglossal canal,** ***dark green arrow*** **intrajugular process of the temporal bone,** ***violet arrow*** **opening of the musculo-tubal canal**

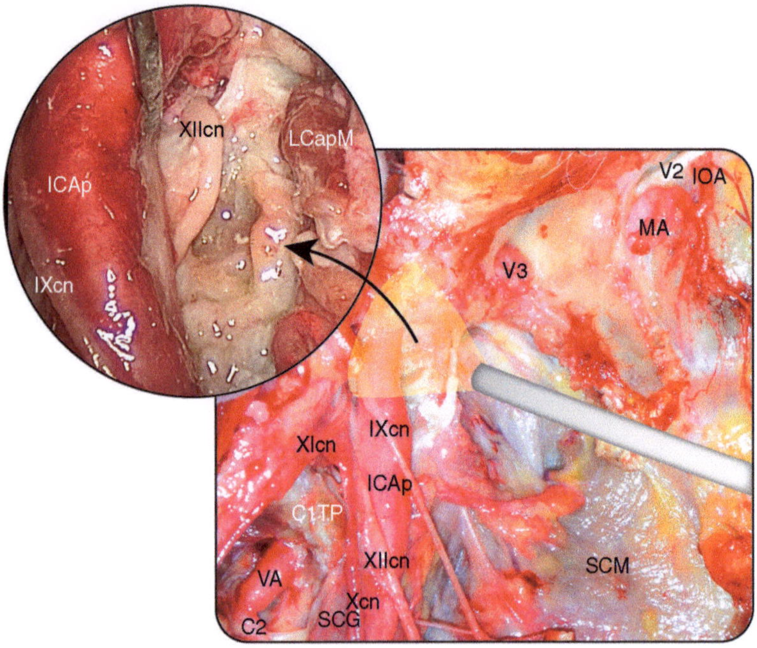

Fig. 1.52 External view of the extracranial segment of the hypoglossal nerve

C1TP **transverse process of C1,** ***C2*** **second cervical nerve root,** ***ICAp*** **parapharyngeal portion of the internal carotid artery,** ***IOA*** **infraorbital artery,** ***LCapM*** **longus capitis muscle,** ***MA*** **maxillary artery,** ***SCG*** **superior cervical ganglion,** ***SCM*** **superior constrictor muscle,** ***VA*** **vertebral artery,** ***V2*** **second branch of the trigeminal nerve,** ***V3*** **third branch of the trigeminal nerve,** ***IXcn*** **glossopharyngeal nerve,** ***Xcn*** **vagus nerve,** ***XIcn*** **accessory nerve,** ***XIIcn*** **hypoglossal nerve**

The hypoglossal nerve exits from the hypoglossal canal medial to the carotid sheath. It lies posterior to the vagus nerve and runs laterally between the IJV and the ICAp (enclosed within the carotid sheath). Coursing inferiorly, it is lateral to the internal and external carotid artery and covered by the styloid process.

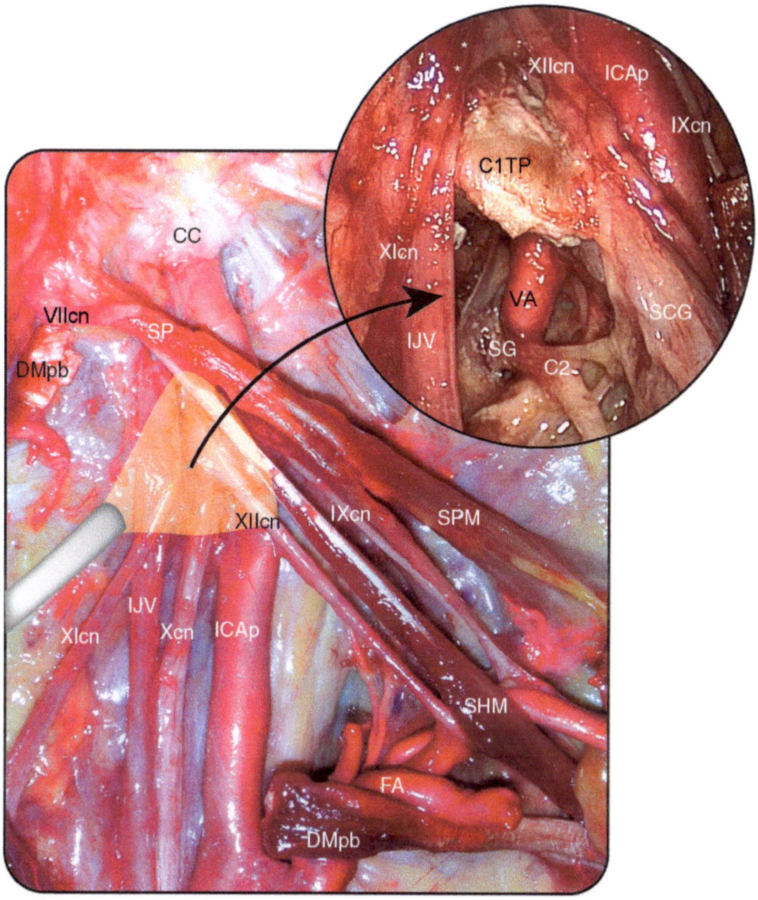

Fig. 1.53 External view of the relationship between the parapharyngeal portion of the internal carotid artery and the vertebral artery. A vertebral window between the transverse processes is needed to visualize the vertebral bed. Note that the posterior belly of the digastric muscle has been cut

C1TP **transverse process of C1, C2 second cervical root,** ***CC*** **carotid canal,** ***DMpb*** **posterior belly of the digastric muscle,** ***FA*** **facial artery,** ***ICAp*** **parapharyngeal portion of the internal carotid artery,** ***IJV*** **internal jugular vein,** ***SCG*** **superior cervical ganglion,** ***SG*** **spinal ganglion,** ***SHM*** **stylohyoid muscle,** ***SP*** **styloid process,** ***SPM*** **stylopharyngeus muscle,** ***VA*** **vertebral artery,** ***VIIcn*** **facial nerve,** ***IXcn*** **glossopharyngeal nerve,** ***Xcn*** **vagus nerve,** ***XIcn*** **accessory nerve,** ***XIIcn*** **hypoglossal nerve**

The medial segment of the styloid diaphgram consists of the stylopharyngeal fascia and is medial to the styloid process and attached muscles (Bejjani et al. 1998). It is a thick fascia inserting superiorly at the cranial base and medially at the pharyngeal wall.

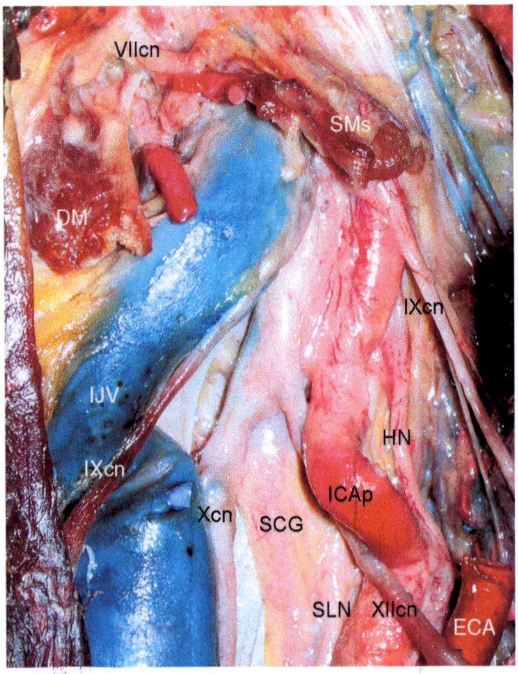

Fig. 1.54 External view of the jugular foramen region

DM **digastric muscle,** ***ECA*** **external carotid artery,** ***HN*** **Hering's nerve,** ***ICAp*** **parapharyngeal portion of the internal carotid artery,** ***IJV*** **internal jugular vein,** ***SCG*** **superior cervical ganglion,** ***SLN*** **superior laryngeal nerve,** ***SMs*** **styloid muscles,** ***VIIcn*** **facial nerve,** ***IXcn*** **glossopharyngeal nerve,** ***Xcn*** **vagus nerve,** ***XIcn*** **accessory nerve,** ***XIIcn*** **hypoglossal nerve**

On the outer skull base, the hypoglossal nerve runs on the medial surface of the IJV and on the lateral surface of the vagus nerve in more than 90 % of cases (Lang 1995). Then, it curves around the occipital artery and runs first to the lateral and then to the anterior surface of the ECA. In most cases, there are anastomoses between the inferior ganglion of the vagus nerve and the sympathetic ganglion. The SLN branched off from the vagus nerve a little bit inferior to the inferior ganglion. It lies posterior to the vagus nerve and passes laterally between the IJV and ICAp. Inferiorly, it lies lateral to ICA and ECA and deep to styloid process. The nerve of Hering, carotid branch of IXcn, descends between the ICAp and ECA to reach the carotid body and sinus (Janfaza and Fabian 2001b).

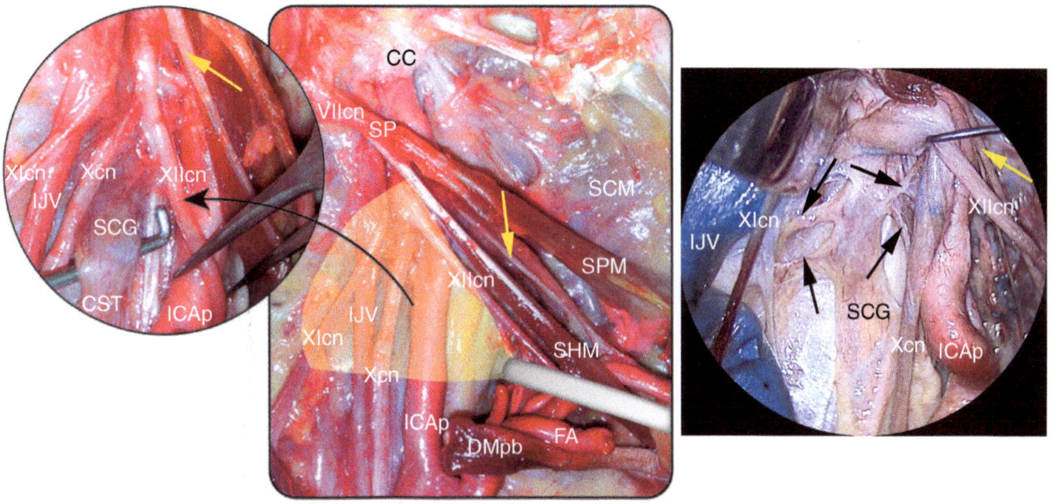

Fig. 1.55 External views of the upper parapharyngeal region and focus on superior cervical ganglion

CC **carotid canal,** ***CST*** **cervical sympathetic trunk,** ***DMpb*** **posterior belly of the digastric muscle,** ***FA*** **facial artery,** ***ICAp*** **parapharyngeal portion of the internal carotid artery,** ***IJV*** **internal jugular vein,** ***LC*** **longus capitis,** ***SCG*** **superior cervical ganglion,** ***SCM*** **superior constrictor muscle,** ***SHM*** **stylohyoid muscle,** ***SP*** **styloid process,** ***SPM*** **stylopharyngeus muscle,** ***VIIcn*** **facial nerve,** ***X*** **vagus nerve,** ***XIcn*** **accessory nerve,** ***XIIcn*** **hypoglossal nerve,** ***yellow arrow*** **glossopharyngeal nerve,** ***black arrows*** **anastomosis between the superior cervical ganglion and lower cranial nerves**

The cervical sympathetic trunk lies posterior to the carotid sheath, within a duplication of the prevertebral fascia and medial to the vagus nerve (Janfaza and Fabian 2001a). It is located in a fascial reflection from the posterior wall of the carotid sheath.

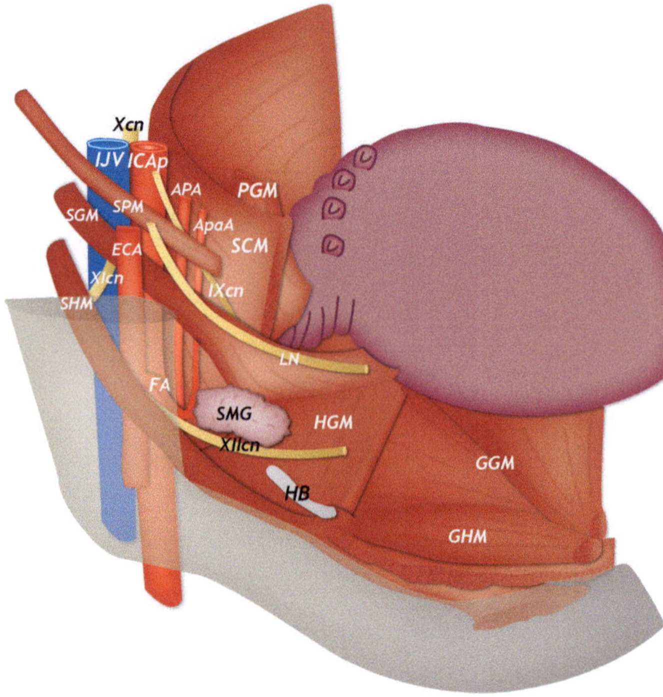

Fig. 1.56 Lateral view of the parapharyngeal region. 3D reconstruction

APA **ascending pharyngeal artery,** ***ApaA*** **ascending palatine artery,** ***ECA*** **external carotid artery,** ***FA*** **facial artery,** ***GGM*** **genioglossus muscle,** ***GHM*** **geniohyoid muscle,** ***HB*** **hyoid bone,** ***HGM*** **hyoglossus muscle,** ***ICAp*** **parapharyngeal portion of the internal carotid artery,** ***IJV*** **internal jugular vein,** ***LN*** **lingual nerve,** ***MHM*** **mylohyoid muscle,** ***PGM*** **palatoglossus muscle,** ***SCM*** **superior constrictor muscle,** ***SGM*** **styloglossus muscle,** ***SHM*** **stylohyoid muscle,** ***SMG*** **submandibular gland,** ***SPM*** **stylopharyngeus muscle,** ***IXcn*** **glossopharyngeal nerve,** ***Xcn*** **vagus nerve,** ***XIcn*** **accessory nerve,** ***XIIcn*** **hypoglossal nerve**

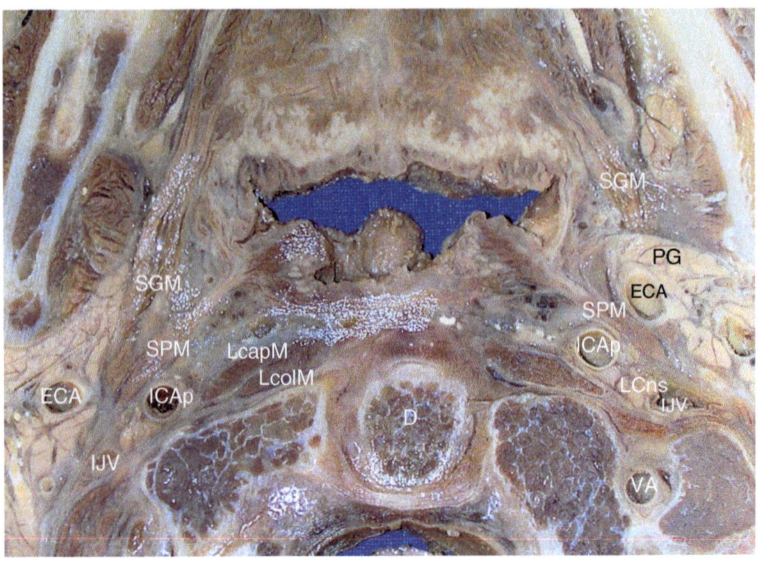

Fig. 1.57 Axial view of the parapharyngeal region

D **dens,** ***ECA*** **external carotid artery,** ***ICAp*** **parapharyngeal portion of the internal carotid artery,** ***IJV*** **internal jugular vein,** ***LCapM*** **longus capitis muscle,** ***LCns*** **lower cranial nerves,** ***LcolM*** **longus colli muscle,** ***PG*** **parotid gland,** ***SGM*** **styloglossus muscle,** ***SPM*** **stylopharyngeus muscle,** ***VA*** **vertebral artery**

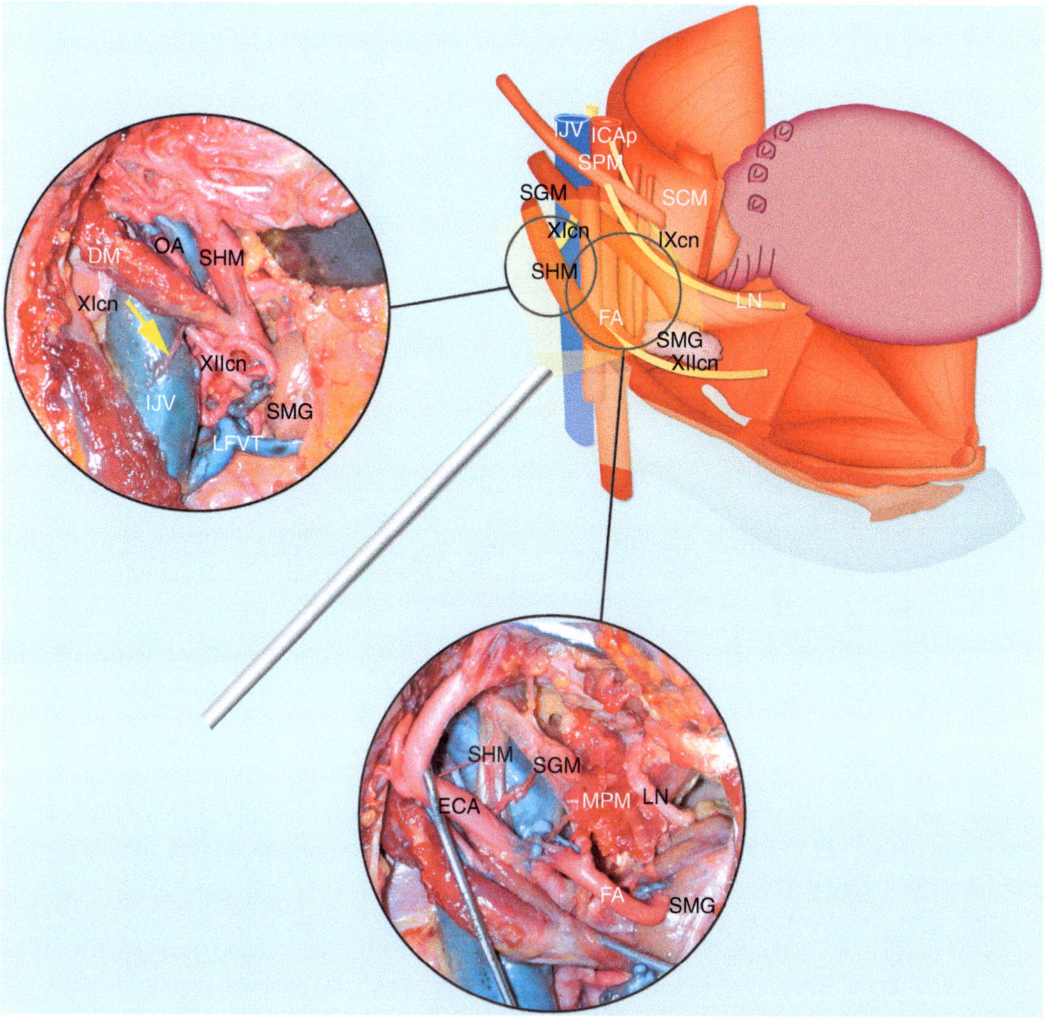

Fig. 1.58 Lateral vision of the upper cervical and lower parapharyngeal regions. The vertical branch of the mandible has been removed

DM **digastric muscle,** ***ECA*** **external carotid artery,** ***FA*** **facial artery,** ***ICAp*** **parapharyngeal portion of the internal carotid artery,** ***IJV*** **internal jugular vein,** ***LFVT*** **linguofacial venous trunk,** ***LN*** **lingual nerve,** ***MPM*** **medial pterygoid muscle,** ***OA*** **occipital artery,** ***SCM*** **superior constrictor muscle,** ***SGM*** **styloglossus muscle,** ***SHM*** **stylohyoid muscle,** ***SMG*** **submandibular gland,** ***SPM*** **stylopharyngeus muscle,** ***IXcn*** **glossopharyngeal nerve,** ***XIcn*** **accessory nerve,** ***XIIcn*** **hypoglossal nerve,** ***yellow arrow*** **ansa cervicalis profunda**

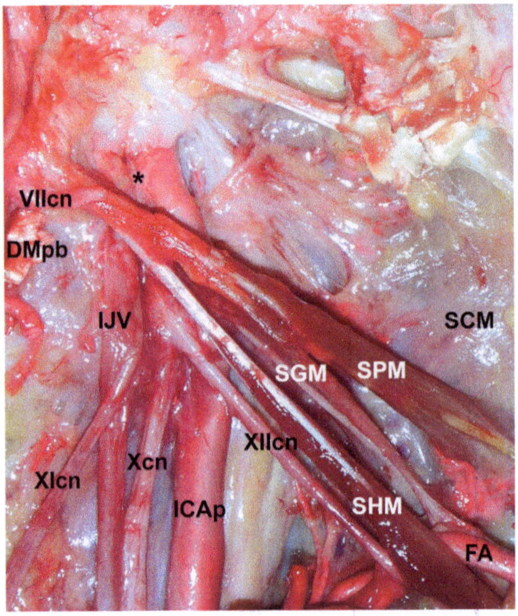

Fig. 1.59 External view of the styloid muscles and their relationship to great cervical vessels. The vertical portion of the mandible has been removed and the ITF content subtotally cleaned

DMpb **posterior belly of the digastric muscle,** ***FA*** **facial artery,** ***ICAp*** **parapharyngeal portion of the internal carotid artery,** ***IJV*** **internal jugular vein,** ***SCM*** **superior constrictor muscle,** ***SGM*** **styloglossus muscle,** ***SHM*** **stylohyoid muscle,** ***SPM*** **stylopharyngeus muscle,** ***VIIcn*** **facial nerve,** ***Xcn*** **vagus nerve,** ***XIcn*** **accessory nerve,** ***XIIcn*** **hypoglossal nerve,** ***black asterisk*** **glossopharyngeal nerve at the skull base**

The SPM runs inferiorly on the lateral aspect of the ICAp. The SHM is lateral to the ECA. The SGM passes lateral to the ICAp, medially to the ECA. The stylomandibular ligament is a condensation of the deep layer of the parotid fascia. It connects the styloid process with the angle of the mandible.

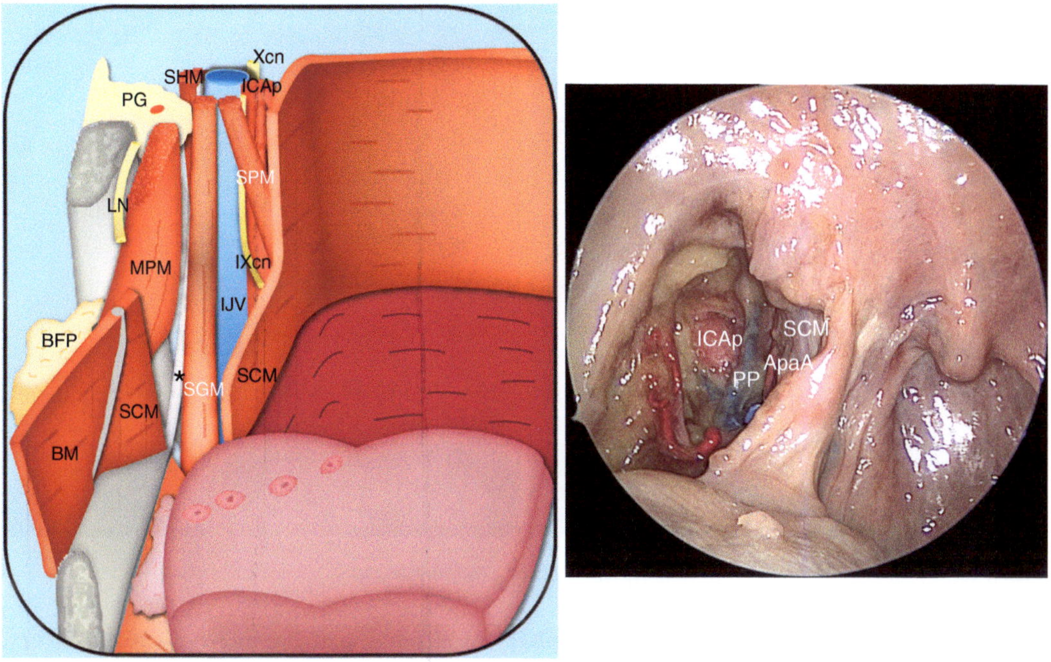

Fig. 1.60 Transoral endoscopic view of the parapharyngeal region

***ApaA* ascending palatine artery, *BFP* buccal fat pad, *BM* buccinator muscle, *ICAp* parapharyngeal portion of the internal carotid artery, *IJV* internal jugular vein, *LN* lingual nerve, *MPM* medial pterygoid muscle, *PG* parotid gland, *PP* pharyngeal plexus, *SCM* superior constrictor muscle, *SGM* styloglossus muscle, *SHM* stylohyoid muscle, *SPM* stylopharyngeus muscle, *IXcn* glossopharyngeal nerve, *Xcn* vagus nerve, *black asterisk* stylomandibular ligament**

The pterygomandibular raphe is tied between the hamulus of the medial pterygoid plate and the posterior part of the mylohyoid line of the mandible. The buccinator muscle attaches to it.

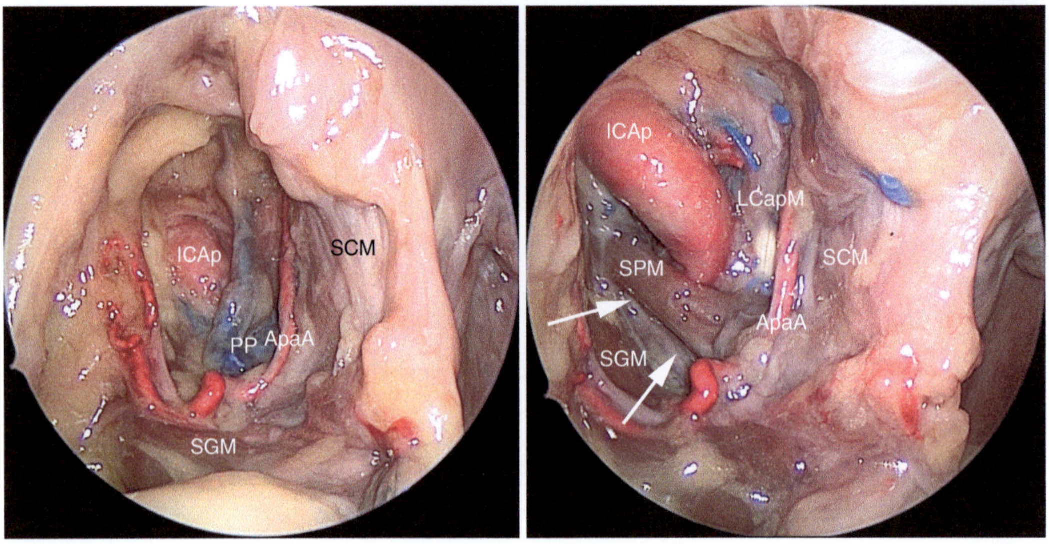

Fig. 1.61 Transoral endoscopic view of the parapharyngeal region

ApaA **ascending palatine artery,** ***ICAp*** **parapharyngeal portion of the internal carotid artery,** ***LCapM*** **longus capitis muscle,** ***PP*** **pharyngeal plexus,** ***SCM*** **superior constrictor muscle,** ***SGM*** **styloglossus muscle,** ***SPM*** **stylopharyngeus muscle,** ***white arrows*** **glossopharyngeal nerve**

The external carotid artery passes deeply to the digastric and stylohyoid muscles, but superficially to the stylopharyngeus and styloglossal muscle when running toward the parotid gland (Janfaza et al. 2001). With a transoral window it is possible to control the space between the medial pterygoid muscle laterally and the superior constrictor muscle medially. The stylopharyngeus and styloglossus muscles are critical landmarks, being usually placed anterior to the great vessels (Dallan et al. 2011). Note that the presence of kinking or looping of the ICAp could make this statement untrue.

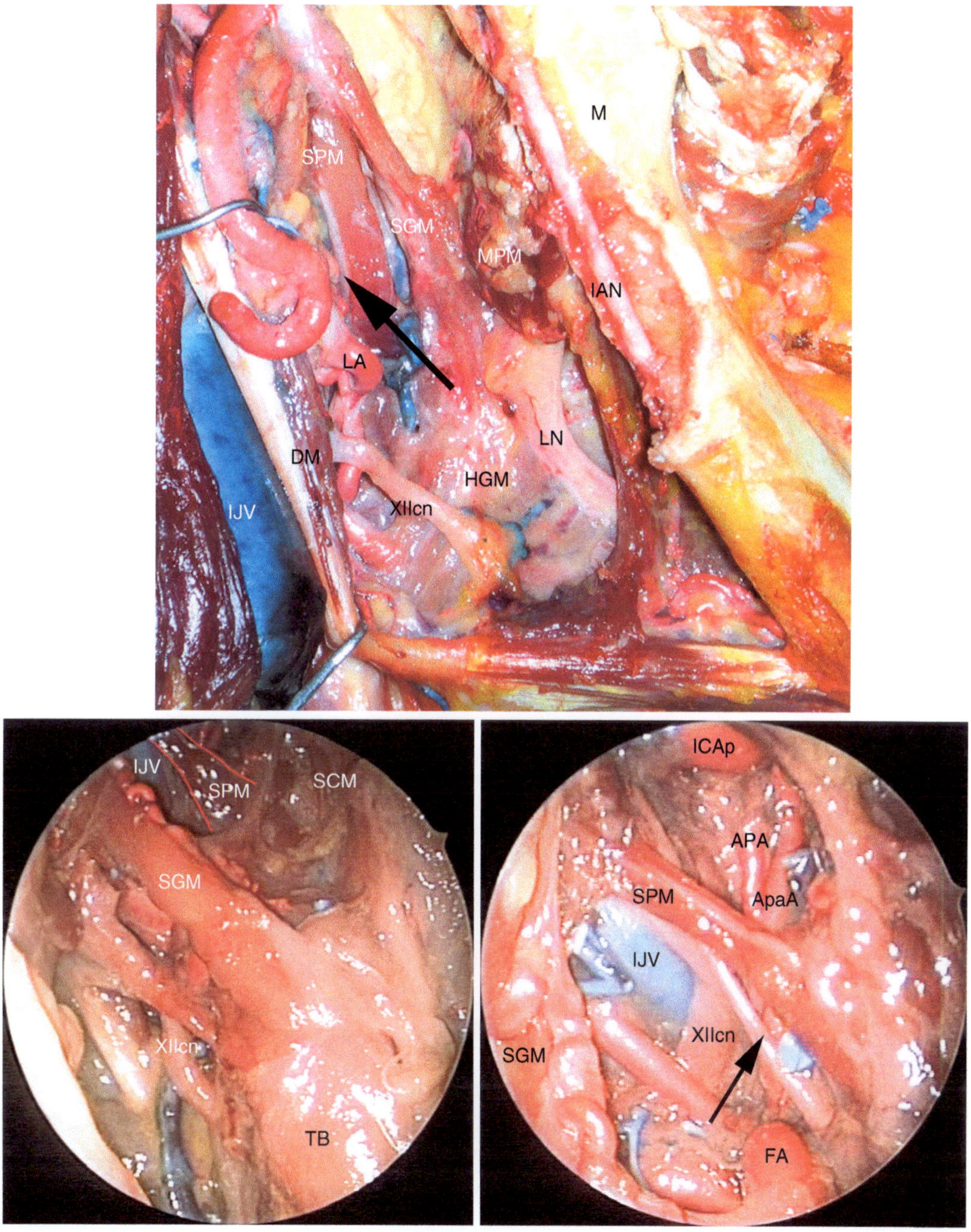

Fig. 1.62 Lateral external and transoral endoscopic views of the tongue base and parapharyngeal regions

APA **ascending pharyngeal artery,** ***ApaA*** **ascending palatine artery,** ***DM*** **digastric muscle,** ***FA*** **facial artery,** ***HGM*** **hyoglossus muscle,** ***IAN*** **inferior alveolar nerve,** ***ICAp*** **parapharyngeal portion of the internal carotid artery,** ***IJV*** **internal jugular vein,** ***LA*** **lingual artery,** ***LN*** **lingual nerve,** ***M*** **mandible,** ***MPM*** **medial pterygoid muscle,** ***SCM*** **superior constrictor muscle,** ***SGM*** **styloglossus muscle,** ***SPM*** **stylopharyngeus muscle,** ***TB*** **tongue base,** ***XIIcn*** **hypoglossal nerve,** ***black arrows*** **glossopharyngeal nerve**

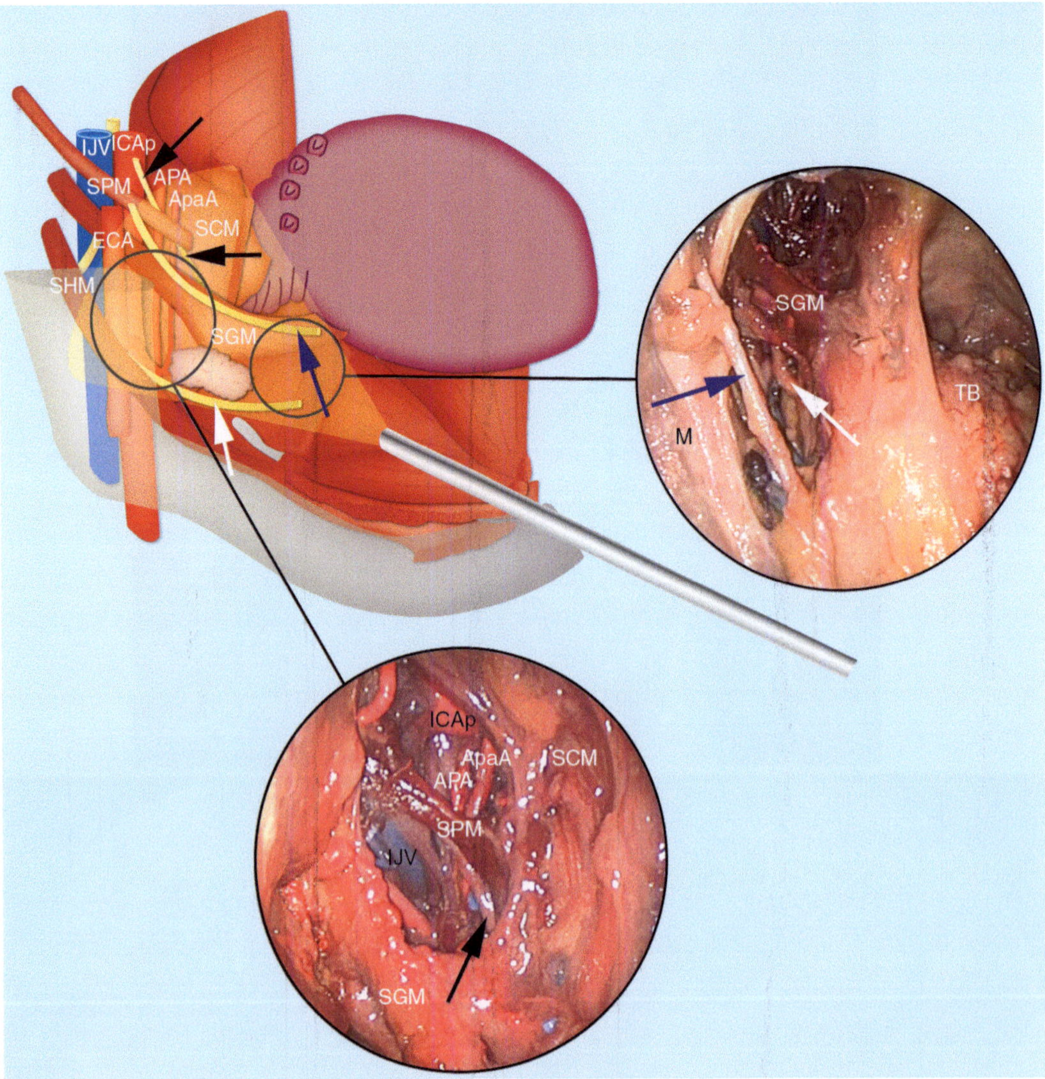

Fig. 1.63 Transoral endoscopic view of the parapharyngeal region

APA **ascending pharyngeal artery,** ***ApaA*** **ascending palatine artery,** ***ICAp*** **parapharyngeal portion of the internal carotid artery,** ***IJV*** **internal jugular vein,** ***LN*** **lingual nerve,** ***M*** **mandible,** ***SCM*** **superior constrictor muscle,** ***SGM*** **styloglossus muscle,** ***SHM*** **stylohyoid muscle,** ***SPM*** **stylopharyngeus muscle,** ***TB*** **tongue base,** ***white arrow*** **hypoglossal nerve,** ***black arrows*** **glossopharyngeal nerve,** ***blue arrows*** **lingual nerve**

References

Bejjani GK, Sullivan B, Salas-Lopez E et al (1998) Surgical anatomy of the infratemporal fossa: the styloid diaphragm revisited. Neurosurgery 43:842–852

Beretta F, Hemida SA, Andaluz N et al (2006) Exposure of the Cervical Internal Carotid Artery: Surgical Steps to the Cranial Base and Morphometric Study. Neurosurgery 59 (Suppl 1):25–34

Cavalcanti DD, Garcia-Gonzalez U, Agrawal A et al (2010) A clear map of the lower cranial nerves at the superior carotid triangle. World Neurosurg 74: 188–194

Dallan I, Bignami M, Battaglia P et al (2010) Fully endoscopic transnasal approach to the jugular foramen: anatomic study and clinical considerations. Neurosurgery 67(3 Suppl):1–7

Dallan I, Lenzi R, Bignami M et al (2010) Endoscopic transnasal anatomy of the infratemporal fossa and upper parapharyngeal regions: correlations with traditional perspectives and surgical implications. Minim Invasive Neurosurg 53(5–6):261–269

Dallan I, Seccia V, Muscatello L et al (2011) Transoral endoscopic anatomy of the parapharyngeal space: a step-by-step logical approach with surgical considerations. Head Neck 33(4):557–561

Falcon RT, Rivera-Serrano CM, Miranda JF et al (2011) Endoscopic endonasal dissection of the infratemporal fossa: anatomic relationships and importance of Eustachian tube in the endoscopic skull base surgery. Laryngoscope 121(1):31–41

Janfaza P, Fabian RL (2001a) Anatomy of the neck: general considerations. In: Janfaza P, Nadol JB Jr, Galla R, Fabian RL, Montgomery WW (eds) Surgical anatomy of the head and neck. Lippincott Williams & Wilkins, Philadelphia

Janfaza P, Fabian RL (2001b) Temporalis and infratemporal fossae. In: Janfaza P, Nadol JB Jr, Galla R, Fabian RL, Montgomery WW (eds) Surgical anatomy of the head and neck. Lippincott Williams & Wilkins, Philadelphia

Janfaza P, Montgomery WW (2001) Pterygomaxillary (pterygopalatine) fossa and the autonomic nervous system. In: Janfaza P, Nadol JB Jr, Galla R, Fabian RL, Montgomery WW (eds) Surgical anatomy of the head and neck. Lippincott Williams & Wilkins, Philadelphia

Janfaza P, Nadol JB Jr, Montgomery WW et al (2001) Surgical anatomy of the cranial base. In: Janfaza P, Nadol JB Jr, Galla R, Fabian RL, Montgomery WW (eds) Surgical anatomy of the head and neck. Lippincott Williams & Wilkins, Philadelphia

Katsuta T, Rhoton AL Jr, Matsushima T (1997) The jugular foramen: microsurgical anatomy and operative approaches. Neurosurgery 41:149–202

Lang J (1995) Skull base and related structures: atlas of clinical anatomy. Schattauer, Stuttgart

Osawa S, Rhoton AL Jr, Tanriover N et al (2008) Microsurgical anatomy and surgical exposure of the petrous segment of the internal carotid artery. Neurosurgery 63(ONS Suppl 2):ONS210–ONS239

Rhoton AL Jr (2000) The temporal bone and transtemporal approaches. Neurosurgery 47(3 Suppl): S211–S265

Rhoton AL Jr (2003) Cranial anatomy and surgical approaches. Lippincott Williams & Wilkins, Philadelphia

Roche PH, Mercier P, Sameshima T et al (2008) Surgical anatomy of the jugular foramen. Adv Tech Stand Neurosurg 33:233–263

Stambuk HE, Patel SG (2008) Imaging of the parapharyngeal space. Otolaryngol Clin North Am 41:77–101

2 Skull Base Segment

2.1 Anatomic Layout

The petrous portion of the internal carotid artery (ICA) is extradural and intraosseous. It extends from the carotid foramen to the superior margin of the *petrolingual ligament* (PLL). The carotid foramen is anteromedial to the styloid process, posteromedial to the temporomandibular joint. The PLL, placed between the sphenoidal lingula and the petrous apex, represents the posteromedial border of the cavernous sinus (CS). Once it enters in the petrous bone, the ICA presents a short vertical course, and then it turns in front of the cochlea, forming the posterior genu. From here, it runs anteriorly and medially. The petrous ICA then curves upward above the foramen lacerum (FL), thus giving the anterior genu. The segment above the FL is not truly intrapetrous, and it has been called the *lacerum segment* by some authors (Bouthillier et al. 1996). These segments, the anterior genu and the anterior vertical segment, are placed above the FL, and the artery does not cross the foramen. In this sense, it is better called the *supralacerum segment* (Herzallah and Casiano 2007). Anatomically, the FL is an opening in the dry skull that in life is filled by fibrocartilagineous tissue (fibrocartilago basalis). Its borders are the petrous apex, the body of the sphenoid, and medially the occipital bone. It is passed by tiny branches of the periosteal branches of the petrous carotid, the meningeal branches of the ascending pharyngeal artery, and small veins (Ziyal et al. 2005). The ICA passes above it and turns superiorly. At this level, the vidian canal is always lateral to the vertical segment. The lateral part of its terminal part is in the extradural space superior to the PLL. A little superior to the PLL, the abducens nerve crosses the lateral surface of the artery (Osawa et al. 2008). As stated, the horizontal portion of the petrous ICA runs within the temporal bone in an anteromedial direction, posterior to the tensor tympanic muscle, eustachian tube (ET) and spinosum and ovale foramina. When the artery enters into the carotid canal, the carotid sheath divides into 2 layers: 1 layer continues with the periostium of the carotid canal and the other as the periostium lining the lower surface of the skull base (Bouthillier et al. 1996). The bone above the horizontal segment thins progressively as the artery runs medially, so that, usually (80 %), only dura separates the horizontal portion of the ICA (ICAh) from the trigeminal ganglion (Osawa et al. 2008). Regarding the nervous network, the carotid branches of the cervical sympathetic ganglia form a plexus on the lateral surface of the artery. The largest bundle of this plexus usually is located anteroinferiorly and gives rise to the deep petrosal nerve (DPN), which joins the greater petrosal nerve (GPN) to become the vidian nerve. The vidian nerve passes through the pterygoid canal running from the anterior genu of the ICA to reach the pterygopalatine

P. Castelnuovo et al., *Surgical Anatomy of the Internal Carotid Artery*,
DOI 10.1007/978-3-642-29664-2_2, © Springer-Verlag Berlin Heidelberg 2013

ganglion in the upper portion of the pterygopalatine fossa. Within the carotid canal, the horizontal portion of the ICA is surrounded by a venous plexus (Bouthillier et al. 1996; Osawa et al. 2008), in direct continuity with the CS.

2.1.1 Gross Anatomy

The tympanic cavity lies posterolaterally to the posterior vertical segment/posterior genu. Usually, a few millimetres of bone separate the carotid canal and the middle ear. The posterior genu sits directly posterior to the entrance of the ET into the middle ear (Osawa et al. 2008). The cochlea, placed within the petrous bone, is a little bit superior, posterior, and lateral to the posterior genu. The ET and the tensor tympani are located anteriorly to the ICAh. Proceeding medially, the vessel remains within its own canal, while the ET slopes gently downward and the cartilaginous portion of the tube is located within the sulcus tubae. This is located on the outer surface of the cranial base and placed anteriorly to the ICAh. The tensor tympani in most cases (>90 %) is located superiorly or anteriorly to the ET, and it is separated from the carotid canal by a thin bone.

2.1.2 Neural Structures

2.1.2.1 Greater Petrosal Nerve

The GPN originates at the level of the geniculate ganglion, exits through the hiatus Fallopii, and courses under the dura toward the gasserian ganglion. The nerve usually runs anteromedially above the horizontal portion.

2.1.2.2 Geniculate Ganglion

The geniculate ganglion is placed above and usually posterolateral to the posterior genu (Osawa et al. 2008).

2.1.2.3 Lesser Petrosal Nerve

The lesser petrosal nerve crosses the middle cranial fossa floor anterior to the GPN and exits the cranium through the small innominate foramen (Osawa et al. 2008), the foramen spinosum, or the sphenopetrosal fissure (Kakizawa et al. 2007).

2.1.2.4 Gasserian Ganglion

The gasserian ganglion is placed within a depression between the trigeminal impression and the foramen ovale. The stem of the trigeminal nerve is placed within the "trigeminal impression." The inferolateral portion of the sphenopetrosal fissure (SPF) is placed above the medial third of the horizontal portion of the ICA, while the superomedial aspect rests against the ascending limb of the intracavernous segment.

2.1.3 Vascular Branches

In most cases, the skull base segment of the ICA presents branches (Tubbs et al. 2007; Osawa et al. 2008).

2.1.3.1 Caroticotympanic Artery

The caroticotympanic artery seems to arise from the proximal vertical part of the petrous ICA and supplies the tympanic cavity. At the level of promontory, it anastomoses with the tympanic branches of the middle meningeal artery (MMA) and stylomastoid and maxillary arteries. Not all authors agree with this position; Osawa et al. thought that this vessel comes from the ascending pharyngeal artery and not from the ICA (Osawa et al. 2008). Also, previously its presence has been doubted (Paullus et al. 1977).

2.1.3.2 Arteries of the Pterygoid Canal (Vidian Arteries)

The artery of the pterygoid canal (vidian artery) is not always present. Anatomically speaking we can consider an anterior (for ECA system) and a posterior (from ICA system) Vidian artery. The posterior one may arise as a single branch or from a common trunk with a periosteal artery (Osawa et al. 2008). This vessel may arise from the horizontal segment of the petrous part of the ICA and course into the pterygoid canal to anastomose with the same-named branch of the maxillary artery (Jinkins 2000). Furthermore, it is also possible that there is no counterpart from the maxillary artery. In this case, the artery (about 0.5 mm) has been described to transverse the cartilage-filled FL to enter the pterygoid canal.

2.1.3.3 Stapedial Artery

Rarely present in adults, the stapedial artery (SA) is a branch of the second branchial arch. The SA pierces the floor of the middle ear cavity and ascends along the promontory enclosed within a bony canal to pass between the crura of the stapes to enter the facial canal. At the level of the hiatus of the GPN, the vessel enters the middle cranial fossa to become the MMA. If the SA persists, the foramen spinosum is absent (Lasjaunias 1981).

2.1.3.4 Periosteal Branch(es)

The periosteal branches are not always present. When present, most of these originate from the anterior genu and the vertical segment. When it originates as a common trunk with the vidian artery, it arises from the horizontal segment. Most periosteal arteries arising from the inferior surface of the ICA send a branch through the FL (Osawa et al. 2008).

2.1.3.5 Persistent Acoustic Artery

The persistent acoustic artery is really a rare branch connecting the carotid (petrous portion) and basilar arteries (Lang 1995).

2.2 Anatomic Pictures

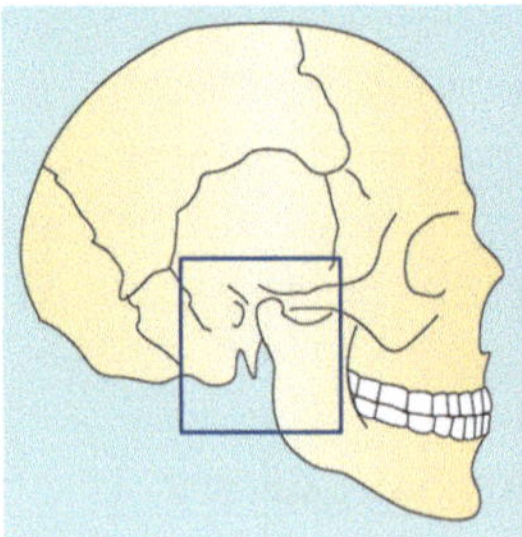

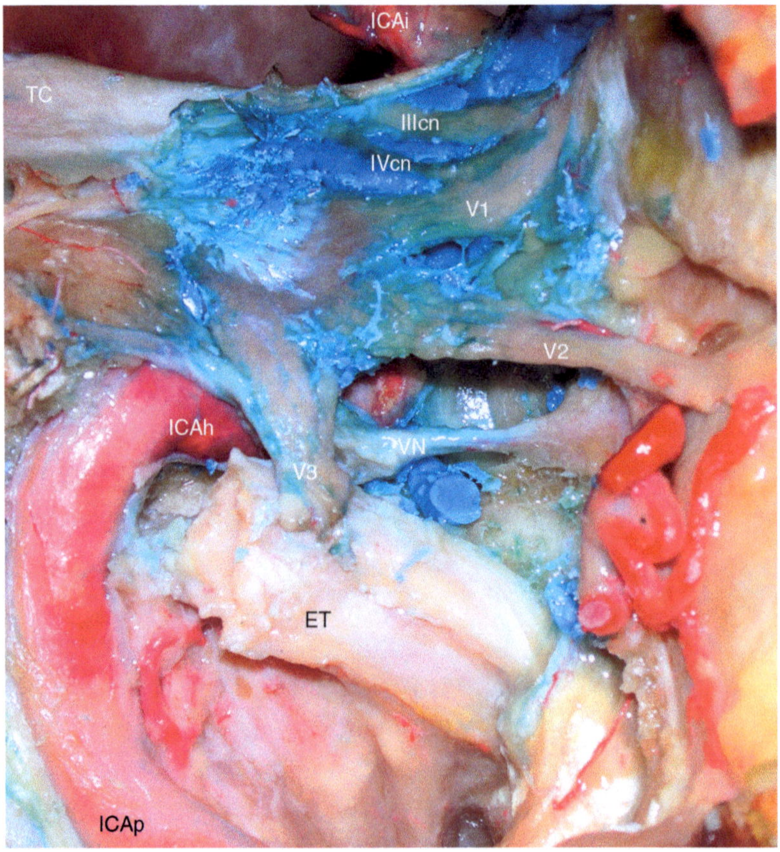

Fig. 2.1 Horizontal segment. Lateral vision of the right cavernous sinus and horizontal portion of the internal carotid artery

ET **eustachian tube,** ***ICAh*** **horizontal portion of the internal carotid artery,** ***ICAi*** **intracranial portion of the internal carotid artery,** ***ICAp*** **parapharyngeal portion of the internal carotid artery,** ***TC*** **tentorium cerebelli,** ***VN*** **vidian nerve,** ***V1*** **first branch of the trigeminal nerve,** ***V2*** **second branch of the trigeminal nerve,** ***V3*** **third branch of the trigeminal nerve,** ***IIIcn*** **oculomotor nerve,** ***IVcn*** **trochlear nerve**

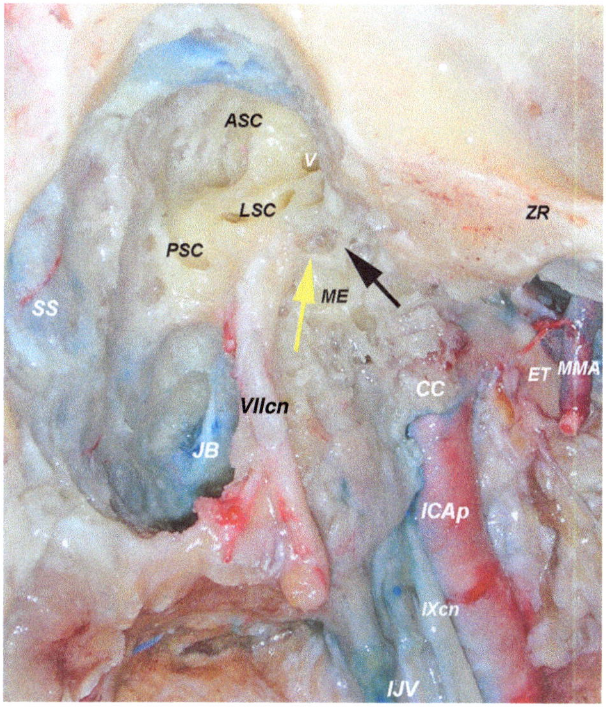

Fig. 2.2 Lateral vision of the right jugulomastoid region

ASC **anterior semicircular canal,** ***CC*** **carotid canal,** ***ET*** **eustachian tube,** ***ICAp*** **parapharyngeal portion of the internal carotid artery,** ***IJV*** **internal jugular vein,** ***JB*** **jugular bulb,** ***LSC*** **lateral semicircular canal,** ***ME*** **middle ear,** ***MMA*** **middle meningeal artery,** ***PSC*** **posterior semicircular canal,** ***SS*** **sigmoid sinus,** ***ZR*** **zygomatic root,** ***VIIcn*** **facial nerve,** ***IXcn*** **glossopharyngeal nerve,** ***V*** **vestibule,** ***yellow arrow*** **stapes,** ***black arrow*** **incus**

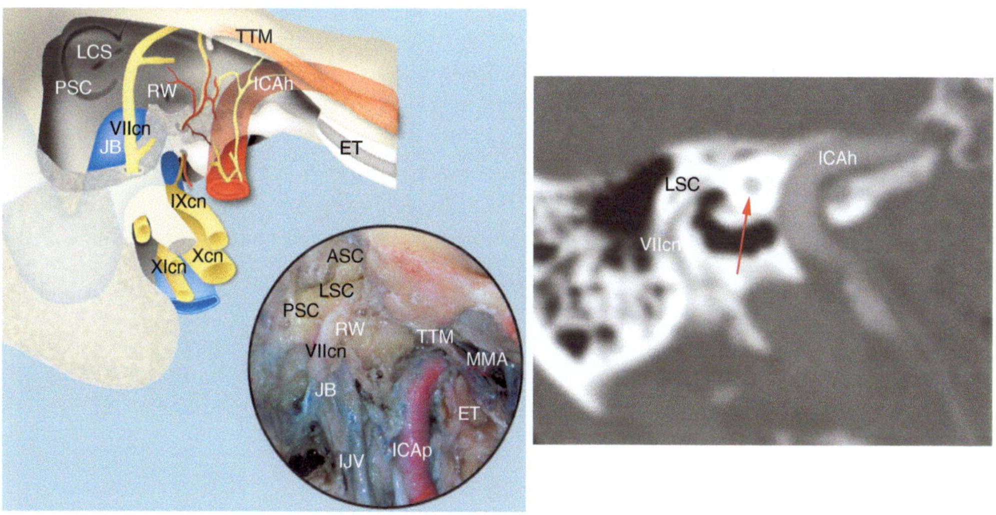

Fig. 2.3 Right exposure of the middle ear and jugular foramen. Note the intimate relationship between the eustachian tube and the carotid canal

ASC **anterior semicircular canal,** ***ET*** **eustachian tube,** ***ICAp*** **parapharyngeal portion of the internal carotid artery,** ***ICAh*** **horizontal portion of the internal carotid artery,** ***IJV*** **internal jugular vein,** ***JB*** **jugular bulb,** ***LSC*** **lateral semicircular canal,** ***MMA*** **middle meningeal artery,** ***PSC*** **posterior semicircular canal,** ***RW*** **round window,** ***TTM*** **tensor tympani muscle,** ***VIIcn*** **facial nerve,** ***IXcn*** **glossopharyngeal nerve,** ***Xcn*** **vagus nerve,** ***XIcn*** **accessory nerve,** ***red arrow*** **cochlea**

The posterior bend of the ICAh within the petrous bone is located just below and anterior to the cochlea. It is separated from the tympanic cavity by a thin bone that may be dehiscent.

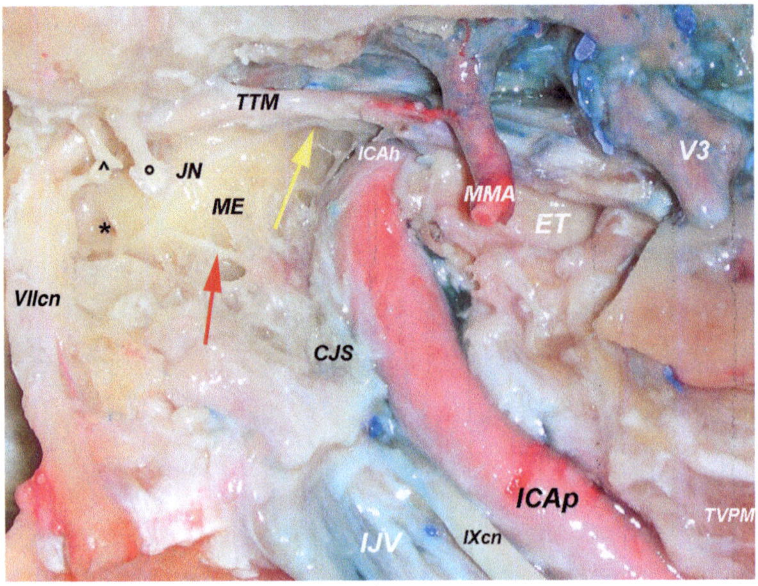

Fig. 2.4 Lateral view of the tympanojugular region

CJS **carotidojugular spine,** ***ET*** **eustachian tube,** ***ICAp*** **parapharyngeal portion of the internal carotid artery,** ***IJV*** **internal jugular vein,** ***JN*** **Jacobson's nerve,** ***ME*** **middle ear,** ***MMA*** **middle meningeal artery,** ***TTM*** **tensor tympani muscle,** ***TVPM*** **tensor veli palatini muscle,** ***V3*** **third branch of the trigeminal nerve,** ***VIIcn*** **facial nerve,** ***IXcn*** **glossopharyngeal nerve,** ***yellow arrow*** **lesser petrosal nerve,** ***red arrow*** **inferior part of the inferior tympanic nerve (Jacobson's nerve),** ***black asterisk*** **round window,** ***black circle*** **malleus,** ***arrowhead*** **incudostapedial joint**

At the level of the jugular foramen area, the ICA moves away from the jugular bulb below the middle ear, and it is separated from it by the CJS. Jacobson's nerve is joined by the carotidotympanic nerves from the pericarotid sympathetic plexus to form the lesser petrosal nerve (Janfaza and Nadol 2001b).

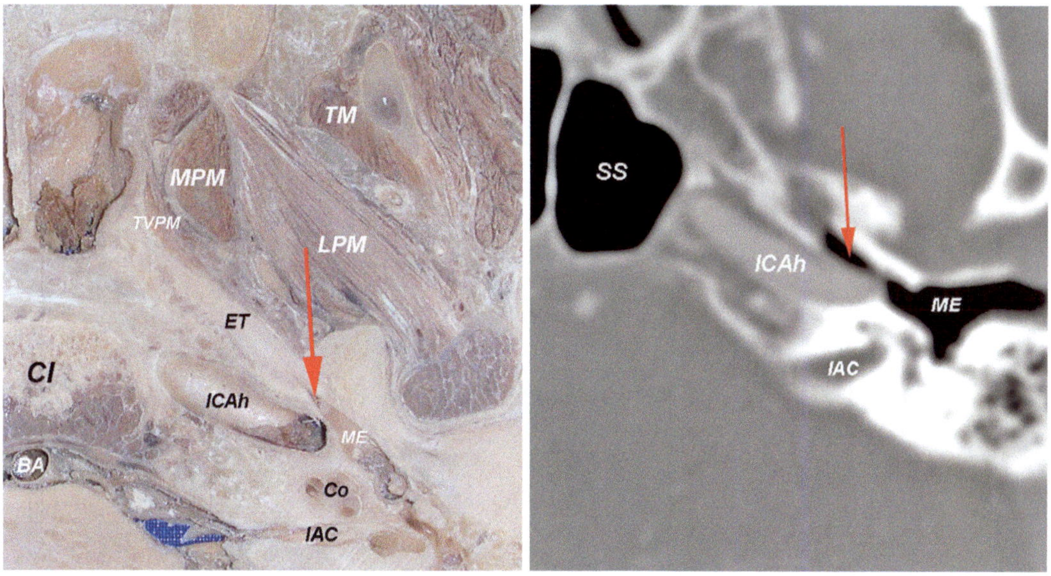

Fig. 2.5 Axial view at the level of the horizontal portion of the internal carotid artery

BA **basilar artery,** ***Cl*** **clivus,** ***Co*** **cochlea,** ***ET*** **eustachian tube,** ***IAC*** **internal acoustic canal,** ***ICAh*** **horizontal portion of the internal carotid artery,** ***LPM*** **lateral pterygoid muscle,** ***ME*** **middle ear,** ***MPM*** **medial pterygoid muscle,** ***SS*** **sphenoid sinus,** ***TM*** **temporal muscle,** ***TVPM*** **tensor veli palatini muscle,** ***red arrow*** **bony segment of the eustachian tube (musculo-tubal canal)**

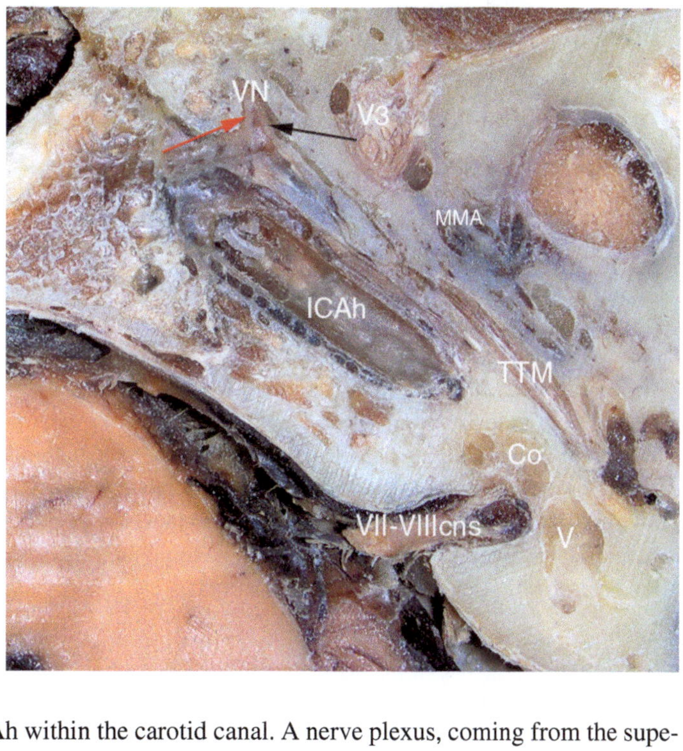

Fig. 2.6 Axial view at the level of the horizontal portion of the internal carotid artery

Co **cochlea,** ***ICAh*** **horizontal portion of the internal carotid artery,** ***MMA*** **middle meningeal artery,** ***TTM*** **tensor tympani muscle,** ***V*** **vestibule,** ***VN*** **vidian nerve,** ***V3*** **third branch of the trigeminal nerve,** ***VII–VIIIcns*** **acoustic-facial bundle,** ***red arrow*** **deep petrosal nerve,** ***black arrow*** **greater petrosal nerve**

A venous plexus surrounds the ICAh within the carotid canal. A nerve plexus, coming from the superior cervical ganglion, accompanies the artery.

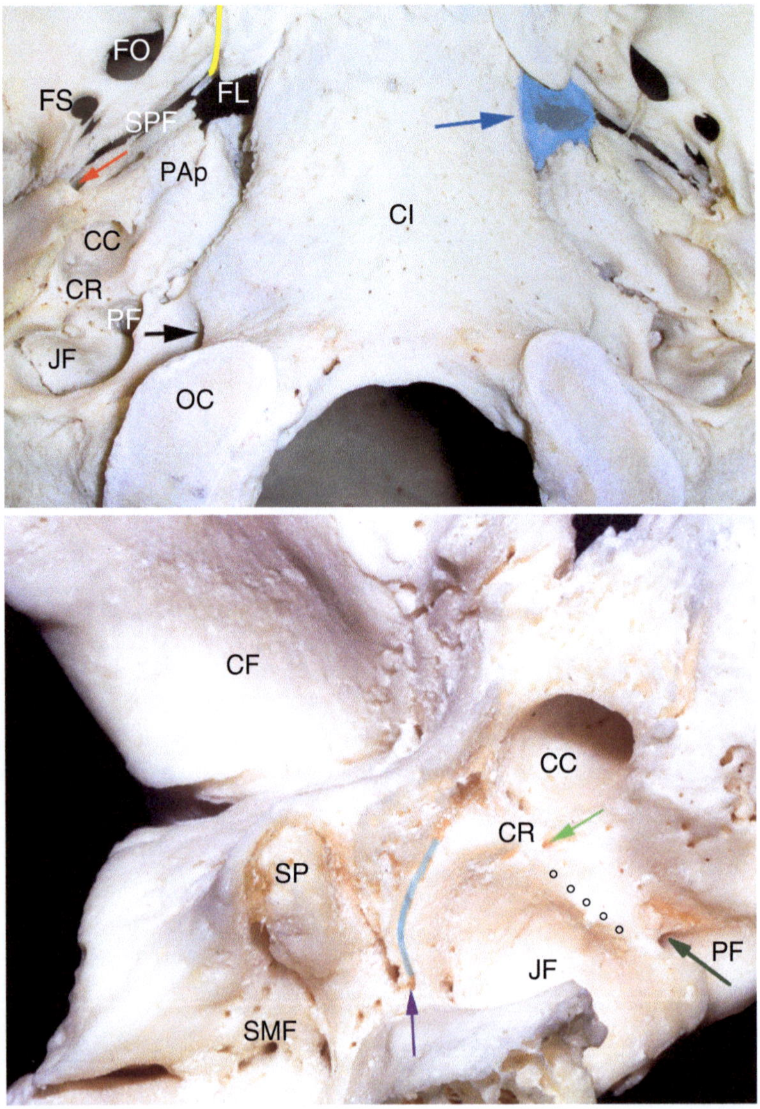

Fig. 2.7 Skull base from below

CC **carotid canal,** ***CF*** **condylar fossa,** ***Cl*** **clivus,** ***CR*** **carotid ridge,** ***FL*** **foramen lacerum,** ***FO*** **foramen ovale,** ***FS*** **foramen spinosum,** ***JF*** **jugular fossa,** ***PAp*** **petrous apex,** ***PF*** **pyramidal fossa,** ***SMF*** **stylomastoid foramen,** ***SP*** **styloid process,** ***SPF*** **sphenopetrosal fissure,** ***dark green arrow*** **external opening of the cochlear aqueduct,** ***violet arrow*** **mastoid canaliculus,** ***red arrow*** **opening of the musculo-tubal canal,** ***blue arrow*** **foramen lacerum region,** ***green arrow*** **tympanic canaliculus,** ***black circles*** **intrajugular ridge,** ***black arrow*** **hypoglossal canal,** ***blue-sky line*** **groove for the auricular branch of vagus nerve (Arnold's nerve)**

The FL is a hole in the dry skull; it is closed by fibrocartilaginous tissue in living patients. It is passed by meningeal branches of the ascending pharyngeal artery and emissary veins. The FO transmits the V3 and accessory meningeal artery and sometimes the lesser superficial petrosal nerve. The FS transmits the middle meningeal artery and veins and the recurrent branch of V3 (for the dura of the middle cranial fossa). The mastoid canaliculus transmits Arnold's nerve (of the vagus nerve). This nerve passes through the mastoid and exits at the level of the tympanomastoid suture. The tympanic canaliculus transmits Jacobson's nerve and the inferior tympanic artery (from the ascending pharyngeal artery).

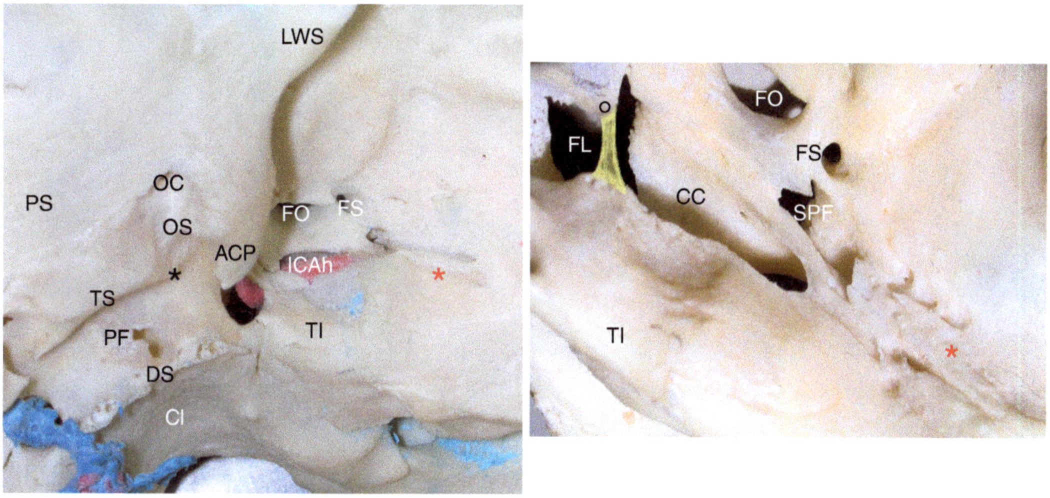

Fig. 2.8 Right middle cranial fossa and clivus from above

ACP **anterior clinoid process,** ***CC*** **carotid canal,** ***Cl*** **clivus,** ***DS*** **dorsum sellae,** ***FL*** **foramen lacerum,** ***FO*** **foramen ovale,** ***FS*** **foramen spinosum,** ***ICAh*** **horizontal portion of the internal carotid artery,** ***LWS*** **lesser wing of the sphenoid,** ***OC*** **optic canal,** ***OS*** **optic strut,** ***PF*** **pituitary fossa,** ***PS*** **planum sphenoidale,** ***SPF*** **sphenopetrosal fissure,** ***TI*** **trigeminal impression,** ***TS*** **tuberculum sellae,** ***yellow drawing*** **petrolingual ligament,** ***black circle*** **lingual process of the sphenoid,** ***red asterisk*** **groove for the greater petrosal nerve,** ***black asterisk*** **middle clinoid process**

The petrolingual ligament can be considered as a continuation of the periostium of the carotid canal (Osawa et al. 2008). In most cases, the medial aspect of the horizontal portion of the internal carotid artery is not covered by bone, but simply by dura. The hiatus of the facial canal transmits the greater superficial petrosal nerve and the superficial petrosal branch of the middle meningeal artery (*MMA*) to the facial nerve.

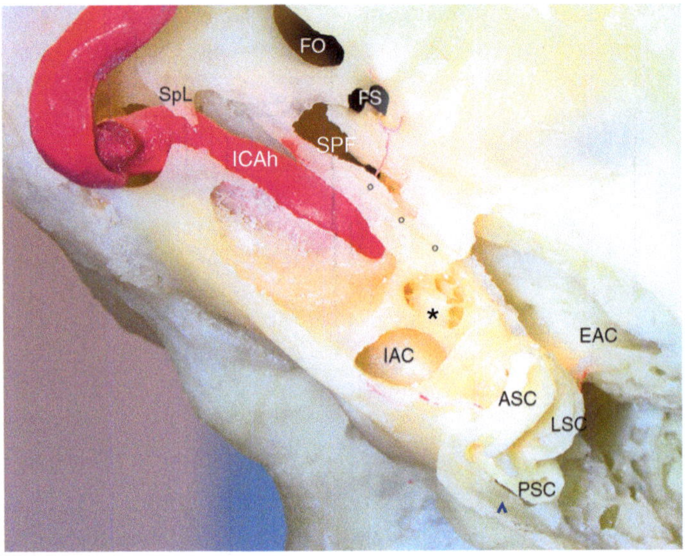

Fig. 2.9 Relationship between the horizontal portion of the internal carotid artery and the cochlea (vision from above)

ASC **anterior semicircular canal,** ***EAC*** **external auditory canal,** ***FO*** **foramen ovale,** ***FS*** **foramen spinosum,** ***IAC*** **internal auditory canal,** ***ICAh*** **horizontal segment of the internal carotid artery,** ***LSC*** **lateral semicircular canal,** ***PSC*** **posterior semicircular canal,** ***SPF*** **sphenopetrosal fissure,** ***SpL*** **lingula of the sphenoid,** ***blue arrowhead*** **vestibular aqueduct,** ***black asterisk*** **cochlea,** ***black circles*** **groove for the greater petrosal nerve**

The cochlea is posterosuperiorly and laterally located in respect to the posterior bend of the horizontal portion of the internal carotid artery.

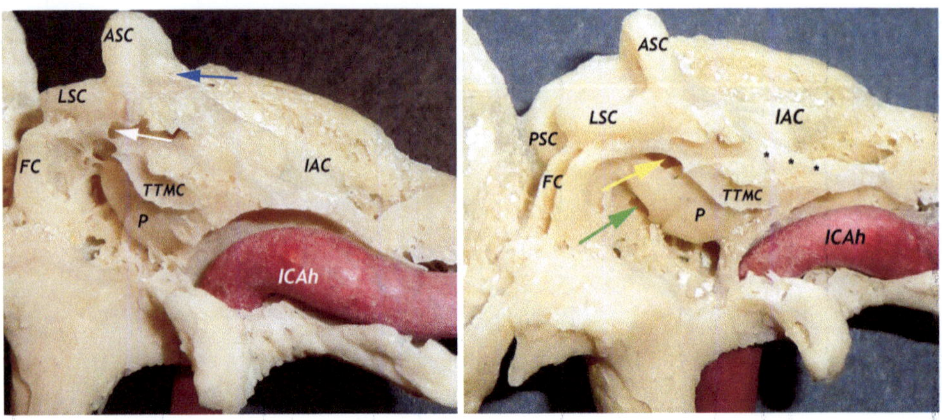

Fig. 2.10 Relationship between the horizontal portion of the internal carotid artery and the inner ear (anterior view)

ASC **anterior semicircular canal,** ***FC*** **facial canal (mastoid segment),** ***IAC*** **internal acoustic canal,** ***ICAh*** **horizontal portion of the internal carotid artery,** ***LSC*** **lateral semicircular canal,** ***P*** **promontory,** ***PSC*** **posterior semicircular canal,** ***TTMC*** **tensor tympani muscle canal,** ***blue arrow*** **canal for the subarcuate artery,** ***white arrow*** **tympanic segment of the facial canal,** ***yellow arrow*** **oval window,** ***green arrow*** **round window,** ***black asterisks*** **groove for the greater petrosal nerve**

The subarcuate artery usually originates medial to the internal acoustic meatus, and penetrates the subarcuate canal (petromastoid canal). It can send branches to the petrous apex and to the bone of the semicircular canals and of the vestibule.

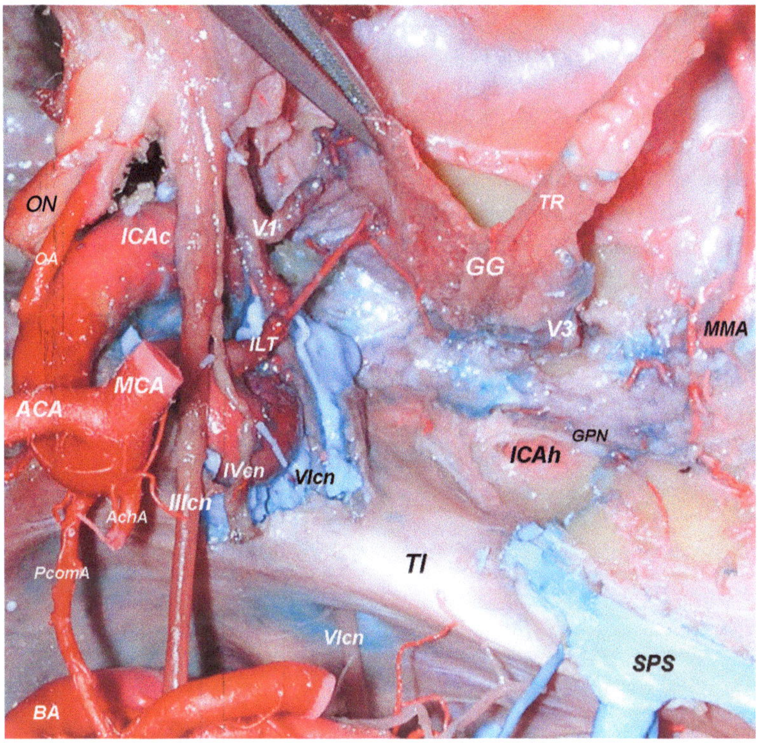

Fig. 2.11 Right middle cranial fossa from above. The gasserian ganglion has been reflected upward to show the position of the petrous portion of the internal carotid artery

***ACA* anterior cerebral artery, *AchA* anterior choroidal artery, *BA* basilar artery, *GG* gasserian ganglion, *GPN* greater petrosal nerve, *ICAc* cavernous portion of the internal carotid artery, *ICAh* horizontal portion of the internal carotid artery, *ILT* inferolateral trunk, *MCA* middle cerebral artery, *MMA* middle meningeal artery, *OA* ophthalmic artery, *ON* optic nerve, *PcomA* posterior communicating artery, *SPS* superior petrosal sinus, *TI* trigeminal impression, *TR* trigeminal root, *V1* first branch of the trigeminal nerve, *V3* third branch of the trigeminal nerve, *IIIcn* oculomotor nerve, *IV* trochlear nerve, *VIcn* abducens nerve**

Usually, the superior petrosal sinus is superior to the roots of the trigeminal nerve. Sometimes, the sinus divides and lies superior and inferior to the roots (Janfaza and Nadol 2001a).

It connects the cavernous sinus to the sigmoid sinus. It drains blood from the veins of the brainstem (including the petrosal vein of Dandy), inferior cerebral vein and superior cerebellar vein.

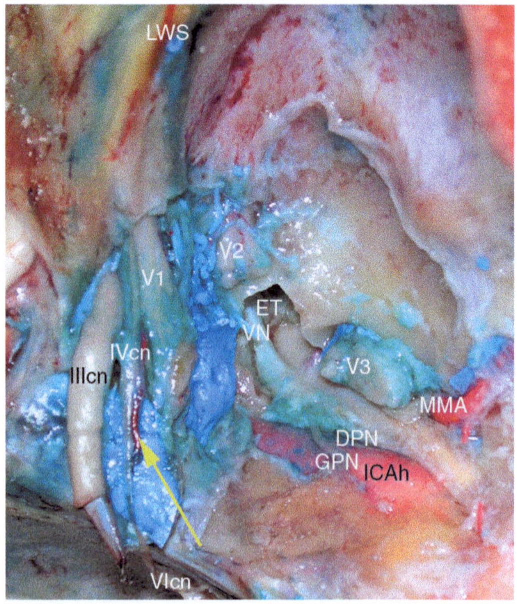

Fig. 2.12 Close vision of the middle cranial fossa. The gasserian ganglion has been removed

DPN **deep petrosal nerve,** ***ET*** **eustachian tube,** ***GPN*** **greater petrosal nerve,** ***ICAh*** **horizontal portion of the internal carotid artery,** ***LWS*** **lesser wing of the sphenoid,** ***MMA*** **middle meningeal artery,** ***VN*** **vidian nerve,** ***V1*** **first branch of the trigeminal nerve,** ***V2*** **second branch of the trigeminal nerve,** ***V3*** **third branch of the trigeminal nerve,** ***IIIcn*** **oculomotor nerve,** ***IVcn*** **trochlear nerve,** ***VIcn*** **abducens nerve,** ***yellow arrow*** **a tentorial branch of the inferolateral trunk**

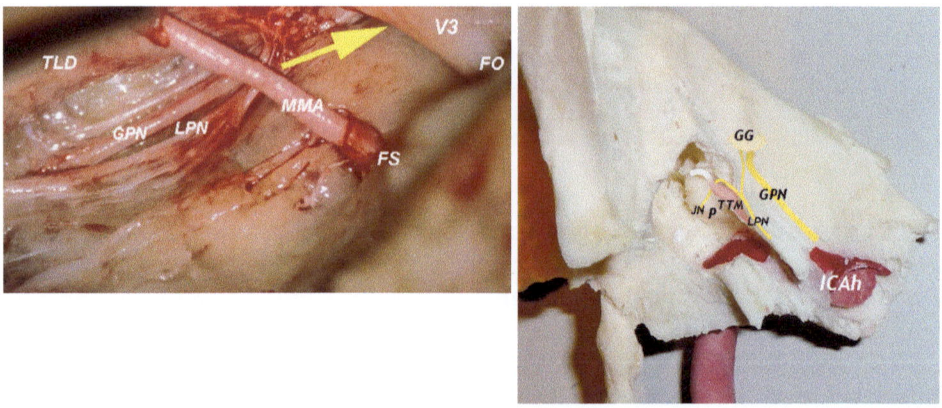

Fig. 2.13 Right middle cranial fossa floor (view through a temporal craniotomy) and reconstruction on petrous bone

GG **geniculate ganglion,** ***GPN*** **greater petrosal nerve,** ***FO*** **foramen ovale,** ***FS*** **foramen spinosum,** ***ICAh*** **horizontal portion of the internal carotid artery,** ***JN*** **Jacobson's nerve,** ***LPN*** **lesser petrosal nerve,** ***MMA*** **middle meningeal artery,** ***P*** **promontory,** ***TLD*** **dura of the temporal lobe,** ***TTM*** **tensor tympani muscle,** ***V3*** **third branch of the trigeminal nerve,** ***yellow arrow*** **petrous apex**

The LPN crosses the floor of the middle cranial fossa (*MCF*) anterior to the GPN (Kakizawa et al. 2007) and exits the cranial cavity most of the time through an innominate canal. The outer surface of this canaliculus is usually located posteriorly to the foramen ovale and spinosum (Kakizawa et al. 2007). This nerve conveys the parasympathetic fibres derived from the superior and inferior salivary nucleus (Porto et al. 1978). It is formed by fibres from cranial nerves VII (nervus intermedius), IX (Jacobson's nerve), and X (Arnolds's nerve). The most important part is due to cranial nerve IX (Jacobson's nerve). This emerges on the MCF posterior to the TTM. While the GPN courses above the ICAh, the LPN courses above the tensor tympani muscle. This muscle occupies a bony canal below the floor of the middle fossa, anterior to the ICAh and above the eustachian tube (*ET*).

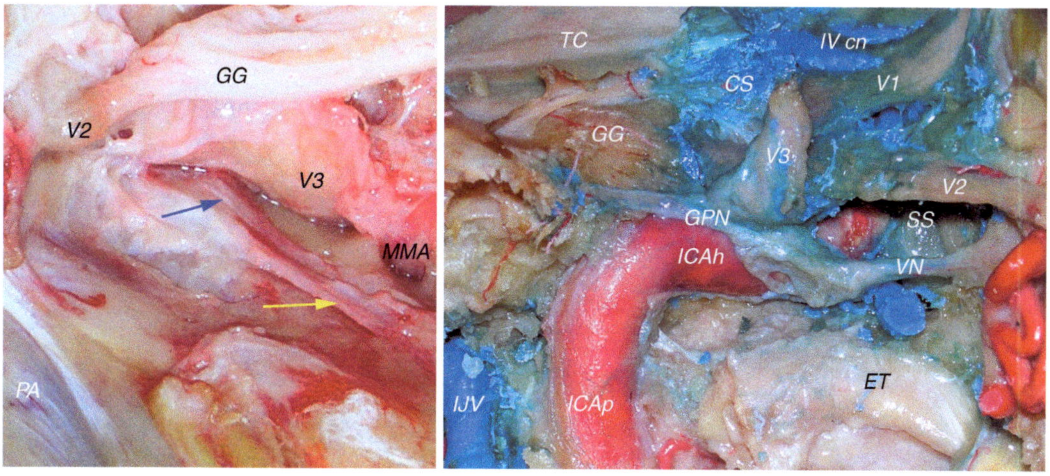

Fig. 2.14 Right anterior petrous apex

CS **cavernous sinus,** ***ET*** **eustachian tube,** ***GG*** **gasserian ganglion,** ***GPN*** **greater petrosal nerve,** ***ICAh*** **horizontal portion of the internal carotid artery,** ***ICAp*** **parapharyngeal portion of the internal carotid artery,** ***IJV*** **internal jugular vein,** ***MMA*** **middle meningeal artery,** ***PA*** **petrous apex,** ***SS*** **sphenoid sinus,** ***TC*** **tentorium cerebelli,** ***VN*** **vidian nerve,** ***V1*** **first branch of the trigeminal nerve,** ***V2*** **second branch of the trigeminal nerve,** ***V3*** **third branch of the trigeminal nerve,** ***IVcn*** **trochlear nerve,** ***blue arrow*** **lesser petrosal nerve,** ***yellow arrow*** **greater petrosal nerve**

The lesser petrosal nerve (LPN) leaves the cranial cavity either through the foramen ovale or via its own canal. Note that in the left picture the medial portion of the ICAh is not covered by bone. This condition is not rare. The LPN is also accompanied by a branch of the middle meningeal artery: the superior tympanic artery. This branch supplies the tensor tympani muscle and part of the mucosa of the tympanic cavity (Lang 1995). LPN and superior tympanic artery enter the tympanic cavity via the superior tympanic canaliculus.

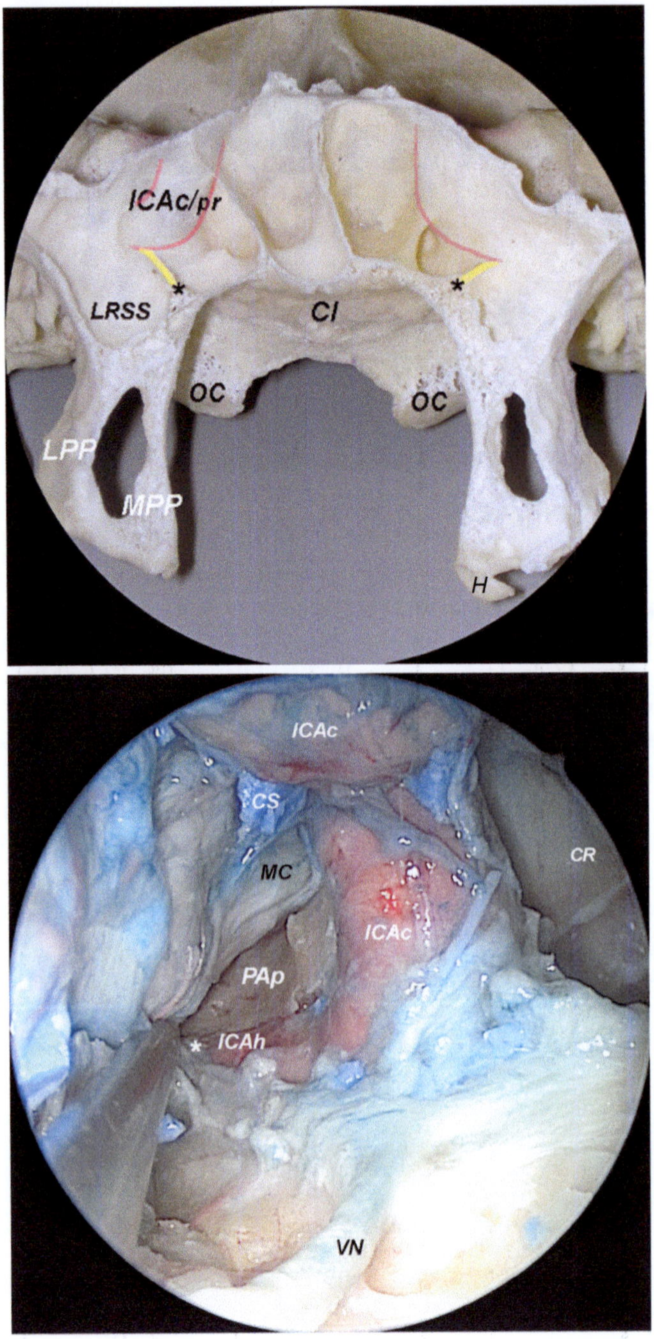

Fig. 2.15 Endoscopic views of sphenoid sinus with particular regard to the so-called front door to Meckel's cave

Cl **clivus,** ***CR*** **clival recess,** ***CS*** **cavernous sinus,** ***H*** **hamulus,** ***ICAc*** **cavernous portion of the internal carotid artery,** ***ICAc/pr*** **protuberance of the cavernous portion of the internal carotid artery,** ***ICAh*** **horizontal portion of the internal carotid artery,** ***LPP*** **lateral pterygoid plate,** ***LRSS*** **lateral recess of the sphenoid sinus,** ***MC*** **Meckel's cave,** ***MPP*** **medial pterygoid plate,** ***OC*** **occipital condyle,** ***PAp*** **petrous apex,** ***VN*** **vidian nerve,** ***yellow line*** **course of the vidian nerve,** ***red lines*** **profile of the carotid artery,** ***white asterisk*** **greater petrosal nerve,** ***black asterisk*** **vidian canal**

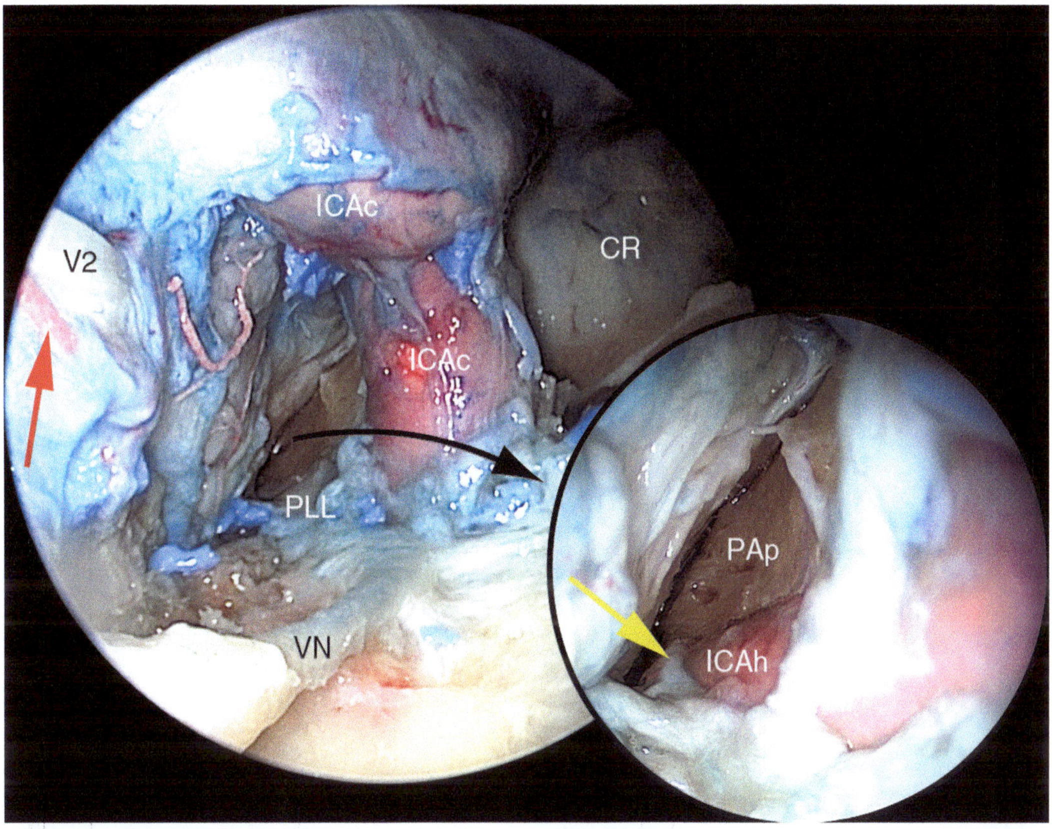

Fig. 2.16 Endoscopic vision of the "front door" to Meckel's cave

CR **clival recess,** ***ET*** **eustachian tube,** ***ICAc*** **cavernous portion of the internal carotid artery,** ***ICAh*** **horizontal portion of the internal carotid artery,** ***PAp*** **petrous apex,** ***PLL*** **petrolingual ligament,** ***VN*** **vidian nerve,** ***V2*** **second branch of the trigeminal nerve,** ***red arrow*** **artery for the foramen rotundum,** ***yellow arrow*** **greater petrosal nerve**

The petrolingual ligament connects the petrous apex and the lingula of the sphenoid. It can be considered the border between the horizontal and cavernous portions of the internal carotid artery.

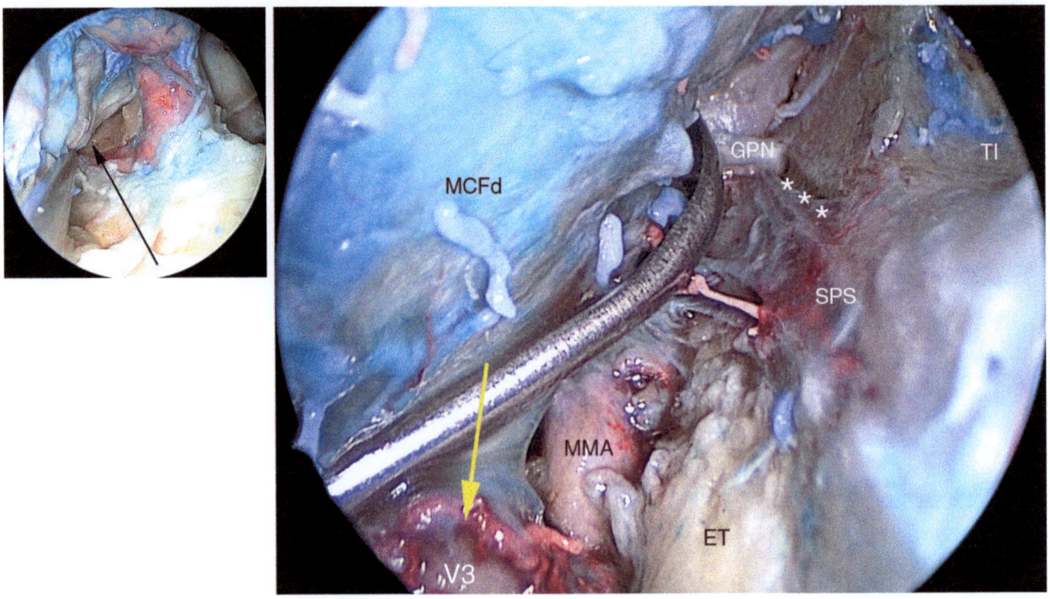

Fig. 2.17 Endoscopic vision of the suprapetrous window. The dura of the middle cranial fossa has been displaced upward, and the greater petrosal nerve coming out from the geniculate ganglion is evident. The *black arrow* in the small picture indicates the perspective of the vision in the bigger image

ET **eustachian tube,** ***GPN*** **greater petrosal nerve,** ***MCFd*** **dura of the middle cranial fossa,** ***MMA*** **middle meningeal artery,** ***SPS*** **superior petrosal surface,** ***TI*** **trigeminal impression,** ***V3*** **third branch of the trigeminal nerve,** ***yellow arrow*** **accessory middle meningeal artery,** ***white asterisks*** **greater petrosal nerve groove**

The skull base given by the sphenoid bone has been drilled away, and the third branch of the trigeminal nerve and the MMA have been freed from their canals. An accessory MMA is seen in close relationship to V3. When present, it passes through the foramen ovale.

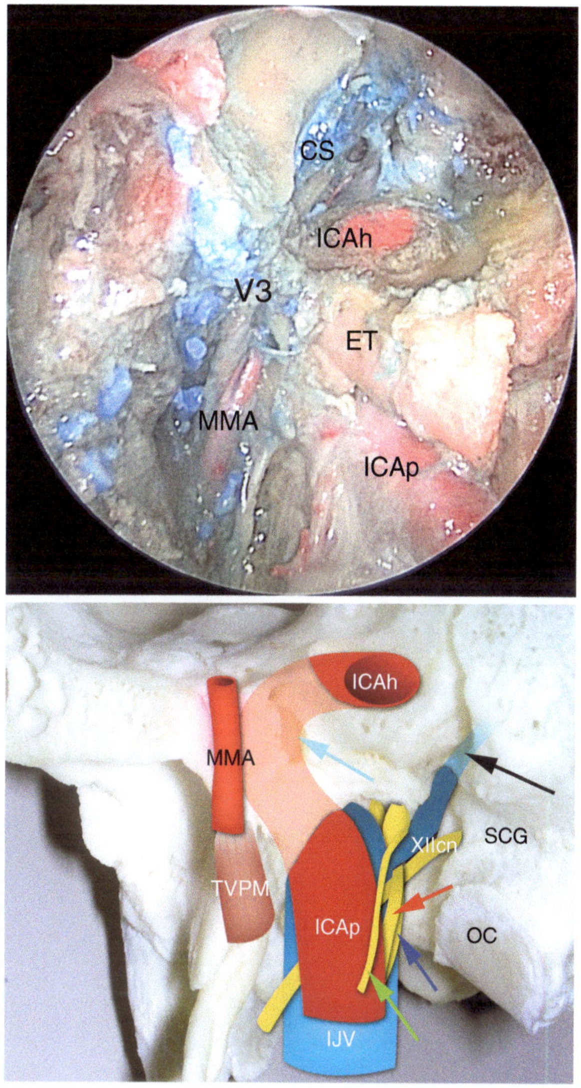

Fig. 2.18 Endoscopic view of the relationship between the eustachian tube and the horizontal segment of the internal carotid artery

CS **cavernous sinus,** ***ET*** **eustachian tube,** ***ICAh*** **horizontal portion of the internal carotid artery,** ***ICAp*** **parapharyngeal portion of the internal carotid artery,** ***IJV*** **internal jugular vein,** ***MMA*** **middle meningeal artery,** ***OC*** **occipital condyle,** ***SCG*** **supracondylar groove,** ***TVPM*** **tensor veli palatini muscle,** ***V3*** **third branch of the trigeminal nerve,** ***XIIcn*** **hypoglossal nerve,** ***green arrow*** **glossopharyngeal nerve,** ***blue arrow*** **accessory nerve,** ***blue-sky arrow*** **isthmus of the ET (musculo-tubal canal),** ***black arrow*** **inferior petrosal sinus,** ***red arrow*** **vagus nerve**

The second genu of the internal carotid artery (ICA) occupies the upper portion of the foramen lacerum. The lower aspect of the foramen lacerum (FL) is covered by fibrocartilaginous tissue, which is firmly attached to the ICA, eustachian tube, clivus, and petrous portion of the temporal bone (Falcon et al. 2011). To reach the skull base attachment of the ET, the insertion of the tensor veli palatine muscle (at the level of the anterior wall of the ET and the spine of the sphenoid) has to be removed. Into the carotid canal, the ICAh is surrounded by a loose venous plexus and by sympathetic plexus.

From the ventral perspective the medial margin of the jugular tubercle is postero-medially located to the lower portion of the foramen lacerum (Fernandez-Miranda 2012).

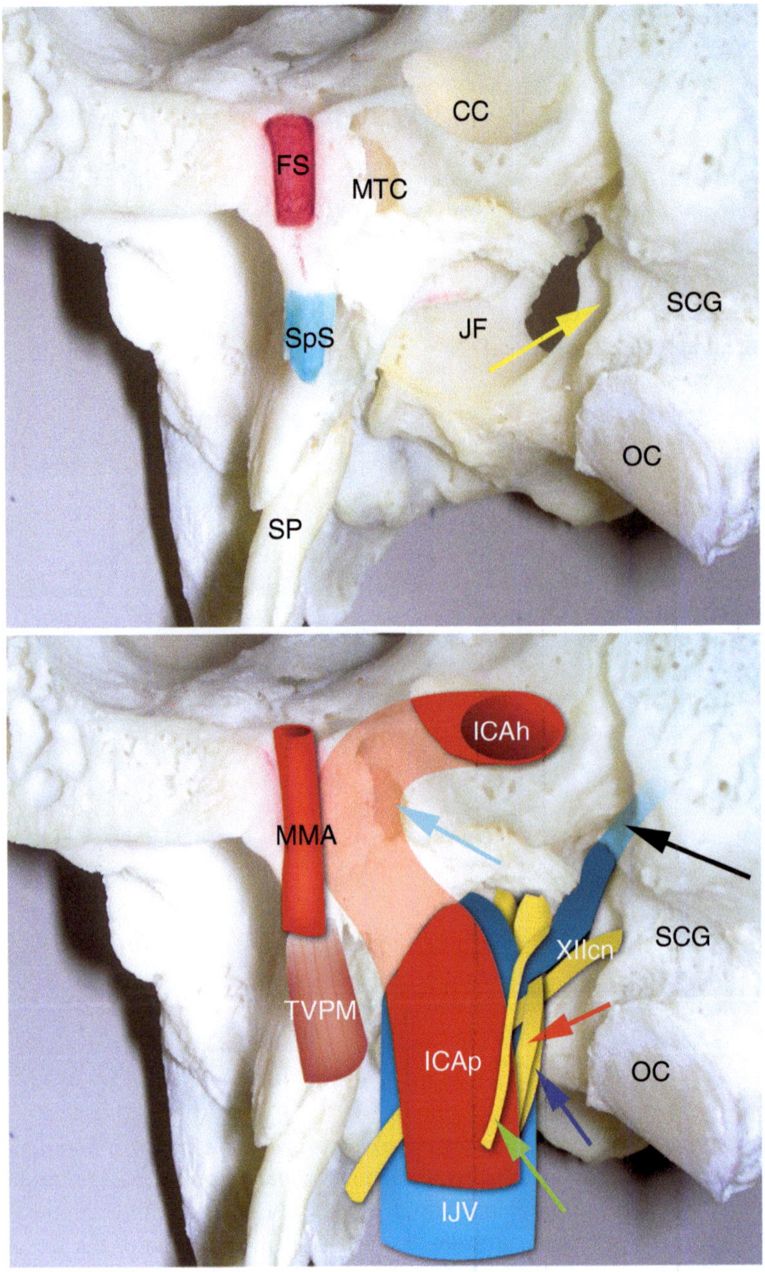

Fig. 2.19 Relationship between the bony eustachian tube and the horizontal segment of the internal carotid artery

CC **carotid canal,** ***FS*** **foramen spinosum,** ***ICAh*** **horizontal portion of the internal carotid artery,** ***ICAp*** **parapharyngeal portion of the internal carotid artery,** ***IJV*** **internal jugular vein,** ***JF*** **jugular foramen,** ***MMA*** **middle meningeal artery,** ***MTC*** **musculo-tubal canal,** ***OC*** **occipital condyle,** ***SCG*** **supracondylar groove,** ***SP*** **styloid process,** ***SpS*** **spine of the sphenoid,** ***TVPM*** **tensor veli palatini muscle,** ***XIIcn*** **hypoglossal nerve,** ***green arrow*** **glossopharyngeal nerve,** ***blue arrow*** **accessory nerve,** ***red arrow*** **vagus nerve,** ***blue-sky arrow*** **isthmus of the ET (musculo-tubal canal),** ***black arrow*** **inferior petrosal sinus,** ***yellow arrow*** **extracranial orifice of the hypoglossal canal**

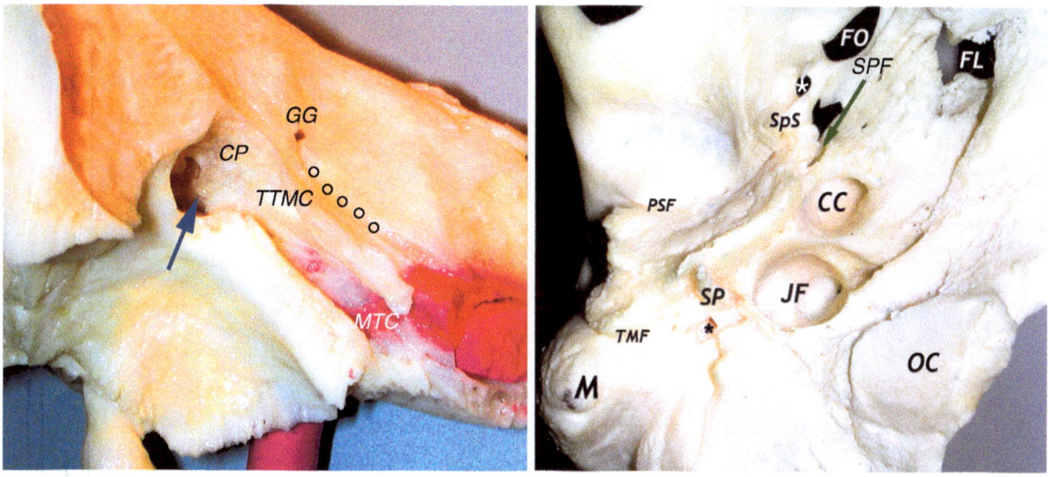

Fig. 2.20 Relationship between the bony eustachian tube and the horizontal segment of the internal carotid artery

CC **carotid canal,** ***CP*** **cochleariform process,** ***FL*** **foramen lacerum,** ***FO*** **foramen ovale,** ***GG*** **geniculate ganglion,** ***JF*** **jugular foramen,** ***M*** **mastoid,** ***MTC*** **musculo-tubal canal,** ***OC*** **occipital condyle,** ***PSF*** **petrosquamous fissure,** ***SP*** **styloid process,** ***SPF*** **sphenopetrosal fissure,** ***SpS*** **spine of the sphenoid,** ***TMF*** **tympanomastoid fissure,** ***TTMC*** **tensor tympani muscle canal,** ***dark green arrow*** **isthmus of the eustachian tube,** ***blue arrow*** **stapes,** ***black asterisk*** **stylomastoid foramen,** ***black circles*** **groove for the greater petrosal nerve,** ***white asterisk*** **foramen spinosum**

Note that the eustachian tube indicates the carotid canal only approximately. In other words, it lies on a different plane in respect of the vessel, and from an anterior viewpoint, it covers the vessel for all its length. Surgeons should have in mind that the external orifice of the carotid canal is not on the same coronal plane of the foramen lacerum (anterior genu). It is by far more posteriorly located.

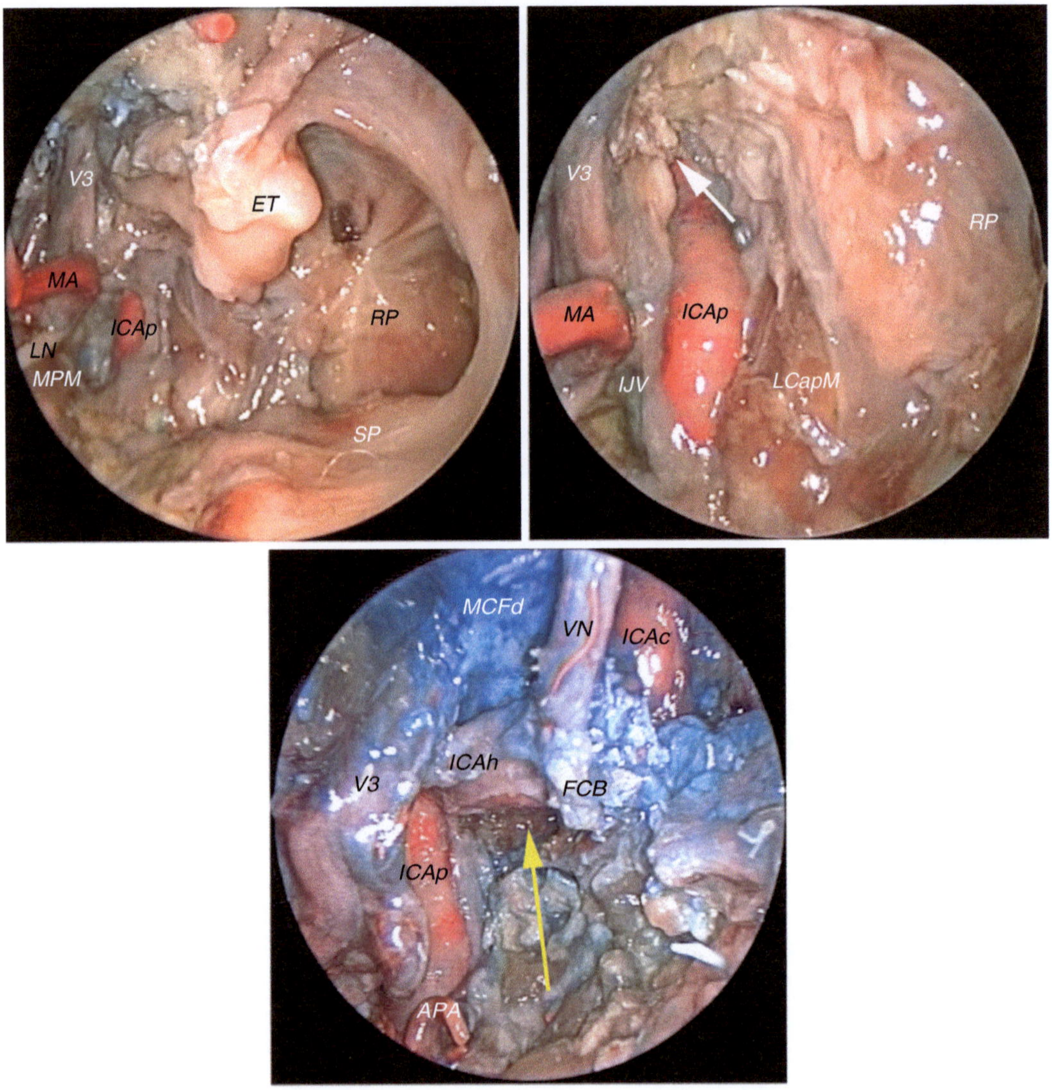

Fig. 2.21 Endoscopic vision of the infratemporal fossa and upper parapharyngeal space

ET **eustachian tube,** ***FCB*** **fibrocartilago basalis,** ***ICAc*** **cavernous portion of the internal carotid artery,** ***ICAh*** **horizontal portion of the internal carotid artery,** ***ICAp*** **parapharyngeal portion of the internal carotid artery,** ***IJV*** **internal jugular vein,** ***LCapM*** **longus capitis muscle,** ***LN*** **lingual nerve,** ***MA*** **maxillary artery,** ***MCFd*** **middle cranial fossa dura,** ***MMA*** **middle meningeal artery,** ***MPM*** **medial pterygoid muscle,** ***RP*** **rhinopharynx,** ***SP*** **soft palate,** ***VN*** **vidian nerve,** ***V3*** **third branch of the trigeminal nerve,** ***white arrow*** **bony portion of the ET (just anterior to the carotid canal),** ***yellow arrow*** **petrous apex and petroclival region**

Although not perfectly, the tube acts like an arrow and helps in the identification of the most cranial part of the parapharyngeal portion of the internal carotid artery. Given the variability of the carotid artery within the parapharyngeal space, the surgeon should be aware of such relationship.

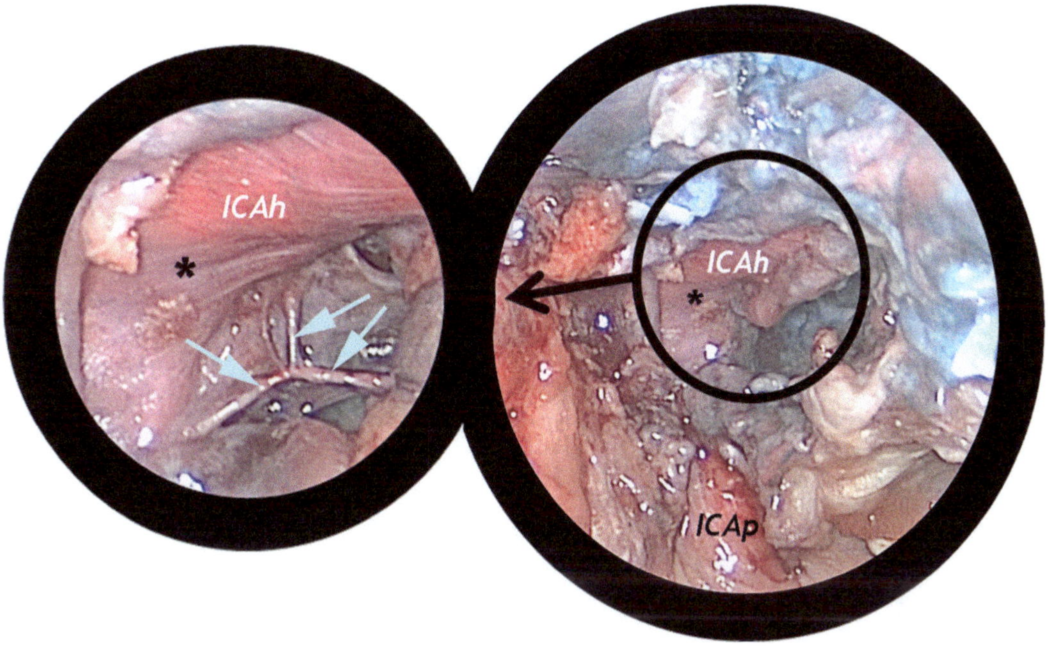

Fig. 2.22 Endoscopic view of the petrous and upper parapharyngeal portion of the internal carotid artery

ICAh **horizontal portion of the internal carotid artery,** ***ICAp*** **parapharyngeal portion of the internal carotid artery,** ***blue-sky arrows*** **periosteal branches,** ***black asterisk*** **posterior genu of the horizontal portion of the internal carotid artery**

The internal carotid artery within the carotid canal offers some branches: vidian, periosteal, and caroticotympanic arteries. The caroticotympanic artery arises from the vertical part of the ICAh and supplies the tympanic cavity. The vidian artery may arise from the horizontal segment of the ICAh, enter the pterygoid canal, and anastomose with the same-named branch from the maxillary artery. Periosteal branches can arise from the ICAh at different levels.

References

Bouthillier A, van Loveren H, Keller J (1996) Segments of the internal carotid artery: a new classification. Neurosurgery 38:425–433

Dallan I, Bignami M, Battaglia P et al (2010) Fully endoscopic transnasal approach to the jugular foramen: anatomic study and clinical considerations. Neurosurgery 67 (3 Suppl): ons1–7

Falcon RT, Rivera-Serrano CM, Miranda JF et al (2011) Endoscopic endonasal dissection of the infratemporal fossa: anatomic relationships and importance of eustachian tube in the endoscopic skull base surgery. Laryngoscope 121:31–41

Fernandez-Miranda JC, Morera VA, Snyderman CH et al (2012) Endoscopic endonasal transclival approach to the jugular tubercle. Neurosurgery 71 (suppl1): ons146–159

Herzallah IR, Casiano RR (2007) Endoscopic endonasal study of the internal carotid artery and variations. Am J Rhinol 21:262–270

Janfaza P, Nadol JB Jr (2001a) Scalp, cranium, and brain. In: Janfaza P, Nadol JB Jr, Galla R, Fabian RL, Montgomery WW (eds) Surgical anatomy of the head and neck. Lippincott Williams & Wilkins, Philadelphia

Janfaza P, Nadol JB Jr (2001b) Temporal bone and ear. In: Janfaza P, Nadol JB Jr, Galla R, Fabian RL, Montgomery WW (eds) Surgical anatomy of the head and neck. Lippincott Williams & Wilkins, Philadelphia

Jinkins JR (2000) Atlas of neuroradiologic embryology, anatomy, and variants. Lippincott Williams & Wilkins, Philadelphia

Kakizawa Y, Abe H, Fukushima Y et al (2007) The course of the lesser petrosal nerve on the middle cranial fossa. Neurosurgery 61(3 Suppl):15–23

Lang J (1995) Skull base and related structures: atlas of clinical anatomy. Schattauer, Stuttgart

Lasjaunias PL (1981) Craniofacial and upper cervical arteries: functional, clinical and angiographic aspects. Lippincott Williams & Wilkins, Baltimore

Osawa S, Rhoton AL Jr, Tanriover N et al (2008) Microsurgical anatomy and surgical exposure of the petrous segment of the internal carotid artery. Neurosurgery 63(4 Suppl 2):210–238

Paullus WS, Pait TG, Rhoton AL Jr (1977) Microsurgical exposure of the petrous portion of the carotid artery. J Neurosurg 47:713–726

Porto AF Jr, Whicker J, Proud GO (1978) An anatomic study of the hypotympanic branch of Jacobson's nerve. Laryngoscope 88:56–60

Tubbs RS, Hansasuta A, Loukas M et al (2007) Branches of the petrous and cavernous segments of the internal carotid artery. Clin Anat 20:596–601

Ziyal IM, Ozgen T, Sekhar LN et al (2005) Proposed classification of segments of the internal carotid artery: anatomical study with angiographical interpretation. Neurol Med Chir (Tokyo) 45:184–191

Intracranial Segment 3

Cavernous Segment

3.1 Anatomic Layout

Above the petrolingual ligament, the internal carotid artery (ICA) can be considered to be intracavernous. From an endoscopic anterior viewpoint, we can define a *paraclival* and a *parasellar* segment, especially evident in well-pneumatised sphenoid sinuses. The paraclival segment corresponds to the vertical segment of the ICAc (cavernous portion of the ICA). Endoscopically speaking, this portion of the vessel represents the lateral border of the clival window. Although some authors have divided the paraclival portion in subsegments (Herzallah and Casiano 2007), we do not consider this further classification as having surgical utility. At a variable distance from the posterior clinoid process, the vertical segment—paraclival—bends forward, forming the *posterior bend* of the ICAc. Then, the artery usually runs horizontally for a short distance (*horizontal segment*) and curves upward, thus giving the *anterior bend* that reaches the anterior clinoid process. For this reason, the cavernous portion in the typical neurosurgical literature has been divided into five segments: *posterior vertical*, *posterior bend*, *horizontal*, *anterior bend*, and *anterior vertical* (Inoue et al. 1990). It must be underlined that the configuration of the posterior bend varies significantly, and that sometimes it can bulge upward into and deform the dura of the cavernous sinus (CS) roof just lateral to the posterior clinoid process. The last segment, the anterior vertical, also named the *clinoid*, *infraclinoid* or *paraclinoid*, is not completely intracavernous, but in "endoscopic" practice, it can be considered so; for this reason, we have included it in this section.

Different authors have tried to classify the ICAc, using different names but with similar conclusions (Herzallah and Casiano 2007; Jittapiromsak et al. 2010). These works both described two types of intracavernous ICA. Notwithstanding this, such differentiation appears of limited utility from an endosurgical viewpoint. Looking through a sphenoidal window, the parasellar ICA is positioned on the side of the pituitary gland, thus producing the parasellar ICA prominence on the sphenoid sinus wall. This prominence corresponds, more or less, to the distal part of the horizontal segment, the anterior bend, and the clinoid segment. The intracavernous segment of the ICA presents different branches, the most constant are the *meningohypophyseal* and the *inferolateral trunk* (ILT).

3.1.1 Gross Anatomy

This portion grossly corresponds to the sphenoid sinus. Endoscopic anatomical landmarks are identified once a wide sphenoidal window is performed: the lateral and medial opticocarotid recess (lOCR and mOCR, respectively), the parasellar and paraclival carotid canal, the sellar prominence, the clival recess, and the strut of bone over the interCS. The lOCR is given by the pneumatisation of the optic strut, thus forming a recess that extends between the optic nerve superiorly and

P. Castelnuovo et al., *Surgical Anatomy of the Internal Carotid Artery*,
DOI 10.1007/978-3-642-29664-2_3, © Springer-Verlag Berlin Heidelberg 2013

the intracavernous carotid artery inferiorly. The mOCR corresponds, on the intracranial surface, to the lateral tubercular crest (most lateral part of the tuberculum sellae). The middle clinoid process (MCP) is placed a little bit lateral and inferior to the lateral aspect of the tuberculum sellae. It is a small eminence of the carotid sulcus at the level of the anterior part of the lateral wall of the sella turcica. The base of the MCP is just medial to the anterior genu of the parasellar ICA. And it projects laterally. The mOCR is placed at the confluence of the sella, tuberculum sellae, carotid protuberance, optic canal and planum sphenoidale. So, opening the mOCR permits visualization of the carotid canal, the optic nerve, the sella, and the medial CS. Obviously, these landmarks are easily recognizable in case of a sellar-type sphenoid sinus. In case of a presellar and conchal type, this task is respectively demanding and definitely impossible.

When looking at the lateral wall in well-pneumatised sinuses, 3 bony protrusions and 4 bony depressions can be visualized. Among the protuberances, from rostral to caudal, they correspond to the optic canal, the superior orbital fissure (SOF), and V2. The optic canal is placed above the parasellar ICA, while the SOF lies directly below the lOCR. The bony depressions include the lOCR, the mOCR, the depression between the CS apex and V2, and the depression below V2. In these cases, the vidian nerve, covered or not by bone, can be easily visualized at the level of the floor of the sphenoid sinus.

3.1.2 Neural Structures

Maxillary Nerve

The maxillary nerve corresponds to the inferior limit of the CS, where the lateral wall joins the medial wall of the CS. This nerve also can be identified anteriorly, passing through the foramen rotondum. The nerve crosses the lateral aspect of the trigeminal portion of the paraclival ICA. This landmark is superior and lateral to the vidian canal.

Oculomotor Nerve

Lateral to the intracavernous ICA, within the lateral wall of the CS, it is possible to visualize the oculomotor nerve. This nerve forms the inferior border of the optic struct triangle and runs anteriorly to the upper part of the anterior vertical portion of the parasellar ICA to reach the SOF.

Trochlear Nerve

The trochlear nerve enters the roof of the CS in the posterolateral apex of the oculomotor triangle, a little behind the entrance of the oculomotor nerve. In 20 % of cases, it enters the inferior surface of the tentorium cerebelli (Lang 1995). A small arachnoid pocket is present for a variable length inside the CS. Inside the lateral wall of the CS, it runs alone, slightly inferior to the oculomotor nerve, to gain the SOF. It is usually accompanied by the supero-proximal artery branch of the ILT. Not so rarely, bipartitions of the nerve in the lateral wall can be observed (Lang 1995).

Abducens Nerve

The abducens nerve pierces the dura of the posterior cranial fossa (PCF), on the clivus. Sheaths of dura and arachnoid follow the nerve within the basilar plexus (Lang 1995) and then through the inferior petrosal sinus. The nerve presents a short course superiorly and penetrates the CS, passing through Dorello's canal, at the apex of the petrous bone. The nerve runs anterior and rostrally lateral to the posterior vertical segment of the intracavernous ICA and then along the inferior border of the horizontal portion of the ICAc. It courses inside the lateral part of the CS, medial to the ophthalmic nerve (Yasuda et al. 2005). Most of the time, the nerve is a single trunk, but it must be kept in mind that separated nerve bundles in the prepontine cistern or several bundles within the CS can be present. Typically, anastomoses with sympathetic fibres are present. In the prepontine cistern, in case of separated bundles, the AICA can be found between the bundles.

Ophthalmic Nerve

The ophthalmic (V1) nerve courses within the lateral wall of the CS below the trochlear nerve. It lies lateral to the abducens nerve and runs anterosuperiorly to gain the SOF. A small branch for the tentorium cerebelli has been described

(Lang 1995). Close to the superior orbital fissure, it splits in three nerves: nasociliary, frontal, and lacrimal nerves.

Sympathetic Plexus

The sympathetic plexus fibres diverge from the ICAc to adhere to the abducens nerve while crossing to join the ophthalmic nerve (V1). The main target exit is V1 on the lateral wall of the CS (Jittapiromsak et al. 2010).

3.1.3 Vascular Branches (Isolan et al. 2005; Yasuda et al. 2005; Tubbs et al. 2007)

Meningohypophyseal Trunk

Also called the dorsal main stem artery (Jinkins 2000), the meningohypophyseal trunk (MHT) typically arises from the posterior bend of the ICA. This trunk originates a mean of 10.2 mm distal to the foramen lacerum (Inoue et al. 1990). Two types of the vessel are described: complete and incomplete. In the complete version, there are three branches: the *tentorial artery* (also called the *Bernasconi-Cassinari artery*), the *dorsal meningeal artery* (also called the *dorsal clival artery*) (Conti et al. 2008), and the *inferior hypophyseal artery* (IHA). The incomplete type demonstrates one or more of these three vessels arising directly from the cavernous ICA. More often, it is the dorsal meningeal artery. Rarely, all three vessels arise directly from the ICA. The other two tentorial branches are described by Jinkins (Jinkins 2000) as the *basal meningeal* and the *marginal tentorial arteries* that travel along the attached and free borders of the tentorium cerebelli, respectively. The IHA travels superior and medially toward the pituitary gland and primarily to its posterior lobe. In some cases, the vessel supplies the anterior lobe, mainly on its periphery (Jinkins 2000). The vessel, when approaching the pituitary gland, bifurcates and sometimes trifurcates (Parkinson 1964). The IHA and the dorsal meningeal arteries anastomose with one another on both sides, thus forming a circulus arteriosus around the root of the dorsum sellae. The dorsal meningeal artery, or dorsal clival artery, passes posterior toward Dorello's canal and supplies the dura of the upper clivus and the proximal aspect of the abducens nerve. During its travelling, it contributes, with the artery of Bernasconi-Cassinari, to the blood supply of the proximal part of the cranial nerves inside the CS. The outer circumference of the MHT is 0.75–1 mm (Lang 1995).

Inferolateral Trunk (Artery of the Inferior Cavernous Sinus)

The ILT (also called the artery of the inferior CS) arises from the central one third of the inferior or lateral surface of the horizontal segment of the cavernous ICA, distal to the origin of the MHT (3–13 mm) (Tubbs 2007). It is also called the lateral main stem. Usually, it travels superior to the abducens nerve and then downward between the abducens nerve and V1 to reach the area around the foramina ovale and rotundum. The ILT usually divides into two branches (Krisht et al. 1994). The superior one curves posteriorly along the trochlear nerve and the edge of the tentorium. The second branch is the *artery of the SOF*, which runs under the first two trigeminal branches and provides vascularizaton for the foramen ovale and rotundum. The SOF artery is critical for the blood supply of the distal portion of cranial nerves III, IV, V1, and VI (Conti et al. 2008). When the MHT does not provide a tentorial branch, the artery of the inferior CS provides a marginal tentorial artery. The ILT has been described as arising from the MHT (Jinkins 2000).

McConnell's Capsular Artery

McConnel's capsular artery is not always present (30–50 % of the cases) (Reisch et al. 2002). The vessel(s) may come from the most superior segment of the intracavernous ICA. In less than 10 % of cases, it arises from the medial aspect of the horizontal segment of the cavernous ICA. When present, it supplies the inferior and peripheral aspect of the anterior lobe of the pituitary gland and the diaphragma sellae (Jinkins 2000). McConnell's arteries may give branches that penetrate the sella turcica to enter the sphenoid sinus via the craniopharyngeal canal (when present).

Persistent Trigeminal Artery

When present, the persistent trigeminal artery (PTA) arises from the central middle third of the posterior bend of the ICAc. Its incidence is described as between 0.06 % and 0.6 % (Fields 1968; Silver and Wilkins 1991). In more than half of the cases, the PTA penetrates the sella turcica near the clivus to join the basilar artery. In the remaining cases, the artery travels lateral to the sella turcica (Suttner et al. 2000). There are two types of PTA, according to the relationship to the abducens nerve: a lateral or petrosal and a medial or sphenoidal. If the artery arises from the posterolateral aspect of the cavernous ICA, it runs lateral to the abducens nerve intradurally and inferior to cranial nerve VI within the CS and thus displaces the nerve superiorly. When the PTA arises from the posteromedial aspect of the intracavernous ICA, it pierces the dura over the dorsum sellae and courses medial to the abducens nerve (Salas et al. 1998).

Ophthalmic Artery

The ophthalmic artery can arise from the cavernous portion in 1–7.5 % of cases (Yasargil 1984; Dolenc 1989; Inoue et al. 1990). When coming from the intracavernous segment, it arises from the anterior bend.

Superior Hypophyseal Artery (Arteries)

In rare cases, some perforating branches for the superior aspect of the pituitary gland (superior hypophyseal arteries, SHAs) originate from the intracavernous segment of the ICA (more commonly from the paraclinoid segment). It is also possible to observe several branches, some arising in the intracavernous segment and others coming from the cisternal one.

Recurrent Artery of the Foramen Lacerum

The recurrent artery of the foramen lacerum seems to supply the pericarotid autonomic nervous plexus (Lasjaunias 1981). It forms an anastomosis with the ascending pharyngeal artery. It can be considered a periosteal branch.

Artery of the Gasserian Ganglion

The branches of the artery of the Gasserian ganglion cross the abducens nerve within the CS as they travel laterally.

3.2 Anatomic Pictures

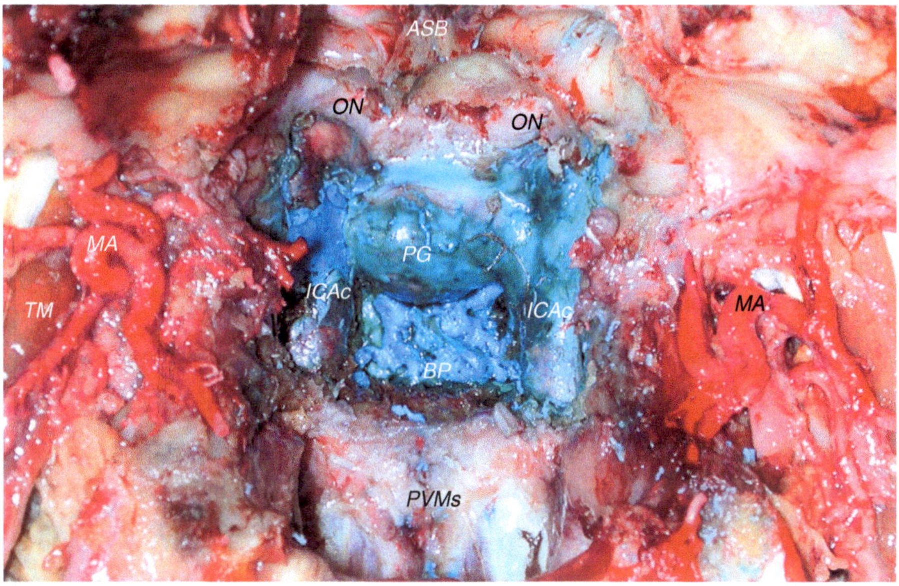

Fig. 3.1 Anterior view of the midline structures

ASB **anterior skull base,** ***BP*** **basilar plexus,** ***ICAc*** **cavernous portion of the internal carotid artery (vertical segment),** ***MA*** **maxillary artery,** ***ON*** **optic nerve,** ***PG*** **pituitary gland,** ***PVMs*** **prevertebral muscles,** ***TM*** **temporal muscle**

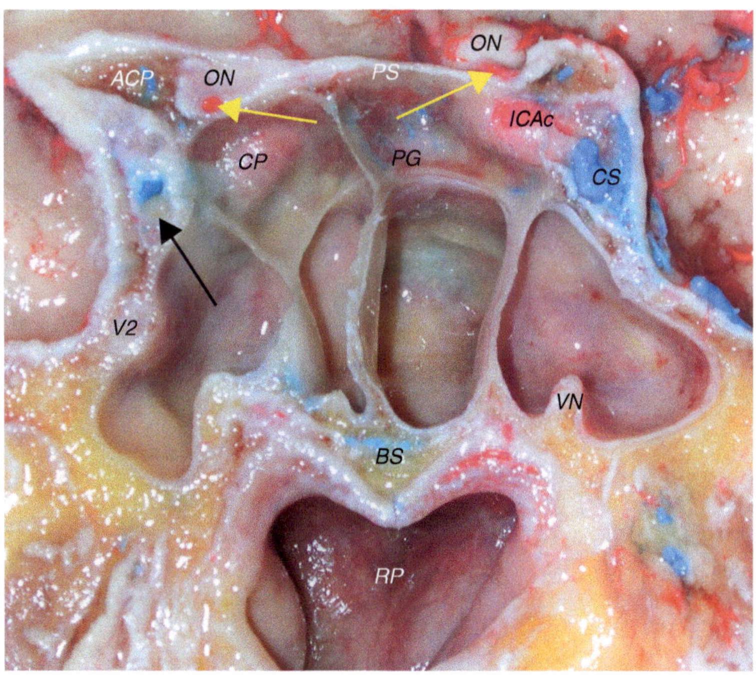

Fig. 3.2 Anterior view of the sphenoid sinus and the rhinopharynx

ACP **anterior clinoid process,** ***BS*** **basisphenoid,** ***CP*** **carotid protuberance,** ***CS*** **cavernous sinus,** ***ICAc*** **cavernous portion of the internal carotid artery,** ***ON*** **optic nerve,** ***PG*** **pituitary gland,** ***RP*** **rhinopharynx,** ***VN*** **vidian nerve,** ***V2*** **second branch of the trigeminal nerve,** ***black arrow*** **first branch of the trigeminal nerve,** ***yellow arrows*** **ophthalmic artery**

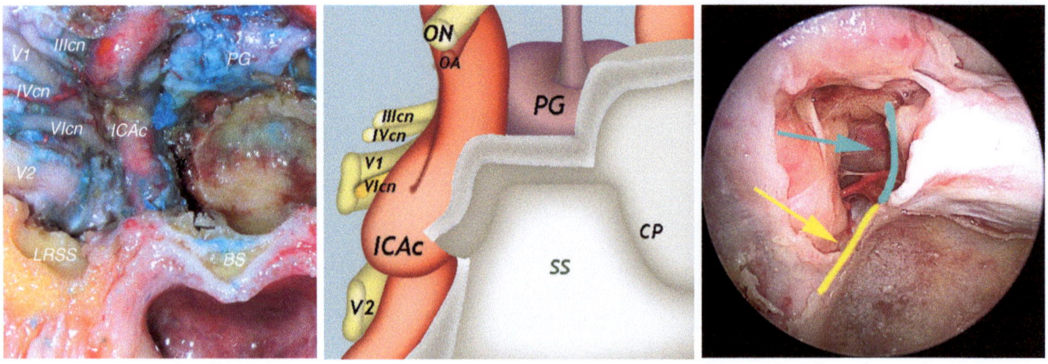

Fig. 3.3 Anterior vision of the right cavernous sinus

BS **basisphenoid,** ***CP*** **carotid protuberance,** ***ICAc*** **cavernous portion of the internal carotid artery (vertical segment),** ***LRSS*** **lateral recess of the sphenoid sinus,** ***OA*** **ophthalmic artery,** ***ON*** **optic nerve,** ***PG*** **pituitary gland,** ***SS*** **sphenoid sinus,** ***V1*** **first branch of the trigeminal nerve,** ***V2*** **second branch of the trigeminal nerve,** ***IIIcn*** **oculomotor nerve,** ***IVcn*** **trochlear nerve,** ***VIcn*** **abducens nerve,** ***yellow arrow*** **inferior part of the medial wall of the cavernous sinus (*****yellow line*****),** ***blue-sky arrow*** **superior part of the medial wall of the cavernous sinus (*****blue-sky line*****)**

The inferior part of the medial wall of the CS faces the lateral part of the body of the sphenoid, while the upper part of the medial wall is directly related to the PG (Martins et al. 2011). In the upper part, the medial wall is given by the meningeal layer, that is a continuation of the diaphragma sellae, which surrounds the pituitary capsule inferiorly (Yasuda et al. 2005; Martins et al. 2011). In the inferior part, the medial wall is given by the endosteal layer that covers the body of the sphenoid bone. So, a sellar (superior) and a sphenoidal (inferior) part can be described. The limits of the medial wall of the cavernous sinus are the superior orbital fissure anteriorly, the dorsum sellae posteriorly, the superior margin of the maxillary nerve inferiorly and the diaphragma sellae superiorly (Yasuda 2005). The presellar segment of the ICAc corresponds to the anterior bend of the ICAc and to the clinoidal segment of the internal carotid artery.

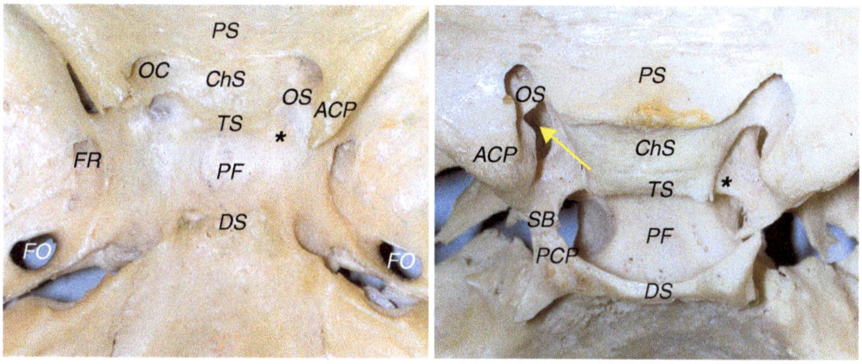

Fig. 3.4 Sphenoid sinus and bone

ACP **anterior clinoid process,** ***ChS*** **chiasmatic sulcus,** ***DS*** **dorsum sellae,** ***FO*** **foramen ovale,** ***FR*** **foramen rotundum,** ***OC*** **optic canal,** ***OS*** **optic strut,** ***PCP*** **posterior clinoid process,** ***PF*** **pituitary fossa,** ***PS*** **planum sphenoidale,** ***SB*** **sellar bridge,** ***TS*** **tuberculum sellae,** ***yellow arrow*** **carotid-clinoid foramen,** ***black asterisk*** **middle clinoid process**

ACPs project posteriorly and laterally to the optic canal and carotid sulcus. The TS separates the chiasmatic sulcus from the pituitary fossa. This is closed posteriorly by the DS. On each side of DS are the PCPs. The OS links the ACP with the sphenoid bone and separates the optic canal from the superior orbital fissure. When anterior and middle clinoid processes fuse, a "carotid-clinoid" foramen is formed. This circumstance is present in about 10 % of adults. The bony connection between anterior and posterior clinoid processes is called the "sellar bridge." This is found in about 6 % of cases (Lang 1995). The base of the middle clinoid process is just medial to the anterior genu of the (parasellar) cavernous ICA, while the apex extends in a dorsolateral direction. The middle clinoid process is, when present, a small eminence of the carotid sulcus at the level of the anterior part of the lateral wall of the sella turcica (Labib et al. 2013). The lateral tubercular crest is a bony eminence placed on the lateral part of the tuberculum sellae.

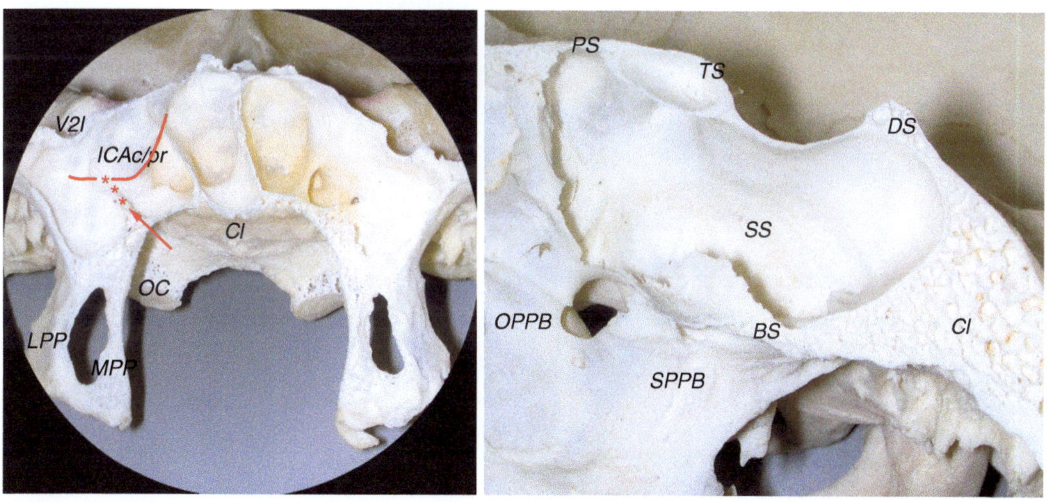

Fig. 3.5 Sphenoid sinus and bone

BS **basisphenoid,** ***Cl*** **clivus,** ***DS*** **dorsum sellae,** ***ICAc/pr*** **protuberance of the cavernous portion of the internal carotid artery,** ***LPP*** **lateral pterygoid plate,** ***MPP*** **medial pterygoid plate,** ***OC*** **occipital condyle,** ***OPPB*** **orbital process of the palatine bone,** ***PS*** **planum sphenoidale,** ***SPPB*** **sphenoidal process of the palatine bone,** ***SS*** **sphenoid sinus,** ***TS*** **tuberculum sellae,** ***V2I*** **incisure of V2,** ***red arrow*** **opening of the vidian canal,** ***red asterisks*** **vidian canal,** ***red line*** **internal carotid artery**

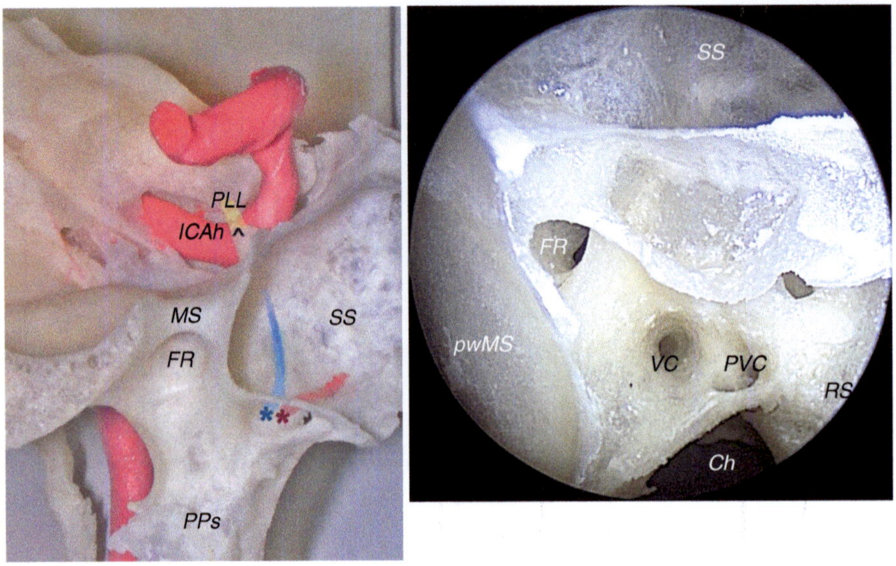

Fig. 3.6 Sphenoid bone and sinus with a focus on the base of the pterygoid region and the relationship with the cavernous portion of the internal carotid artery

Ch **choana,** ***FR*** **foramen rotundum,** ***ICAh*** **horizontal portion of the internal carotid artery,** ***MS*** **maxillary strut,** ***PLL*** **petrolingual ligament,** ***PPs*** **pterygoid plates,** ***PVC*** **palatovaginal canal,** ***pwMS*** **posterior wall of the maxillary sinus,** ***RS*** **rostrum sphenoidale,** ***SS*** **sphenoid sinus,** ***VC*** **vidian canal,** ***black arrowhead*** **lingula of the sphenoid,** ***blue-sky asterisk and line*** **vidian (pterygoid) canal,** ***red asterisk and line*** **palatovaginal (pharyngeal) canal**

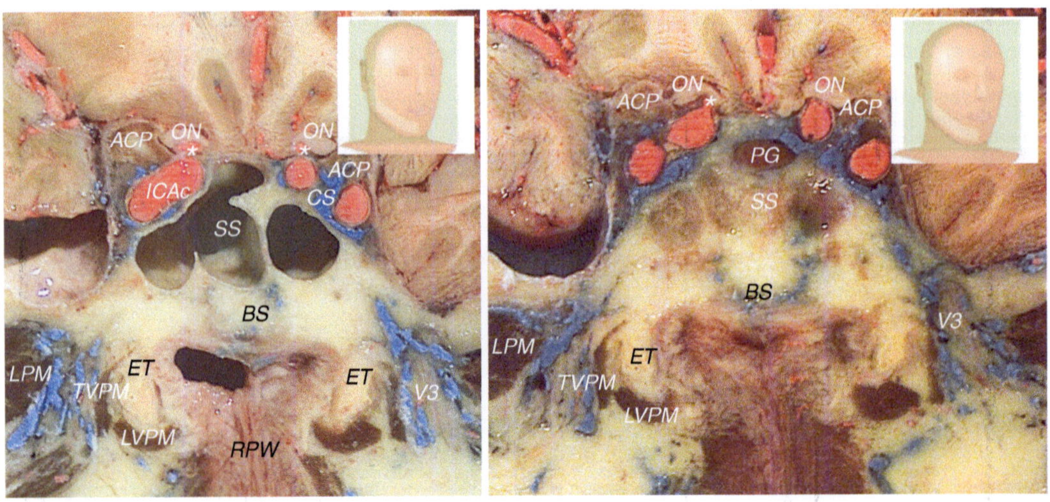

Fig. 3.7 Coronal views at the level of the sphenoidal region. The picture on the left shows a more anterior view than the picture on the right. Note that the picture on the left is seen from posterior, while the picture on the right is seen from anterior

ACP **anterior clinoid process,** ***BS*** **basisphenoid,** ***CS*** **cavernous sinus,** ***ET*** **eustachian tube,** ***ICAc*** **cavernous portion of the internal carotid artery,** ***LPM*** **lateral pterygoid muscle,** ***LVPM*** **levator veli palatini muscle,** ***ON*** **optic nerve,** ***PG*** **pituitary gland,** ***RPW*** **rhinopharyngeal posterior wall,** ***SS*** **sphenoid sinus,** ***TVPM*** **tensor veli palatini muscle,** ***V3*** **third branch of the trigeminal nerve,** ***white asterisk*** **ophthalmic artery**

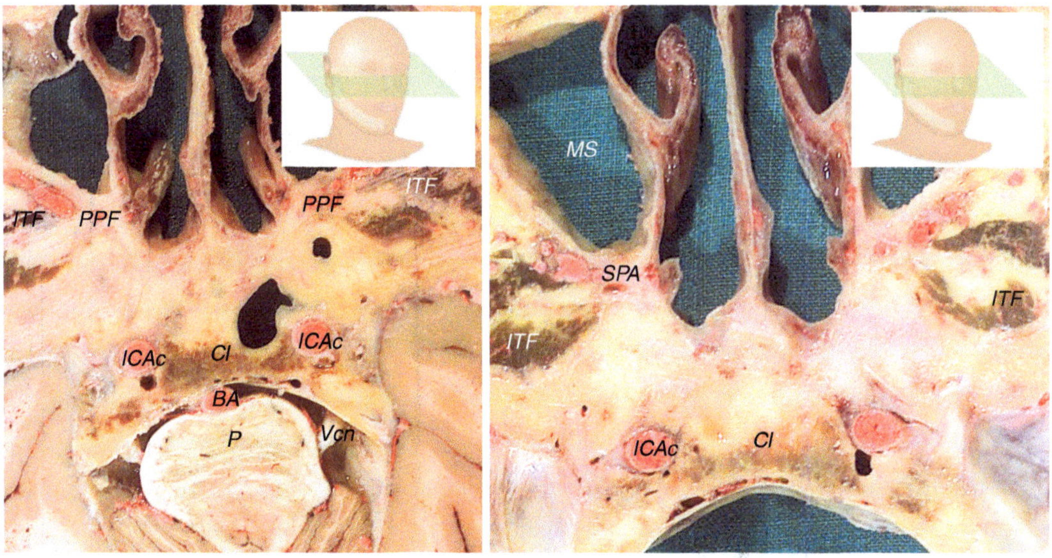

Fig. 3.8 Axial views at the level of the clivus. The picture on the left is seen from below. The picture on the right is seen from above

BA **basilar artery,** ***Cl*** **clivus,** ***ICAc*** **cavernous portion of the internal carotid artery (vertical segment),** ***ITF*** **infratemporal fossa,** ***MS*** **maxillary sinus,** ***P*** **pons,** ***PPF*** **pterygopalatine fossa,** ***SPA*** **sphenopalatine artery,** ***Vcn*** **trigeminal nerve**

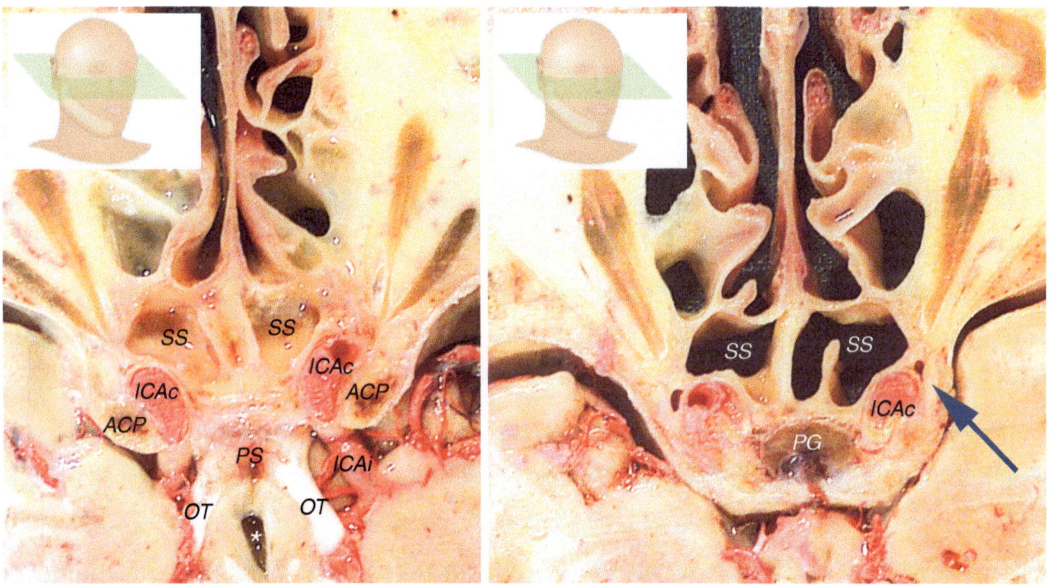

Fig. 3.9 Axial view at the level of the sphenoid sinus. The picture on the left is seen from below. The picture on the right is seen from above. The picture on the left shows a more cranial view

ACP **anterior clinoid process,** ***ICAc*** **cavernous portion of the internal carotid artery,** ***ICAi*** **intracranial portion of the internal carotid artery,** ***OT*** **optic tract,** ***PG*** **pituitary gland,** ***PS*** **pituitary stalk,** ***SS*** **sphenoid sinus,** ***blue arrow*** **abducens nerve,** ***white asterisk*** **third ventricle**

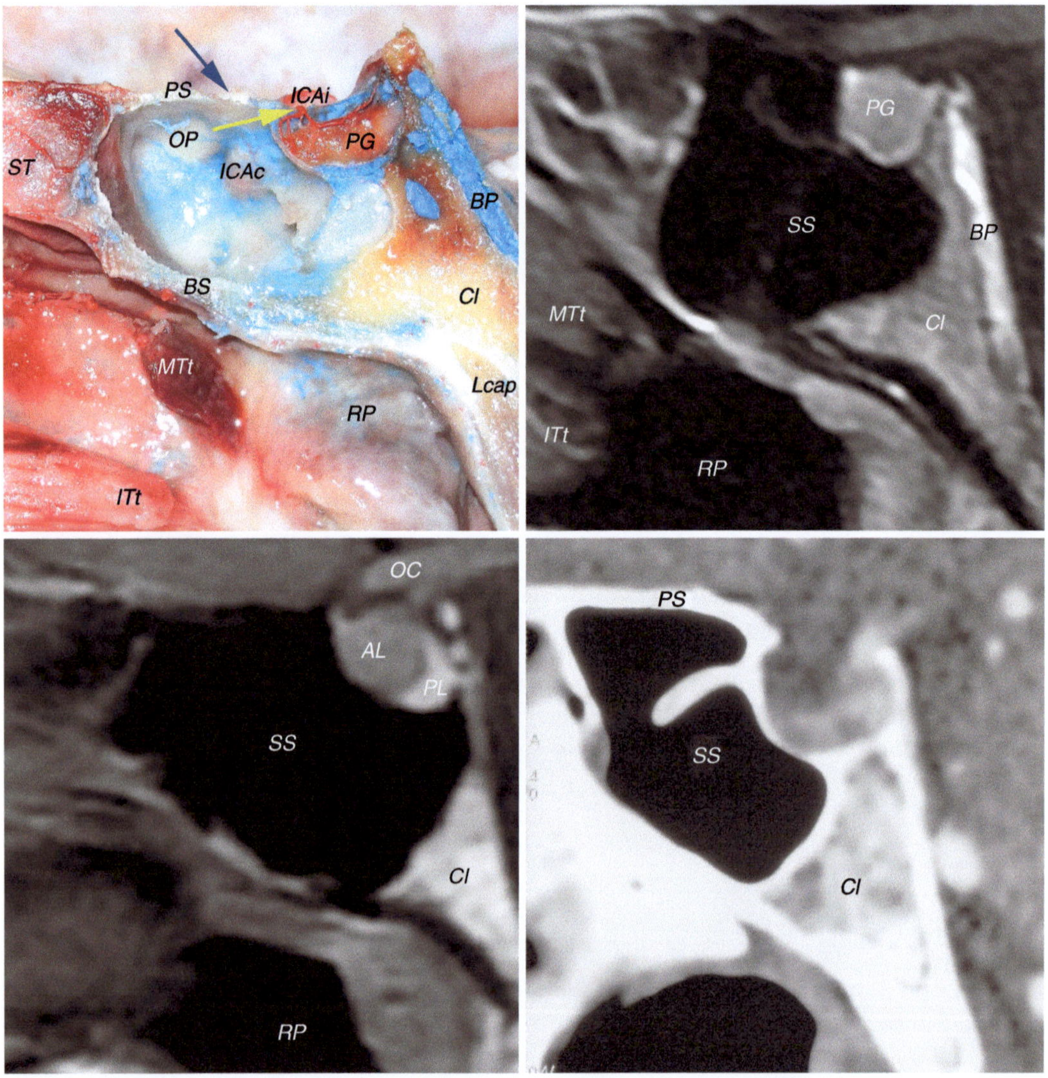

Fig. 3.10 Medial sagittal vision of the sphenoid sinus and its surrounding structures

AL **anterior lobe,** ***BP*** **basilar plexus,** ***BS*** **basisphenoid,** ***Cl*** **clivus,** ***ICAc*** **cavernous portion of the internal carotid artery,** ***ICAi*** **intracranial portion of the internal carotid artery,** ***ITt*** **tail of the inferior turbinate,** ***Lcap*** **longus capitis,** ***MTt*** **tail of the middle turbinate,** ***OC*** **optic chiasm,** ***OP*** **optic protuberance,** ***PG*** **pituitary gland,** ***PL*** **posterior lobe,** ***PS*** **planum sphenoidale,** ***RP*** **rhinopharynx,** ***ST*** **superior turbinate,** ***yellow arrow*** **superior hypophyseal artery(ies),** ***blue arrow*** **optic nerve**

The anterior lobe of the pituitary gland is mainly fed by the superior hypophyseal arteries while the posterior lobe is fed mainly by the inferior hypophyseal artery.

Fig. 3.11 Reconstruction showing the pterygoidal window and the region around the foramen rotundum

CR **clival recess,** ***CS*** **cavernous sinus,** ***ET*** **eustachian tube,** ***ICAc*** **cavernous portion of the internal carotid artery,** ***PG*** **pituitary gland,** ***VN*** **vidian nerve,** ***V2*** **second branch of the trigeminal nerve**

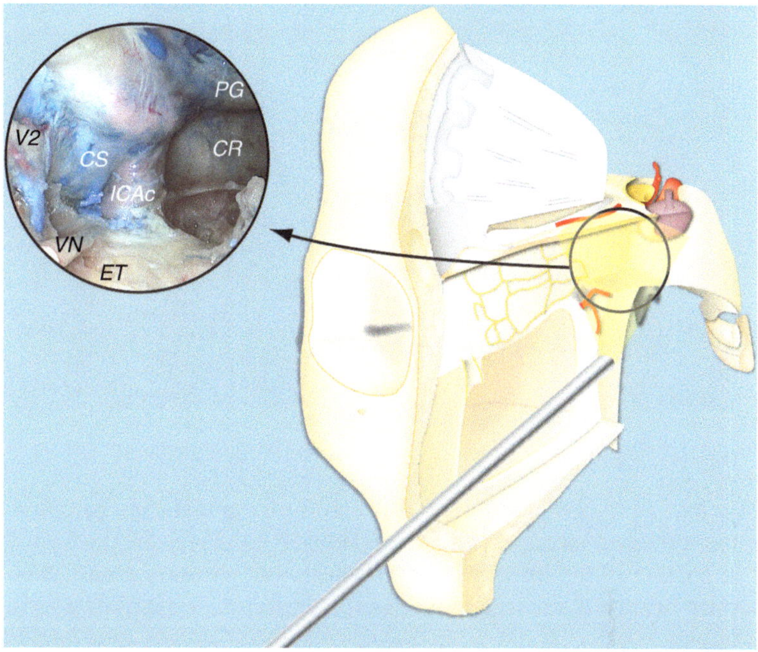

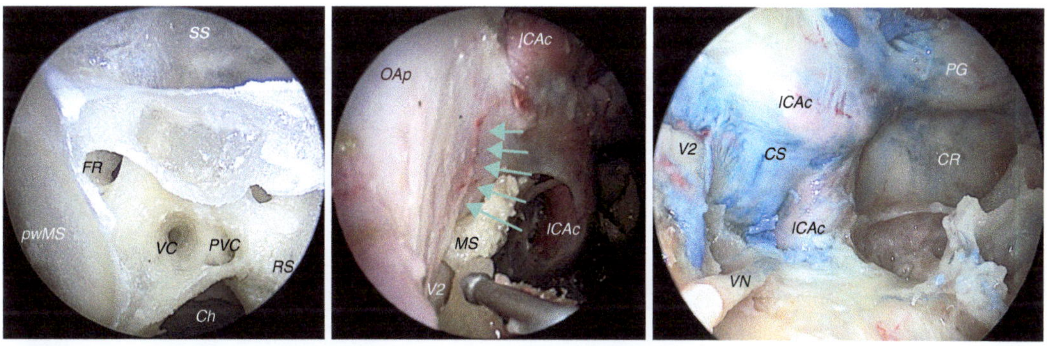

Fig. 3.12 Foramen rotundum region

Ch **choana,** ***CR*** **clival recess,** ***CS*** **cavernous sinus,** ***FR*** **foramen rotundum,** ***ICAc*** **cavernous portion of the internal carotid artery,** ***MS*** **maxillary strut,** ***OAp*** **orbital apex,** ***PG*** **pituitary gland,** ***PVC*** **palatovaginal canal,** ***pwMS*** **posterior wall of the maxillary sinus,** ***RS*** **rostrum sphenoidale,** ***SS*** **sphenoid sinus,** ***VC*** **vidian canal,** ***VN*** **vidian nerve,** ***V2*** **second branch of the trigeminal nerve,** ***blue-sky arrows*** **superior orbital fissure**

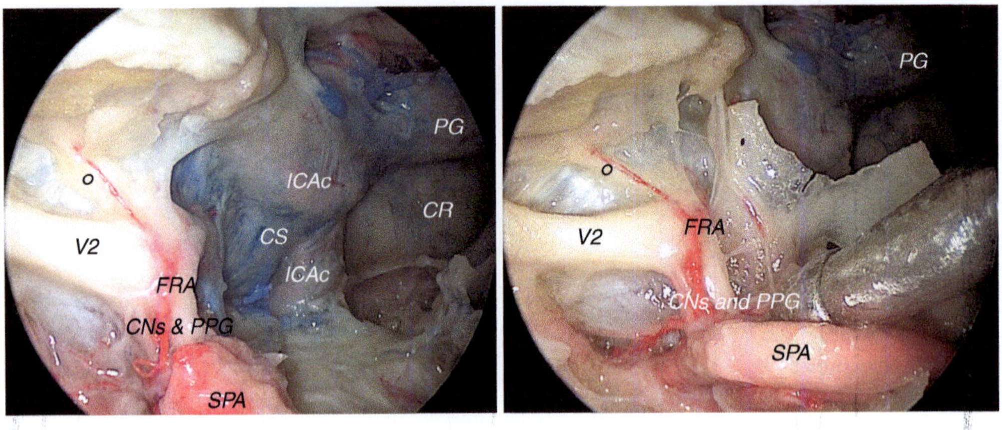

Fig. 3.13 Endoscopic views of the foramen rotundum region

***CNs and PPG* connecting nerves (*V2* and pterygopalatine ganglion) and pterygopalatine ganglion, *CR* clival recess, *CS* cavernous sinus, *FRA* artery for the foramen rotondum, *ICAc* cavernous portion of the internal carotid artery, *PG* pituitary gland, *SPA* sphenopalatine artery, *V2* second branch of the trigeminal nerve, *black circle* zygomatic nerve**

Foramen rotundum transmits the second branch of the trigeminal nerve (maxillary nerve), arteries (foramen rodundum artery), and veins.

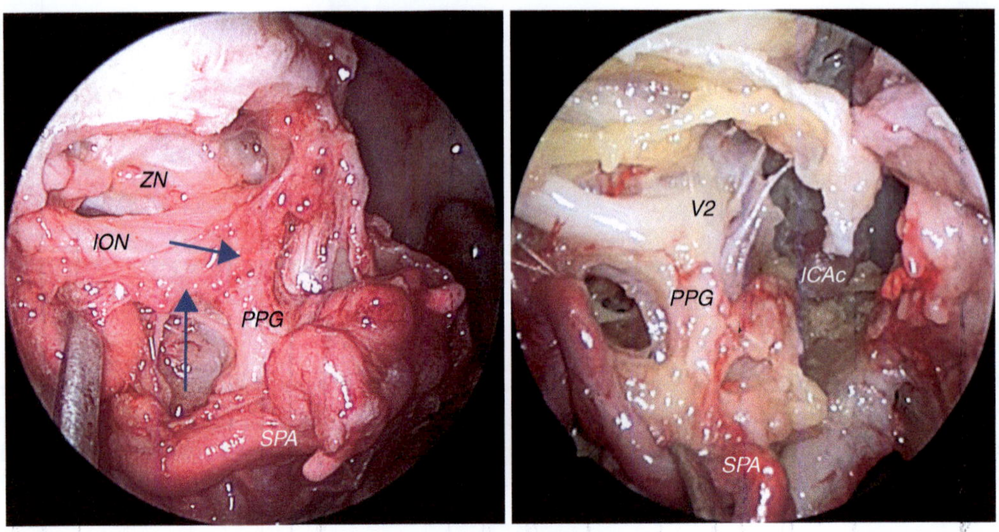

Fig. 3.14 Endoscopic vision of the pterygopalatine ganglion

***ICAc* cavernous portion of the internal carotid artery, *ION* infraorbital nerve, *PPG* pterygopalatine ganglion, *SPA* sphenopalatine artery, *ZN* zygomatic nerve, *V2* second branch of the trigeminal nerve, *blue arrows* artery for the foramen rotundum**

The zygomatic nerve exits the pterygopalatine fossa via the inferior orbital fissure and diverges from the ION to enter the orbit (Janfaza et al. 2001). The PPG is one of the four parasympathetic ganglia of the head (the other are the otic, the submandibular, and the ciliary). It is reached by the vidian nerve (parasympathetic and sympathetic), but only parasympathetic fibres synapse in the ganglion (Janfaza and Montgomery 2001).

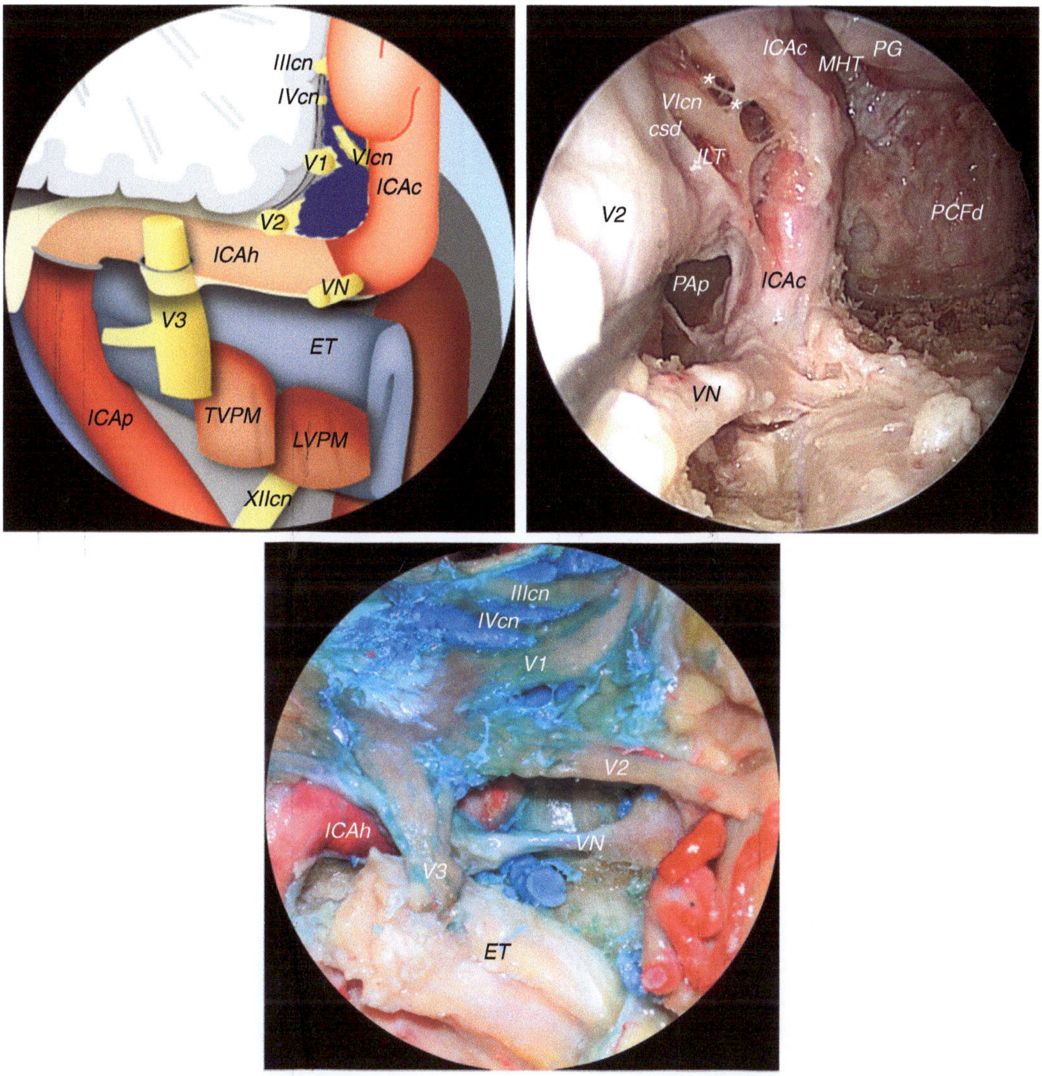

Fig. 3.15 Relationship between the vidian nerve and the anterior genu of the internal carotid artery

BS **basisphenoid,** ***CS*** **cavernous sinus,** ***CSd*** **dura of the cavernous sinus,** ***ET*** **eustachian tube,** ***ICAc*** **cavernous portion of the internal carotid artery,** ***ICAh*** **horizontal portion of the internal carotid artery,** ***ICAp*** **parapharyngeal portion of the internal carotid artery,** ***ILT*** **inferolateral trunk,** ***LVPM*** **levator veli palatini muscle,** ***MHT*** **meningohypophyseal trunk,** ***PAp*** **petrous apex,** ***PCFd*** **posterior cranial fossa dura and periosteum,** ***PG*** **pituitary gland,** ***TVPM*** **tensor veli palatini muscle,** ***VN*** **vidian nerve,** ***IIIcn*** **oculomotor nerve,** ***IVcn*** **trochlear nerve,** ***V1*** **first branch of the trigeminal nerve,** ***V2*** **second branch of the trigeminal nerve,** ***V3*** **third branch of the trigeminal nerve,** ***VIcn*** **abducens nerve,** ***XIIcn*** **hypoglossal nerve,** ***white asterisks*** **sympathetic fibres connecting the** ***VIcn***

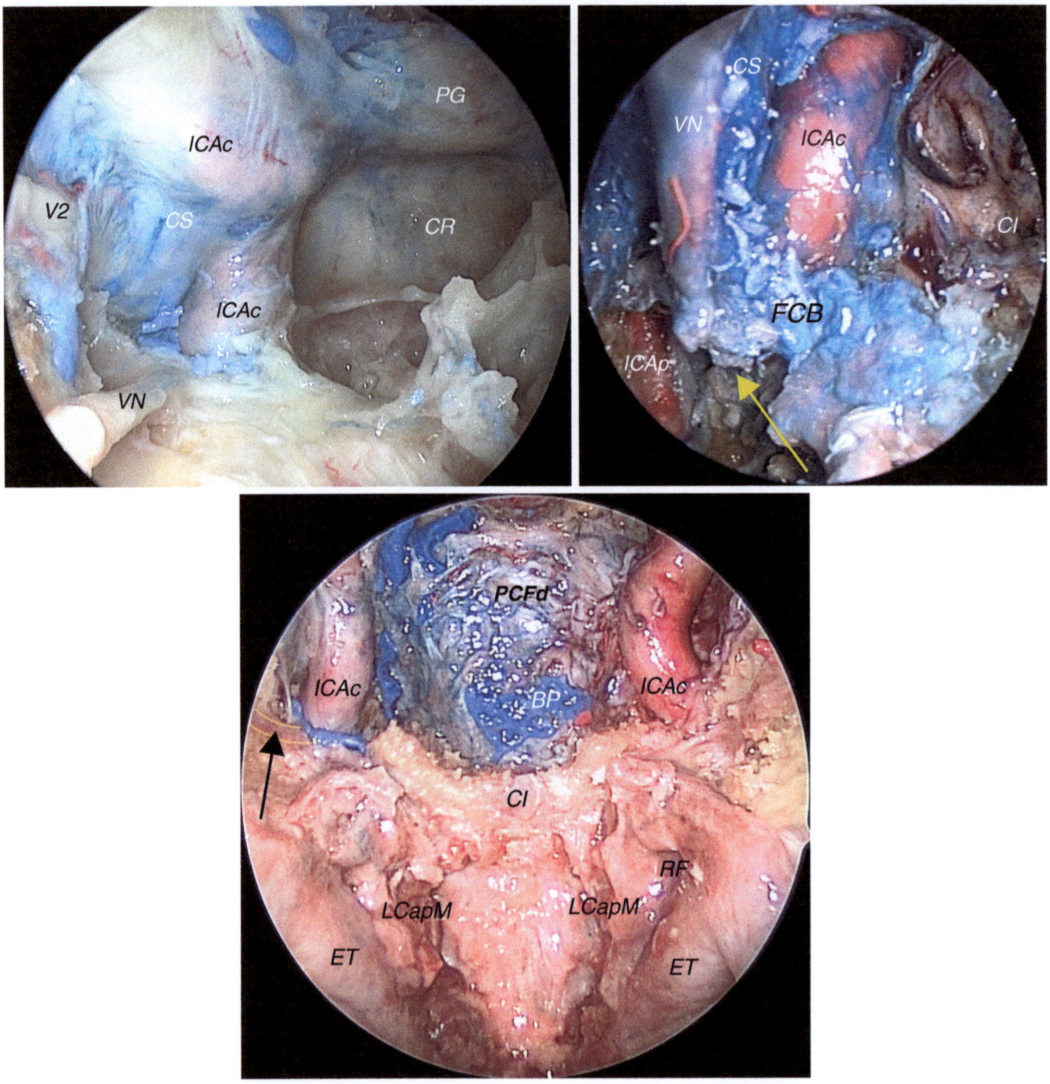

Fig. 3.16 Relationship between the vidian nerve and the anterior genu of the internal carotid artery

BP **basilar plexus,** ***Cl*** **clivus,** ***CR*** **clival recess,** ***CS*** **cavernous sinus,** ***ET*** **eustachian tube,** ***FCB*** **fibrocartilago basalis,** ***ICAc*** **cavernous portion of the internal carotid artery,** ***ICAp*** **parapharyngeal portion of the internal carotid artery,** ***LCapM*** **longus capitis muscle,** ***PCFd*** **dura and periosteum of the posterior cranial fossa,** ***RF*** **Rosenmuller's fossa,** ***VN*** **vidian nerve,** ***V2*** **second branch of the trigeminal nerve,** ***yellow arrow*** **petrous apex and petroclival region (bone removed),** ***black arrow*** **vidian nerve (bordered in** ***yellow*****)**

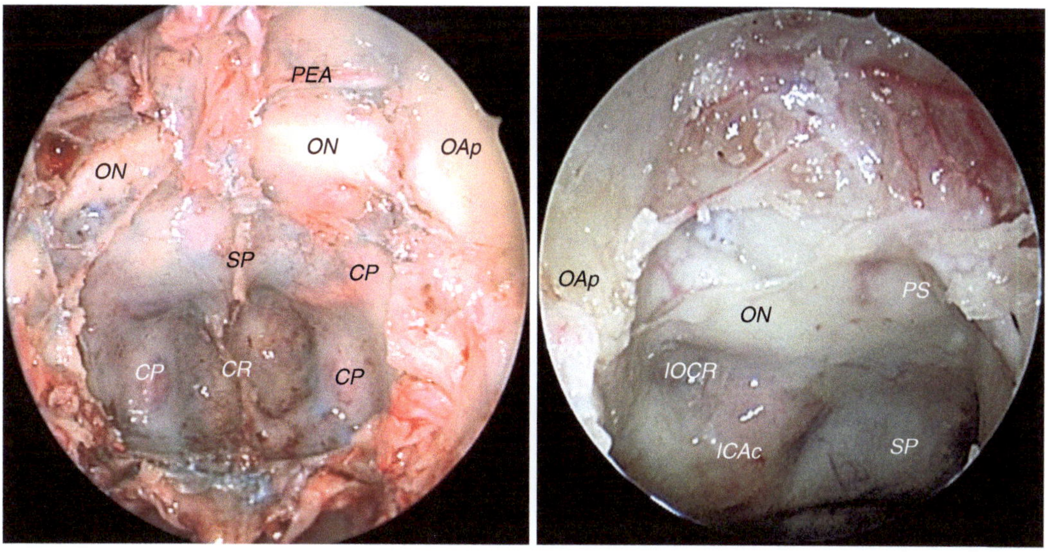

Fig. 3.17 Sphenoidal endoscopic views

CP **carotid prominence,** ***CR*** **clival recess,** ***ICAc*** **cavernous portion of the internal carotid artery,** ***lOCR*** **lateral opticocarotid recess,** ***OAp*** **orbital apex,** ***ON*** **optic nerve,** ***PEA*** **posterior ethmoidal artery,** ***PS*** **planum sphenoidale,** ***SP*** **sellar prominence**

The lOCR corresponds to the pneumatisation of the optic strut. The clinoid segment of the ICA sits against the posterior surface of the optic strut (Yasuda et al. 2005). The endoscopic removal of the bony wall a little bit inferior and lateral to the lOCR exposes the medial aspect of the superior orbital fissure. The middle clinoid process does not corrispond to the medial optico-carotid recess. The MCP is located at the roof of the cavernous sinus, and it indicates the transition between the ICAc and the paraclinoidal ICA. It has no relationship with the optic nerve.

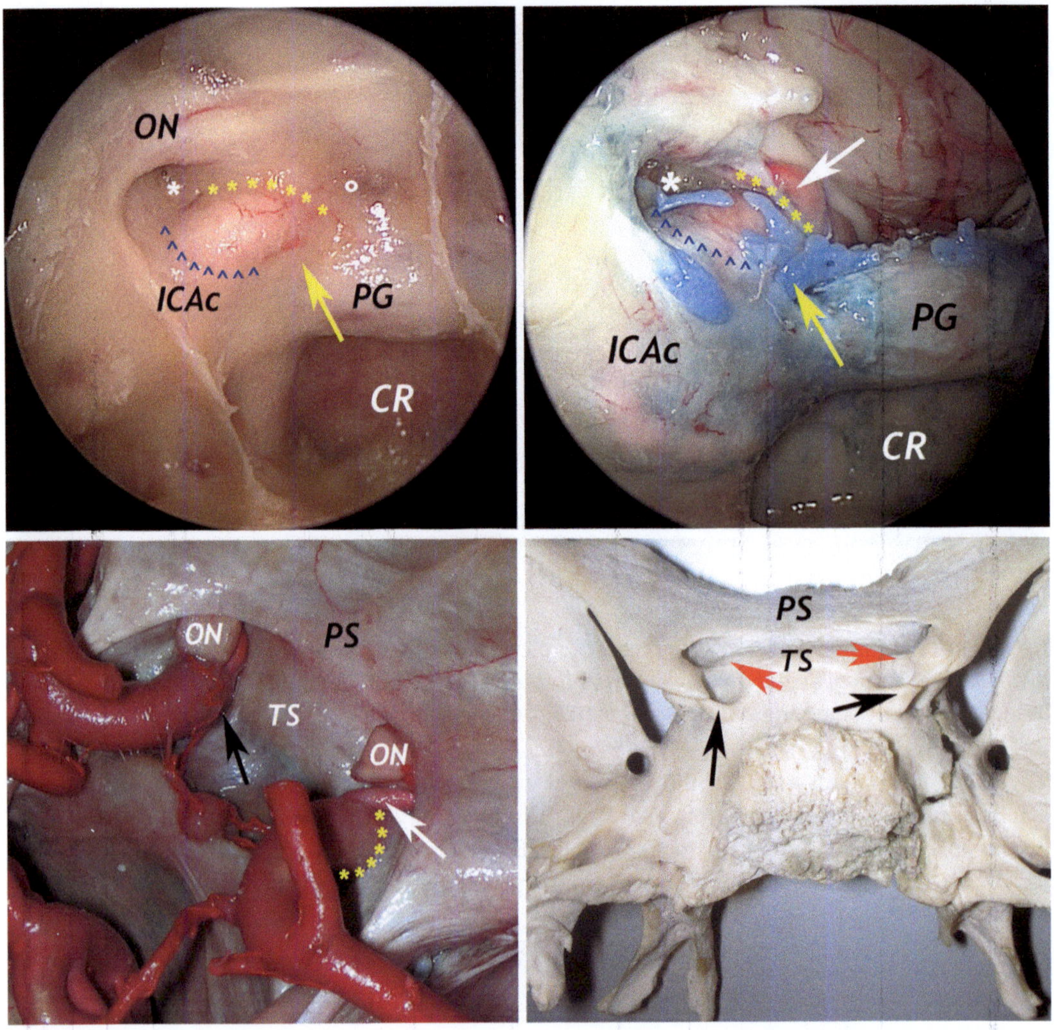

Fig. 3.18 Endoscopic and external views showing the position and relationship of the middle clinoid process and medial optico-carotid recess

Cl **clivus,** ***ICAc*** **cavernous portion of the internal carotid artery,** ***ON*** **optic nerve,** ***PG*** **pituitary gland,** ***PS*** **planum sphenoidale,** ***TS*** **tuberculum sellae,** ***yellow asterisks*** **upper dural ring,** ***blue arrowheads*** **lower dural ring,** ***white asterisk*** **lateral optico-carotid recess,** ***white circle*** **medial optico-carotid recess,** ***white arrow*** **ophthalmic artery,** ***black arrows*** **middle clinoid process,** ***red arrows*** **lateral tubercular crest,** ***yellow arrows*** **endocranial region corresponding to MCP**

The base of the MCP is just medial to the anterior genu of the parasellar ICA. The MCP is present in about half of the cases. And it is located on the medial side of the carotid sulcus at the anterior third of the lateral wall of the sella turcica. At the level of the most lateral part of the tuberculum sellae a small crest can be visualized. The lOCR corresponds to the ventral surface of the optic strut. The superior surface of lOCR is given by the floor of the optic canal. The mOCR is located just medial to the paraclinoidal-supraclinoidal ICA transition and inferior to the distal cisternal segment of the ON (Labib et al. 2013). The dura lining the inferior aspect of the anterior clinoid process forms the lower dural ring. This ring is often incomplete on the medial side and often a venous channel can follow the paraclinoidal ICA to the upper dural ring.

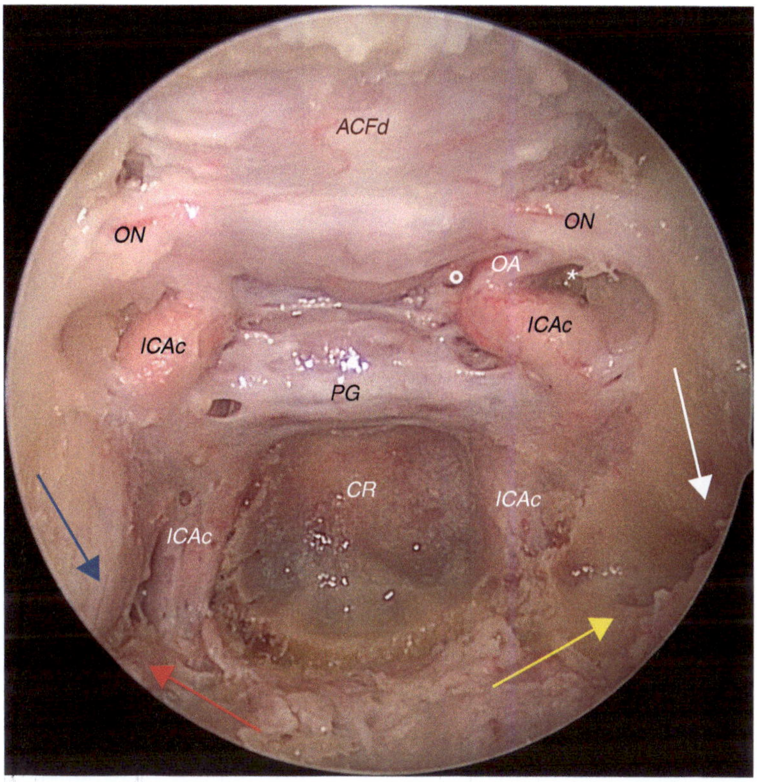

Fig. 3.19 Sphenoidal window

ACFd **anterior cranial fossa dura,** ***CR*** **clival recess,** ***ICAc*** **cavernous portion of the internal carotid artery,** ***OA*** **ophthalmic artery,** ***ON*** **optic nerve,** ***PG*** **pituitary gland,** ***red arrow*** **vidian nerve,** ***blue arrow*** **second branch of the trigeminal nerve,** ***white arrow*** **maxillary prominence,** ***yellow arrow*** **vidian prominence,** ***white asterisk*** **lateral opticocarotid recess,** ***white circle*** **medial opticocarotid recess**

The mOCR is placed at the confluence of the sella, tuberculum sellae, carotid protuberance, optic canal and planum sphenoidale. The mOCR corresponds to the lateral extent of the tuberculum sellae.

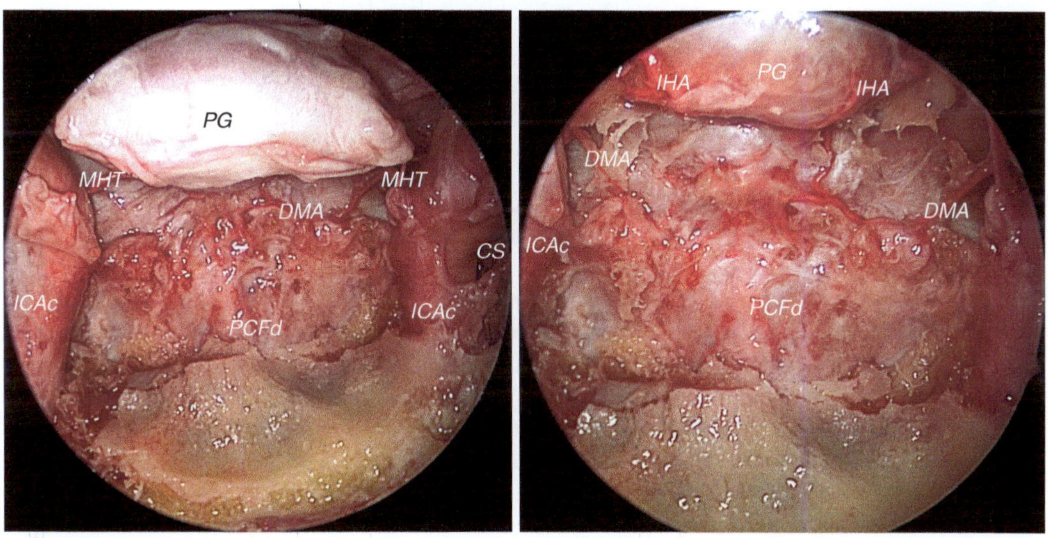

Fig. 3.20 Clival region. The vascularisation of the pituitary gland related to the inferior hypophyseal arteries is clearly visible

CS **cavernous sinus,** ***DMA*** **dorsal meningeal artery,** ***ICAc*** **cavernous portion of the internal carotid artery,** ***IHA*** **inferior hypophyseal artery,** ***MHT*** **meningohypophyseal trunk,** ***PCFd*** **dura and periosteum of the posterior cranial fossa,** ***PG*** **pituitary gland**

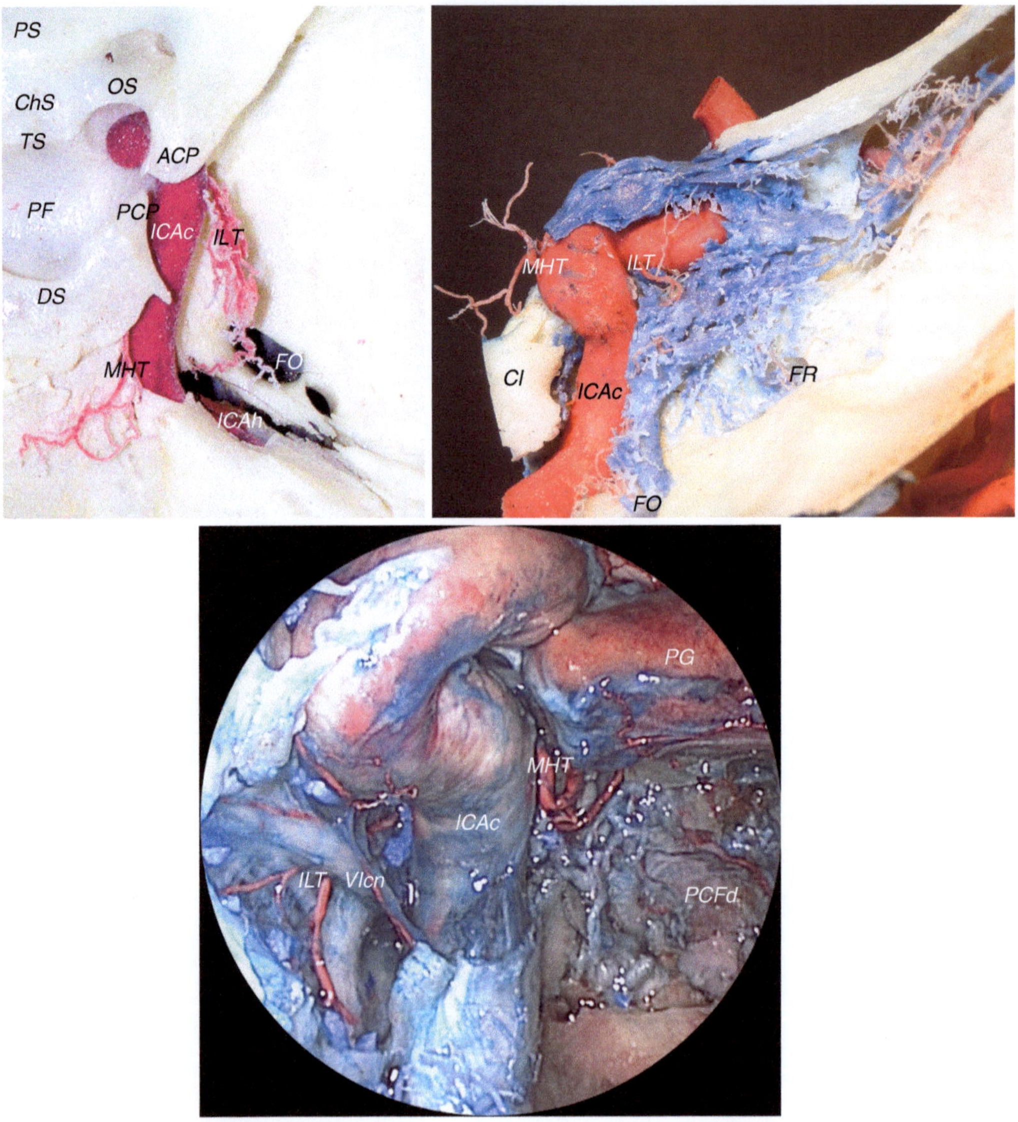

Fig. 3.21 Branches of the cavernous ICA

ACP **anterior clinoid process,** ***ChS*** **chiasmatic sulcus,** ***Cl*** **clivus,** ***DS*** **dorsum sellae,** ***FO*** **foramen ovale,** ***FR*** **foramen rotundum,** ***ICAc*** **cavernous portion of the internal carotid artery,** ***ICAh*** **horizontal portion of the internal carotid artery,** ***ILT*** **inferolateral trunk,** ***MHT*** **meningohypophyseal trunk,** ***OS*** **optic strut,** ***PCFd*** **dura and periosteum of the posterior cranial fossa,** ***PF*** **pituitary fossa,** ***PG*** **pituitary gland,** ***PS*** **planum sphenoidale,** ***TS*** **tuberculum sellae,** ***VIcn*** **abducens nerve**

The most important branches of the cavernous carotid artery are the meningohypophyseal trunk and the inferolateral trunk. When present, capsular arteries arise from the medial wall of the ICAc (horizontal segment), run anteromedially to the hypophyseal capsule, and pass through the medial wall of the CS to join the inferior hypophyseal arteries on the floor of the PF. McConnell's artery has been described in about one-third to one-half of the CS (Rhoton 2002).

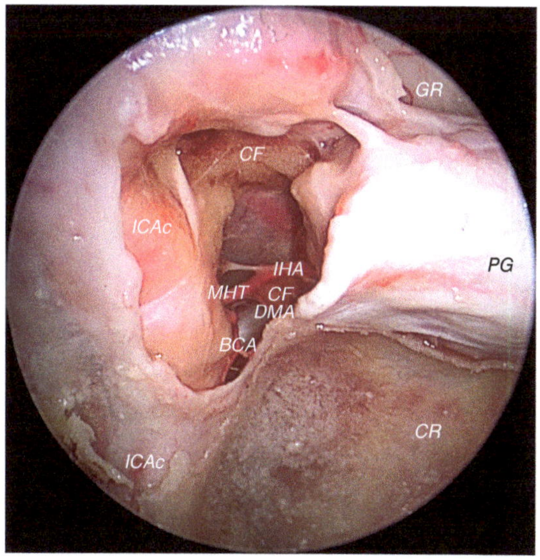

Fig. 3.22
Meningohypophyseal trunk

BCA **Bernasconi-Cassinari artery,** ***CF*** **cavernous fat,** ***CR*** **clival recess,** ***DMA*** **dorsal meningeal artery,** ***GR*** **gyrus rectus,** ***ICAc*** **cavernous portion of the internal carotid artery,** ***IHA*** **inferior hypophyseal artery,** ***MHT*** **meningohypophyseal trunk,** ***PG*** **pituitary gland**

By opening the dura of the medial wall of the cavernous sinus, the space between the internal carotid artery and the PG is exposed. In this space, the MHT is usually evident.

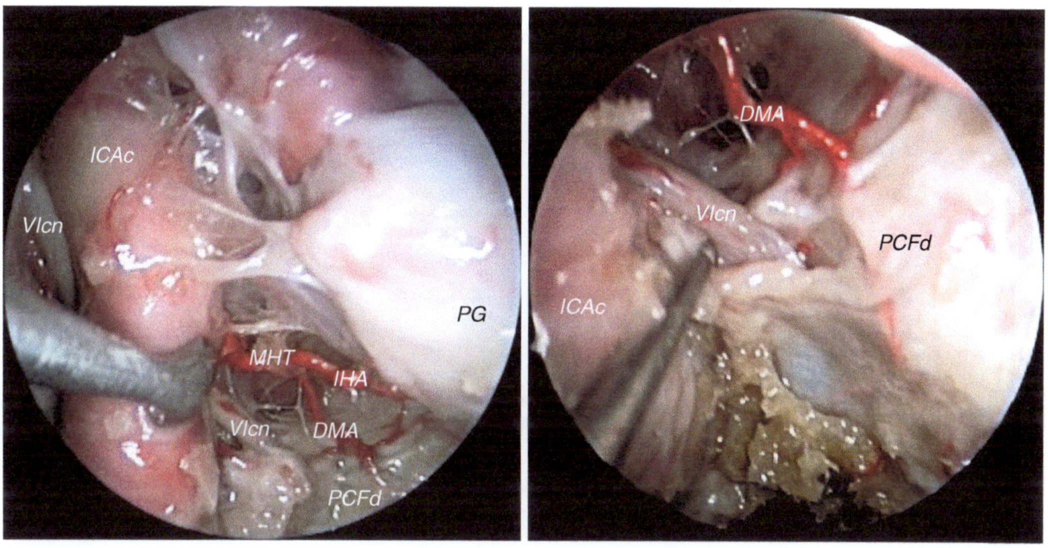

Fig. 3.23 Meningohypophyseal trunk and detail on dorsal meningeal artery

DMA **dorsal meningeal artery,** ***ICAc*** **cavernous portion of internal carotid artery,** ***IHA*** **inferior hypophyseal artery,** ***MHT*** **meningohypophyseal trunk,** ***PCFd*** **dura and periosteum of the posterior cranial fossa,** ***PG*** **pituitary gland,** ***VIcn*** **abducens nerve**

The MHT is traditionally described as having three branches: the inferior hypophyseal artery, the dorsal meningeal artery (also called the dorsal clival artery), and the tentorial artery (also called the Bernasconi-Cassinari artery). The DMA is in close relationship with the abducens nerve at the level of petrous apex (Cavallo et al. 2011). The DMA is the main feeder of the Dorello's segment of VIcn (Martins et al. 2011).

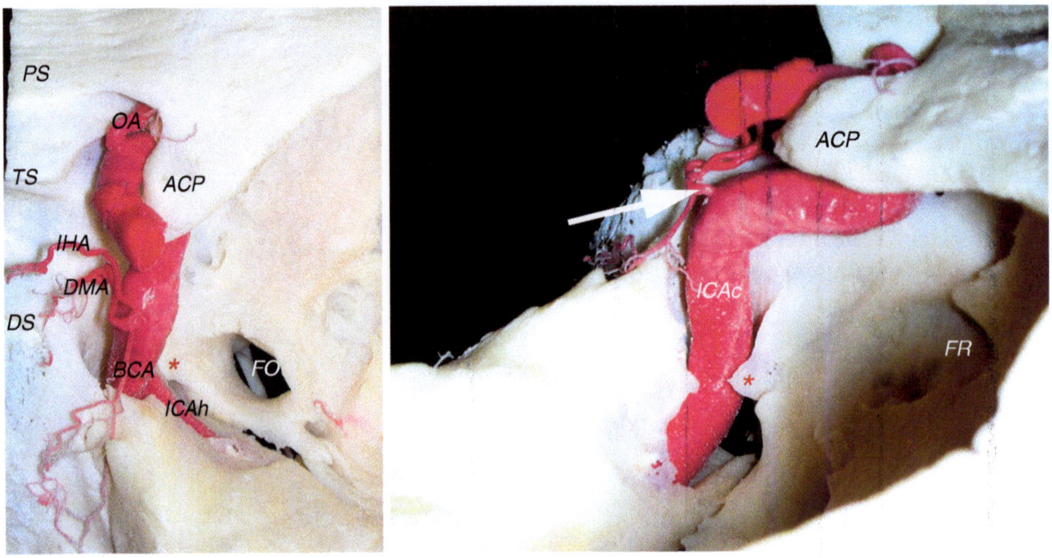

Fig. 3.24 Meningohypophyseal trunk

ACP **anterior clinoid process,** ***BCA*** **Bernasconi-Cassinari artery,** ***DMA*** **dorsal meningeal artery,** ***DS*** **dorsum sellae,** ***FO*** **foramen ovale,** ***FR*** **foramen rotundum,** ***ICAc*** **cavernous portion of the internal carotid artery,** ***ICAh*** **horizontal portion of the internal carotid artery,** ***IHA*** **inferior hypophyseal artery,** ***MHT*** **meningohypophyseal trunk,** ***OA*** **ophthalmic artery,** ***PS*** **planum sphenoiodale,** ***TS*** **tuberculum sellae,** ***white arrow*** **MHT,** ***red asterisk*** **lingula of the sphenoid**

The MHT is present in most cases. Not in all cases does it give off all the typical braches: dorsal meningeal artery (or dorsal clival artery), tentorial artery (or Bernasconi-Cassinari artery), and the inferior hypophyseal arteries. In about half of the cases, some branches arise directly from the ICAc (Jittapiromsak et al. 2010). The tentorial artery is the main feeder of the oculomotor nerve (d'Avella et al. 2008), and usually it is located on the inferior surface of the nerve. Moreover, it can be the feeder of the distal part of the trochlear nerve; in these cases, the vessel runs in close proximity of this nerve to the superior orbital fissure. Other authors show that BCA feeds cranial nerve IV along its course within the tentorium cerebelli (Martins et al. 2011).

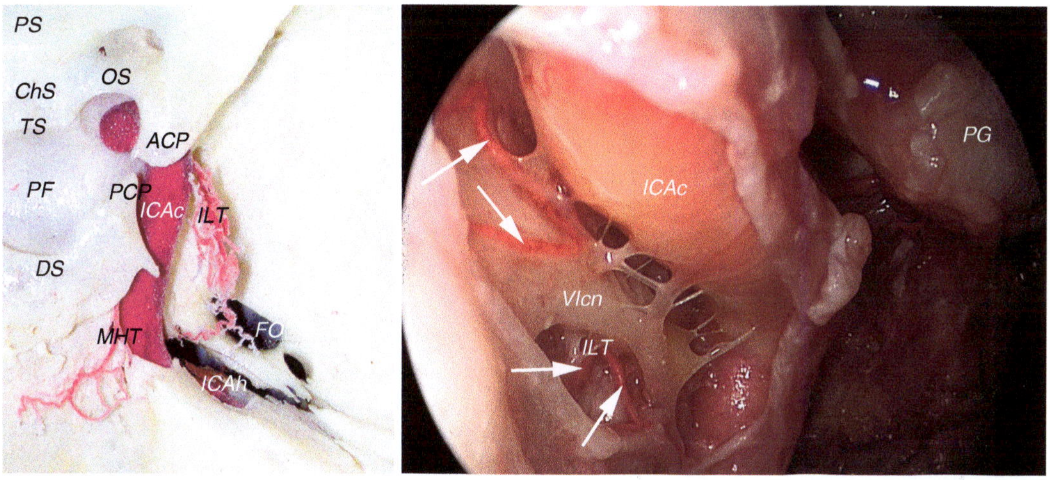

Fig. 3.25 Inferolateral trunk

***ACP* anterior clinoid process, *ChS* chiasmatic sulcus, *DS* dorsum sellae, *FO* foramen ovale, *ICAc* cavernous portion of the internal carotid artery, *ICAh* horizontal portion of the internal carotid artery, *ILT* inferolateral trunk, *MHT* meningohypophyseal trunk, *OS* optic strut, *PCP* posterior clinoid process, *PF* pituitary fossa, *PG* pituitary gland, *TS* tuberculum sellae, *VIcn* abducens nerve, *white arrows* branches of the ILT**

The ILT is present in most cases (Krisht et al. 1994; Tran-Dinh 1987). It may arise as a common trunk with the MHT (Reisch et al. 2002). It is a single trunk in most cases. More often, it arises from the lateral aspect of the horizontal segment of the ICAc, and in most cases it passes superiorly to the abducens nerve (Inoue et al. 1990; Jittapiromsak et al. 2010). It usually gives rise to 3 or 4 branches supplying the dura and the cranial nerves within the cavernous sinus (Lasjaunias et al. 1977; Tran-Dinh 1987). The main trunk of the ILT with small secondary branches is the feeder of the ophthalmic nerve (V1). Usually, these vessels reach the inferior surface of the nerve. Obviously, the ILT also supplies the abducens nerve with several small branches.

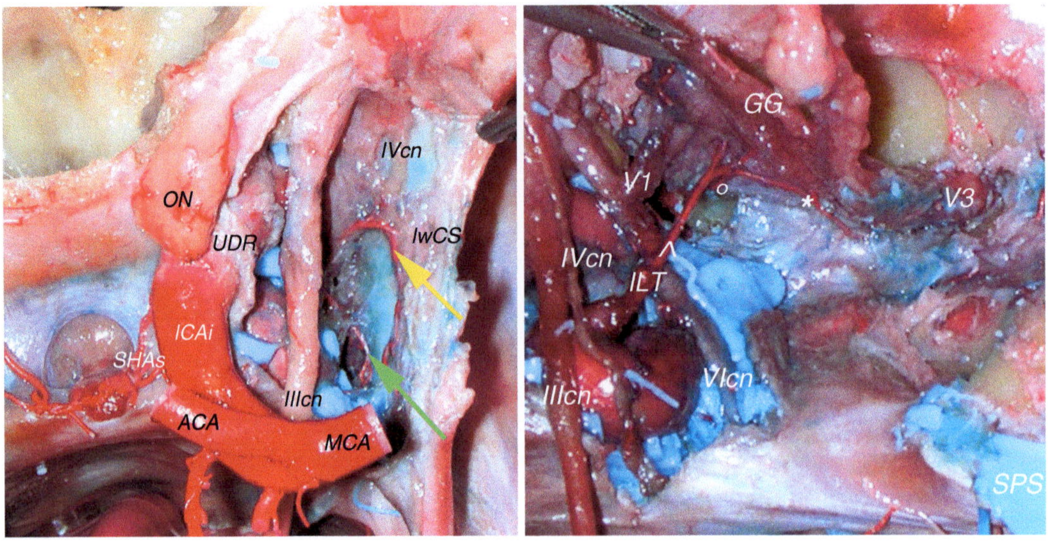

Fig. 3.26 Branches of the inferolateral trunk. In the right picture the gasserian ganglion has been lifted up

ACA **anterior cerebral artery,** ***GG*** **gasserian ganglion,** ***ICAi*** **intracranial portion of the internal carotid artery,** ***ILT*** **inferolateral trunk,** ***lwCS*** **lateral wall of the cavernous sinus,** ***MCA*** **middle cerebral artery,** ***ON*** **optic nerve,** ***SHAs*** **superior hypophyseal arteries,** ***SPS*** **superior petrosal sinus,** ***UDR*** **upper dural ring,** ***IIIcn*** **oculomotor nerve,** ***IVcn*** **trochlear nerve,** ***V1*** **first branch of the trigeminal nerve,** ***V3*** **third branch of the trigeminal nerve,** ***VIcn*** **abducens nerve,** ***yellow arrow*** **superoproximal artery (branch of the ILT),** ***green arrow*** **indicates a tentorial branch of the ILT,** ***white arrowhead*** **artery of the superior orbital fissure,** ***white circle*** **artery for the foramen rotundum,** ***white asterisk*** **artery for the foramen ovale**

The superoproximal artery usually curves superiorly and posteriorly, reaching the IVcn on the lateral wall of the cavernous sinus (*CS*) and goes to the free edge of the tentorium cerebelli (Conti et al. 2008). It is the main feeder of the proximal part of the nerve (d'Avella et al. 2008), but it can also be a supplier of the proximal part of IIIcn and V1 (Conti et al. 2008). Another constant branch is the superior orbital fissure (*SOF*) artery, which runs between V1 and V2 and usually splits in two branches: one for the foramen rotundum and the other for the foramen ovale (Conti et al. 2008). As a whole, the SOF artery can be considered the most important vessel for the blood supply to the distal portion of cranial nerves III, IV, VI, and V1 (Willinsky et al. 1987; Krisht et al. 1994; Tekdemir et al. 1998).

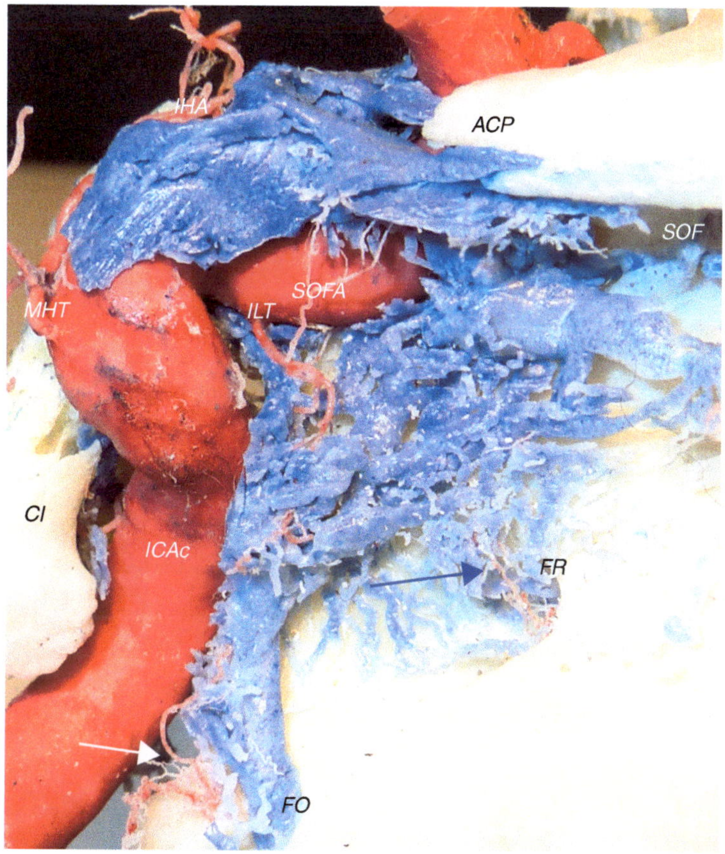

Fig. 3.27 Branches of the inferolateral trunk

ACP **anterior clinoid process,** ***Cl*** **clivus,** ***FO*** **foramen ovale,** ***FR*** **foramen rotundum,** ***ICAc*** **cavernous portion of the internal carotid artery,** ***IHA*** **inferior hypophyseal artery,** ***ILT*** **inferolateral trunk,** ***MHT*** **meningohypophyseal trunk,** ***SOF*** **superior orbital fissure,** ***SOFA*** **superior orbital fissure artery,** ***white arrow*** **artery for the foramen ovale,** ***blue arrow*** **artery for the foramen rotundum**

Obviously, the arborisation for the floor of the middle cranial fossa can be variable, and the arteries for the foramen rotundum and ovale can be given by the main trunk of the ILT. Typically, branches of the ILT anastomose with branches of the middle meningeal artery and accessory middle meningeal artery. It is also possible that tentorial branches arise from the ILT. In this case, their role in feeding neural structures is really critical.

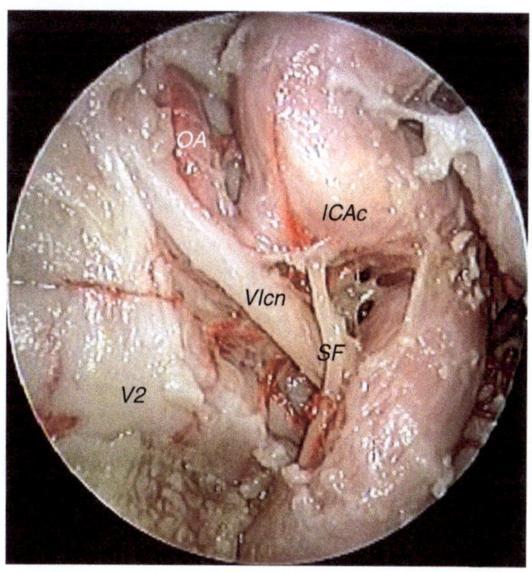

Fig. 3.28 Branches of the cavernous internal carotid artery (*ICA*), a rare variation: ophthalmic artery passing through the superior orbital fissure

ICAc **cavernous portion of the internal carotid artery,** ***OA*** **ophthalmic artery,** ***SF*** **sympathetic fiber,** ***V2*** **second branch of the maxillary nerve,** ***VIcn*** **abducens nerve**

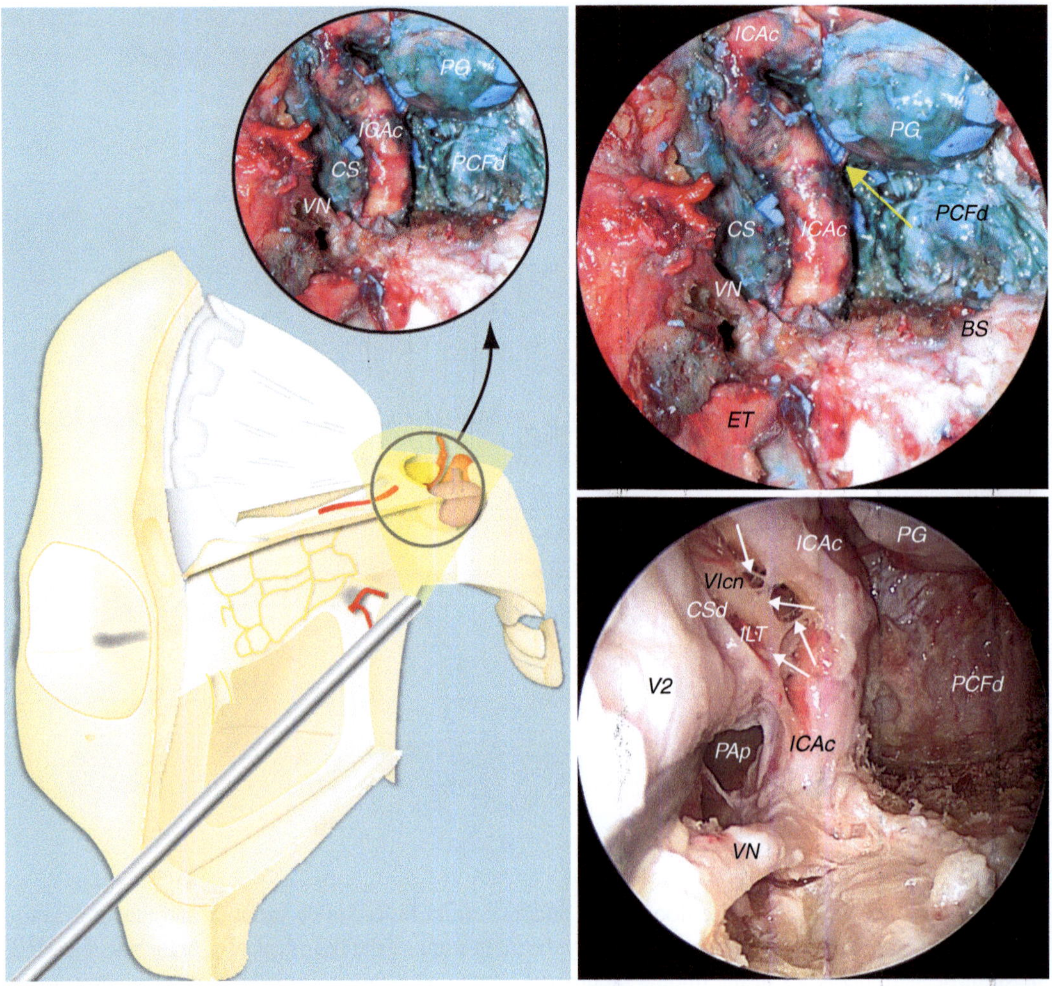

Fig. 3.29 Cavernous window

BS **basisphenoid,** ***CS*** **cavernous sinus,** ***CSd*** **dura of the cavernous sinus,** ***ET*** **eustachian tube,** ***ICAc*** **cavernous portion of the internal carotid artery,** ***ILT*** **inferolateral trunk,** ***PAp*** **petrous apex,** ***PCFd*** **dura and periosteum of the posterior cranial fossa,** ***PG*** **pituitary gland,** ***VN*** **vidian nerve,** ***V2*** **second branch of the trigeminal nerve,** ***VIcn*** **abducens nerve,** ***yellow arrow*** **meningohypophyseal trunk,** ***white arrows*** **sympathetic fibres**

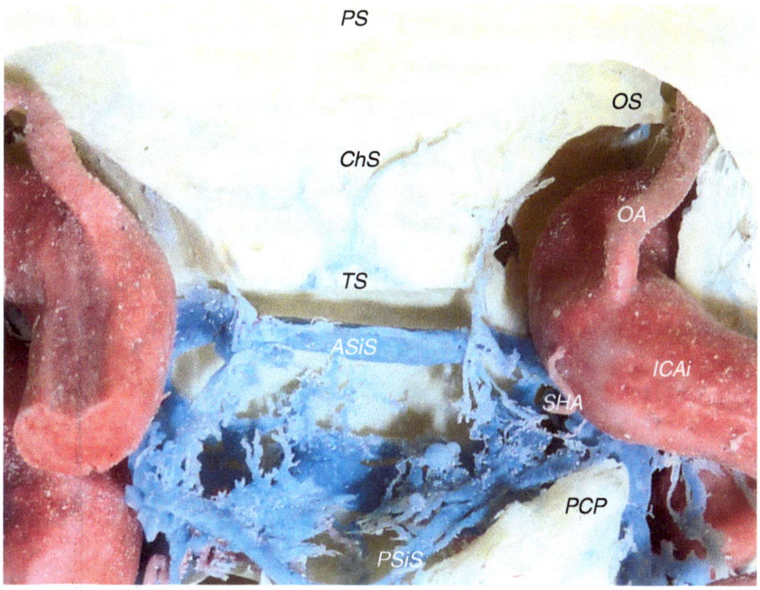

Fig. 3.30
Sellar region

ASiS **anterior superior intercavernous sinus** ***ChS*** **chiasmatic sulcus,** ***ICAi*** **intracranial portion of the internal carotid artery,** ***OA*** **ophthalmic artery,** ***OS*** **optic strut,** ***PCP*** **posterior clinoid process,** ***PSiS*** **posterior superior intercavernous sinus,** ***PS*** **planum sphenoidale,** ***SHA*** **superior hypophyseal artery,** ***TS*** **tuberculum sellae**

The cavernous sinuses are connected to each other via the anterior superior and posterior superior intercavernous sinuses. Together, they are called the circular sinus (Janfaza and Nadol 2001). The superior hypophyseal artery usually arises from the intracranial portion of the internal carotid artery. It supplies the optic chiasm and infundibular region of the hypothalamus. The inferior hypophyseal artery supplies the posterior lobe of the pituitary gland. The OA has been described as having an origin in one-half of the cases above the distal dural ring, in one-third of the cases at the level of the distal dural ring, and in less than 20 % of cases in the paraclinoid area (Lang 1995).

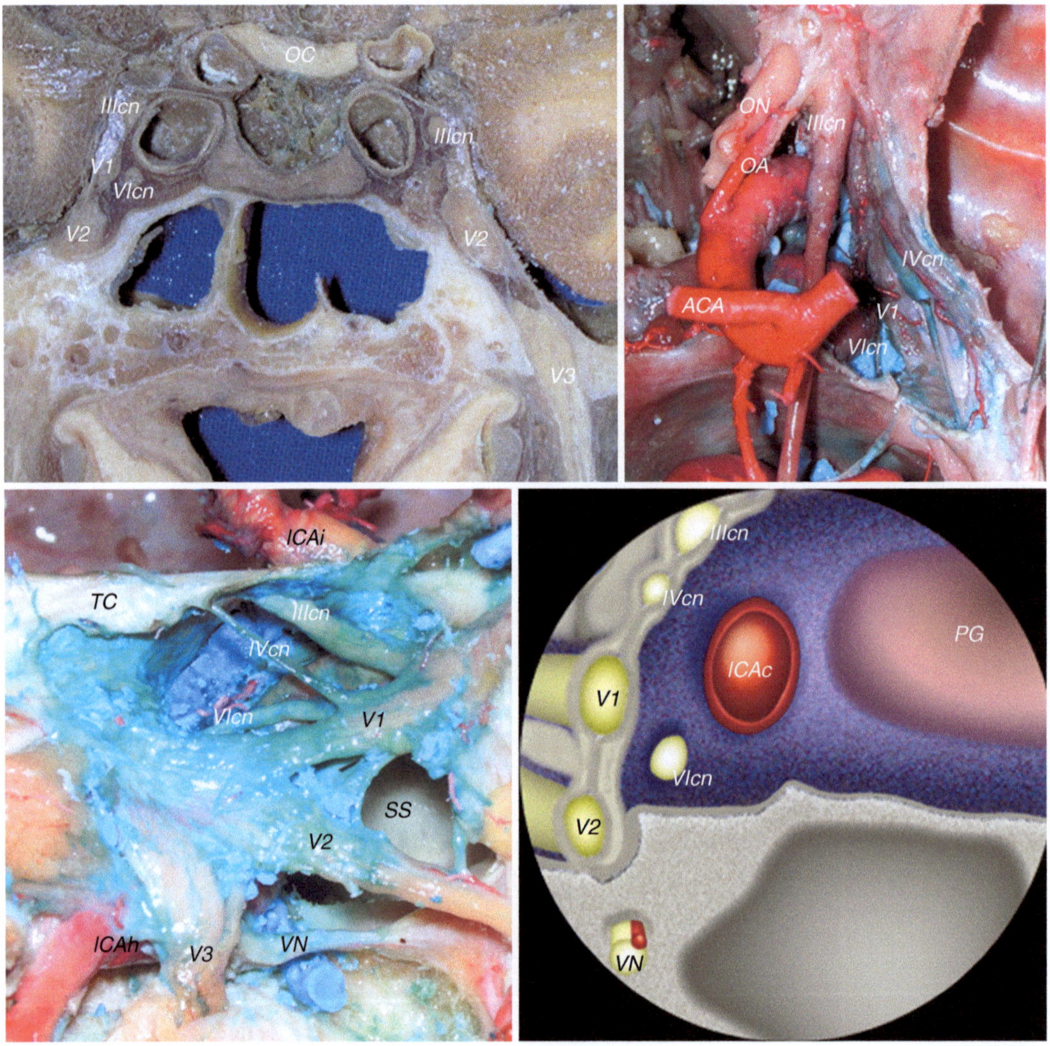

Fig. 3.31 Cavernous sinus

***ACA* anterior cerebral artery, *ICAc* cavernous portion of the internal carotid artery, *ICAh* horizontal portion of the internal carotid artery, *ICAi* intracranial portion of the internal carotid artery, *OA* ophthalmic artery, *OC* optic chiasm, *ON* optic nerve, *PG* pituitary gland, *SS* sphenoid sinus, *TC* tentorium cerebelli, *VN* vidian nerve, *V1* first branch of the trigeminal nerve, *V2* second branch of the trigeminal nerve, *V3* third branch of the trigeminal nerve, *IIIcn* oculomotor nerve, *IVcn* trochlear nerve, *VIcn* abducens nerve**

The CSs are large venous spaces located on both sides of the body of the sphenoid. Probably, the term is too restrictive, neglecting the neural and soft tissue elements. A valuable and rational name is lateral sellar compartment (Parkinson 1990). For the venous compartment, three spaces can be identified: posterosuperior, medial, and inferomedial (Reisch et al. 2002).

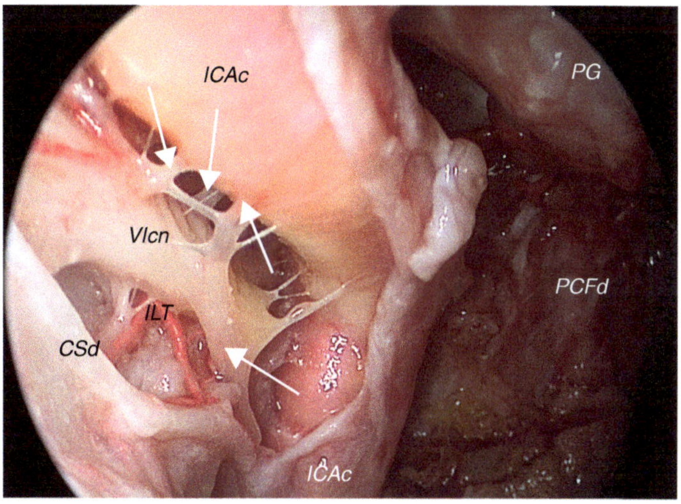

Fig. 3.32
Cavernous sinus

CSd **dura of the cavernous sinus,** ***ICAc*** **cavernous portion of the internal carotid artery,** ***ILT*** **inferolateral trunk,** ***PCFd*** **dura and periosteum of the posterior cranial fossa,** ***PG*** **pituitary gland,** ***VIcn*** **abducens nerve,** ***white arrows*** **sympathetic fibres**

Within the CS, the sympathetic fibres are observed mainly in the anterior part of the artery, and usually they are placed inferiorly. Most of these fibres run together with V1 (Jittapiromsak et al. 2010). The sympathetic fibres diverge from the ICAc to adhere to the abducens nerve while crossing to join the ophthalmic nerve (V1). The main target exit is V1 on the lateral wall of the CS (Jittapiromsak et al. 2010). Within the CS, the abducens nerve typically courses medially to the V1 before it exits through the superior orbital fissure.

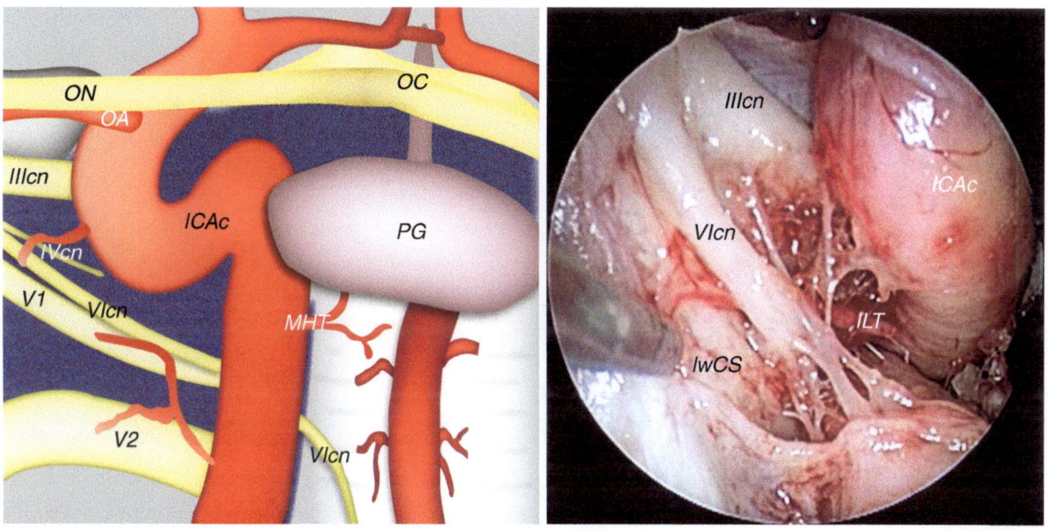

Fig. 3.33 Cavernous sinus: 3D reconstruction and endoscopic endonasal view focusing on the lateral wall

ICAc **cavernous portion of the internal carotid artery,** ***ILT*** **inferolateral trunk,** ***lwCS*** **lateral wall of the cavernous sinus,** ***MHT*** **meningohypophyseal trunk,** ***OA*** **ophthalmic artery,** ***OC*** **optic chiasm,** ***ON*** **optic nerve,** ***PG*** **pituitary gland,** ***IIIcn*** **oculomotor nerve,** ***IVcn*** **trochlear nerve,** ***VIcn*** **abducens nerve,** ***V1*** **first branch of the trigeminal nerve,** ***V2*** **second branch of the trigeminal nerve**

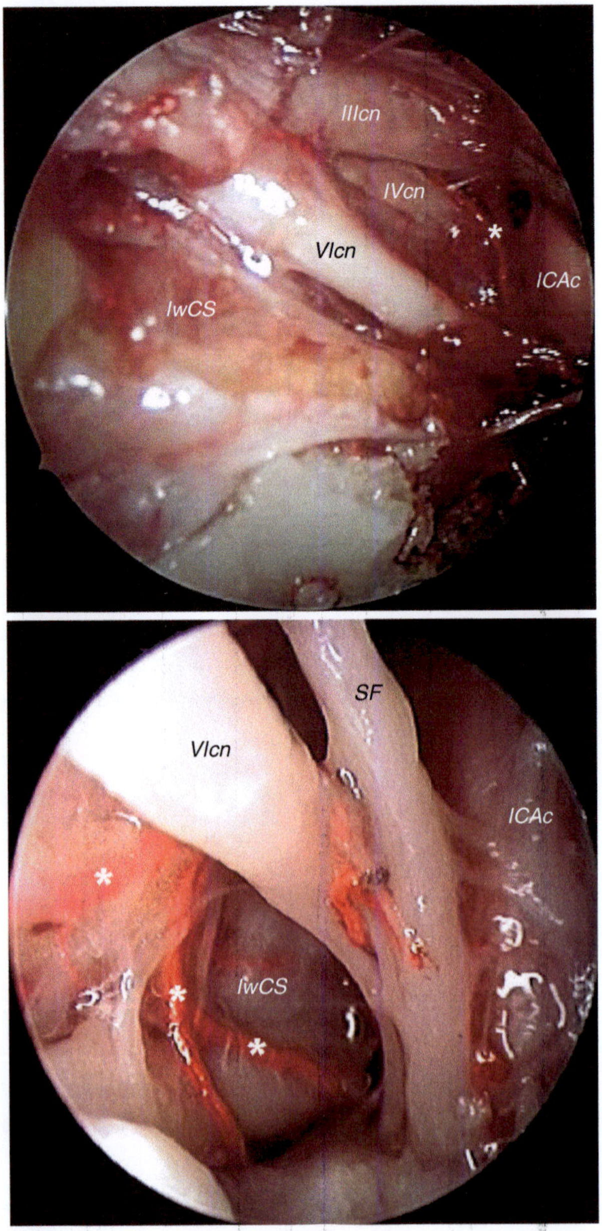

Fig. 3.34 Cavernous sinus with focus on the lateral wall

ICAc **cavernous portion of the internal carotid artery,** ***lwCS*** **lateral wall of the CS,** ***SF*** **sympathetic fiber,** ***IIIcn*** **oculomotor nerve,** ***IVcn*** **trochlear nerve,** ***VIcn*** **abducens nerve,** ***white asterisks*** **branches of the inferolateral trunk**

The largest sympathetic fiber runs close (within 8 mm) to the ILT, posteroinferiorly and medially located to it (Zhang et al. 2012).

After crossing the superior petrosal sinus the trochlear nerve can pierce the roof of the cavernous sinus and runs through its lateral wall. The trochlear nerve, within the cavernous sinus, passes upward the oculomotor nerve (more or less at the level of the optic strut) and becomes the most superior structure of the CS (Iaconetta et al. 2012). Within the CS course the trochlear nerve is surrounded by an arachnoidal sheath (Lang 1995) and it is always superior to V1.

Fig. 3.35 Relationship between the ophthalmic artery and the optic nerve

CBs **chiasmatic branches,** ***Cl*** **clivus,** ***ICAc*** **cavernous portion of the internal carotid artery,** ***IRM*** **inferior rectus muscle,** ***IRMb*** **branch for inferior rectus muscle,** ***MRM*** **medial rectus muscle,** ***OA*** **ophthalmic artery,** ***ON*** **optic nerve,** ***PEA*** **posterior ethmoidal artery,** ***PG*** **pituitary gland,** ***SHA*** **superior hypophyseal artery,** ***SS*** **sphenoid sinus,** ***IIIcn*** **oculomotor nerve**

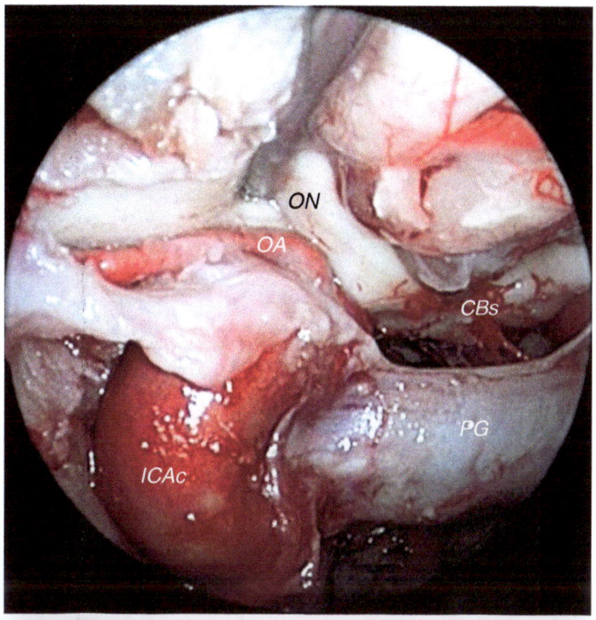

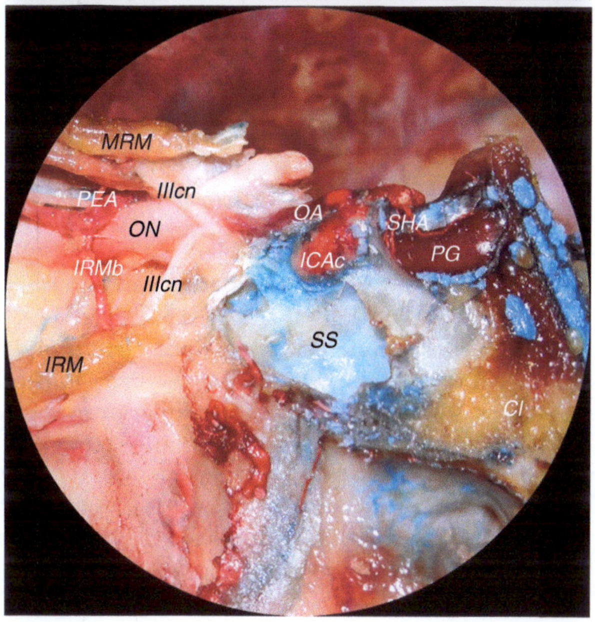

The ophthalmic artery usually arises from the ICAi and accompanies the optic nerve through the optic canal. At this level, the OA may offer small dural branches (Reisch et al. 2002) that may supply the lateral dural structure of the paraclinoid segment. The oculomotor nerve divides into a small superior and large inferior division just before passing through the superior orbital fissure.

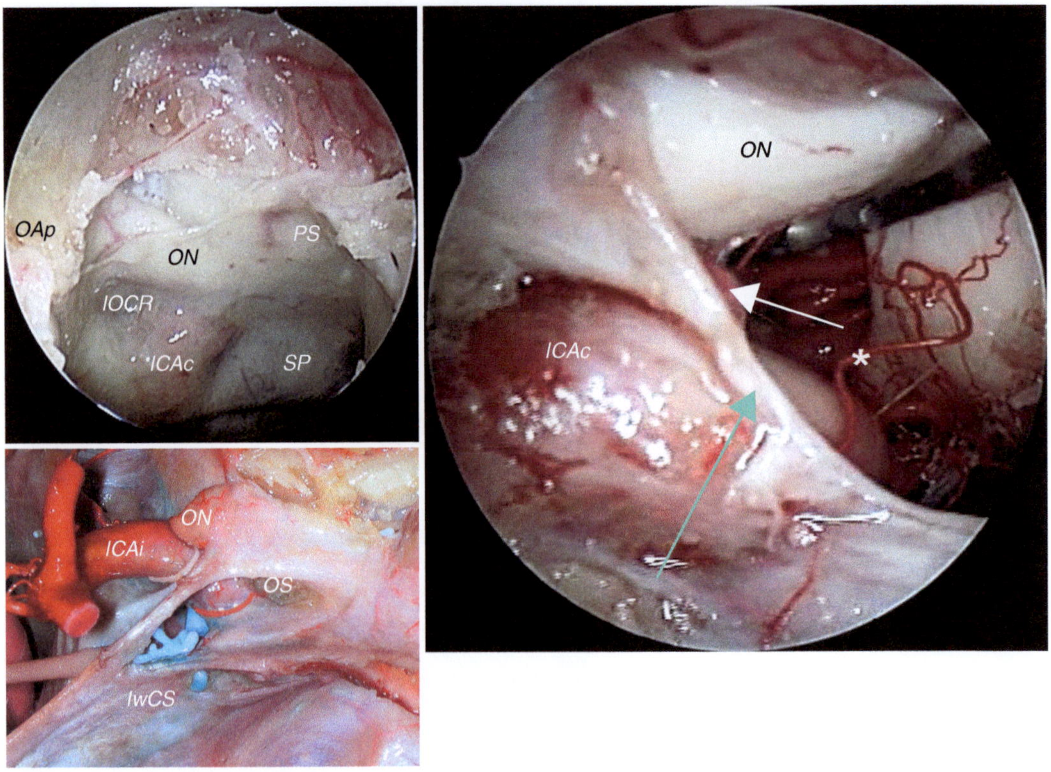

Fig. 3.36 Relationship between the ophthalmic artery and the optic nerve, position and role of the optic strut

***ICAc* cavernous portion of the internal carotid artery, *ICAi* intracranial portion of the internal carotid artery, *lOCR* lateral opticocarotid recess, *lwCS* lateral wall of the cavernous sinus, *OAp* orbital apex, *ON* optic nerve, *OS* optic strut, *PS* planum sphenoidale, *SP* sellar prominence, *white arrow* ophthalmic artery, *blue-sky arrow* upper dural ring, *red line* lower dural ring, *white line* upper dural ring, *white asterisk* superior hypophyseal artery**

Note that the clinoid segment of the ICA is against the optic strut. The lOCR corresponds to the pneumatisation of the optic strut. This structure faces the optic nerve superiorly, the superior orbital fissure inferolaterally, and the clinoid portion of the ICA posteriorly. Within the optic canal, the ON is covered by pia, arachnoid, and dura. Thus, above the lOCR the optic nerve and the ophthalmic artery are surrounded by the dura. The superior and inferior border of the lOCR identify the position of the upper and lower dural rings (Martins et al. 2011). The OA usually passes superiorly to the upper dural ring.

The dura lining the upper and lower surface of the ACP extends medially to form the upper and lower dural rings (these define the upper and lower limits of the clinoid segment of ICA). Posteriorly the upper dural ring joins the lower dural ring to form the apex of the clinoidal triangle of the roof of the cavernous sinus (Yasuda et al. 2005). The upper dural ring is a competent ring that tightly fuses with the adventitia of the artery.

The middle clinoid process (MCP), when present, is located at the transition between the ICAc and the paraclinoidal ICA (that is the continuation of the anterior genu of the ICAc). The MCP covers the anteromedial portion of the roof of the CS and so the proximal dural ring is located just underneath the MCP. The MCP has no anatomical relationship with the optic nerve (Labib et al. 2013). The anterior clinoid process covers the antero-lateral part of the roof of the CS.

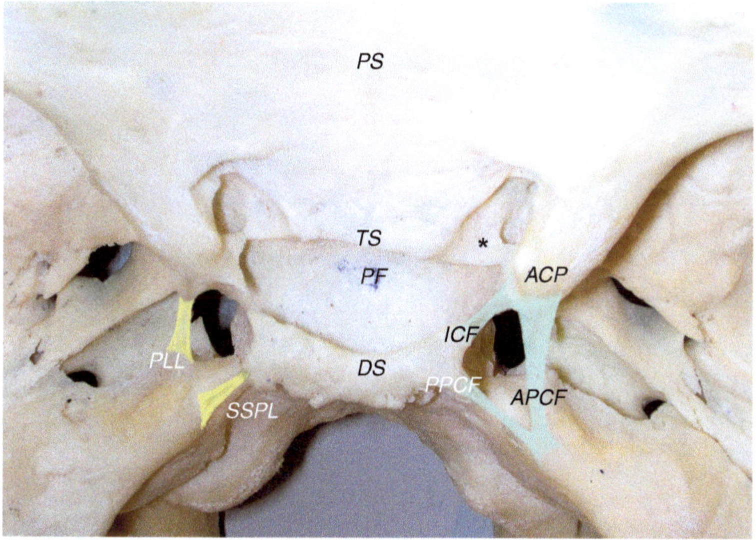

Fig. 3.37 Schematic drawing of folds and ligaments around the sellar region

***ACP* anterior clinoid process, *APCF* anterior petroclinoid fold, *DS* dorsum sellae, *ICF* interclinoid fold, *PF* pituitary fossa, *PLL* petrolingual ligament (inferior sphenopetrosal ligament), *PPCF* posterior petroclinoid fold, *PS* planum sphenoidale, *SSPL* superior sphenopetrosal ligament (Gruber's ligament), *TS* tuberculum sellae, *black asterisk* middle clinoid process**

The dura forming the roof of the cavernous sinus (*CS*) can be divided in two triangles: the clinoid (anterior) and the oculomotor (posterior). The threefolds delineate the oculomotor triangle. The clinoid triangle is placed below the anterior clinoid process. The lateral wall of the cavernous sinus blends into the dura covering Meckel's cave (Yasuda et al. 2005). In the lateral wall, two easily recognizable layers are evident: the meningeal and the endosteal. The meningeal faces the brain and superiorly forms the diaphragma sellae, while the endosteal (outer layer) invests superiorly the nerves in the lateral wall (Yasuda et al. 2005) and inferiorly adheres with the bone. (Martins et al. 2011).

The PLL is between the lingula of the sphenoid and the petrous apex while Gruber's ligament connets the petrous apex and the lower lateral edge of the dorsum sellae. The APCF extends from the petrous apex to ACP, the PPCF extends from the PCP to the petrous apex. The ICF connects the ACP and the PCP (Yasuda et al. 2005). If the Gruber's ligament is ossificated it is called Wegener's bridge.

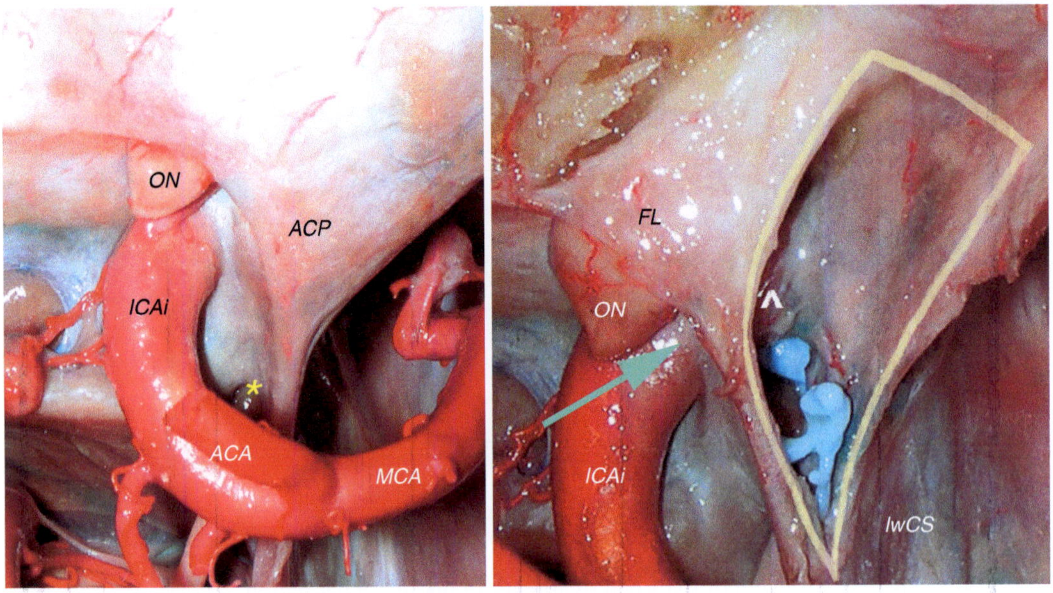

Fig. 3.38 Roof of the cavernous sinus-clinoid triangle

***ACA* anterior cerebral artery, *ACP* anterior clinoid process, *FL* falciform ligament, *ICAi* intracranial portion of the internal carotid artery, *lwCS* lateral wall of the cavernous sinus, *MCA* middle cerebral artery, *ON* optic nerve, *blue-sky arrow* upper dural ring, *white arrowhead* paraclinoid portion of the internal carotid artery, *yellow asterisk* oculomotor nerve entering the roof of the cavernous sinus (*CS*)**

The roof of the CS is located below the level of the ACP (Martins et al. 2011). Cranial nerves III and IV enter the posterior part of the roof of the CS, in strict relationship with the meningohypophyseal trunk, and get the lwCS to enter the superior orbital fissure. Sometimes, cranial nerve IV enters in the tentorium cerebelli (Martins et al. 2011). Cranial nerve III enters the roof included in its own cistern (oculomotor cistern). The dura over the ACP passes over the ON, giving the falciform ligament. Below the ON, the dura surrounds the ICA, forming the upper dural ring, leaving a small posteromedial space called the carotid cave. Not rarely, the superior hypophyseal artery arises in this space.

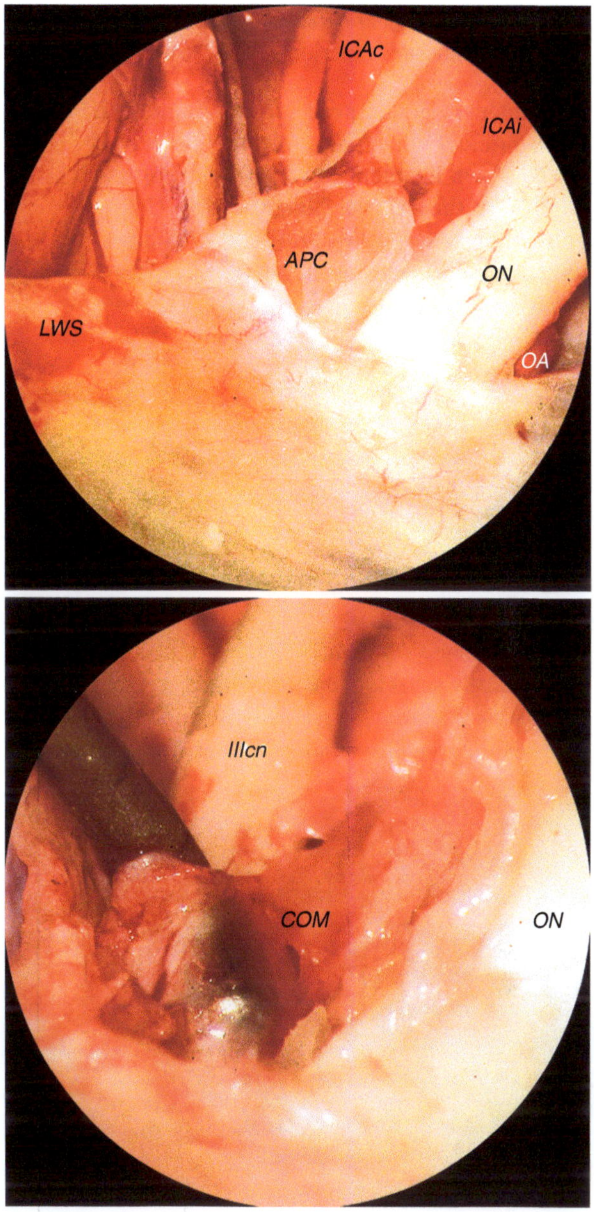

Fig. 3.39 Endoscopic supraorbital view of the anterior clinoid region. The right portion of the planum sphenoidale is seen from above. The anterior clinoid process has been removed. Vision obtained through a right supraorbital approach with a 30° down-facing lens focusing on the cavernous sinus roof

***ACP* anterior clinoid process (removed), *COM* carotid oculomotor membrane, *ICAc* cavernous portion of the internal carotid artery, *ICAi* intracranial portion of the internal carotid artery, *OA* ophthalmic artery, *ON* optic nerve, *LWS* lesser wing of the sphenoid, *IIIcn* oculomotor nerve**

The lower dural ring is given by the COM, that lines the inferior surface of the ACP. It can be visible, through a transcranial route, only by removing the ACP. The lower dural ring is also called Perneczky's ring. Medially the COM blends with the dura that lines the carotid sulcus (Yasuda et al. 2005)

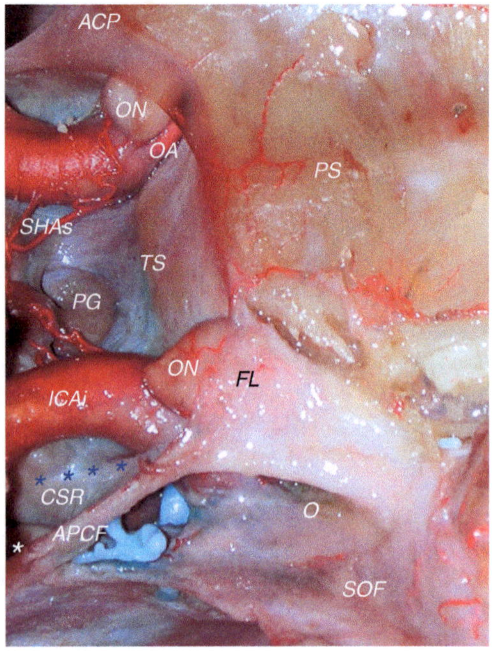

Fig. 3.40 Superolateral vision of the right cavernous sinus and superior orbital fissure

ACP **anterior clinoid process,** ***APCF*** **anterior petroclinoidal fold,** ***CSR*** **cavernous sinus roof,** ***FL*** **falciform ligament,** ***ICAi*** **intracranial segment of the internal carotid artery,** ***OA*** **ophthalmic artery,** ***ON*** **optic nerve,** ***PG*** **pituitary gland,** ***PS*** **planum sphenoidale,** ***SHAs*** **superior hypophyseal arteries,** ***SOF*** **superior orbital fissure,** ***TS*** **tuberculum sellae,** ***white asterisk*** **oculomotor nerve,** ***white circle*** **optic strut area (the optic strut has been removed),** ***blue asterisks*** **interclinoid fold**

Anatomically speaking, the paraclinoid segment of the internal carotid artery is not fully intracavernous, and it is separated from the cavernous sinus by the extension of the dura covering the inferior surface of the anterior clinoid process (Reisch et al. 2002).

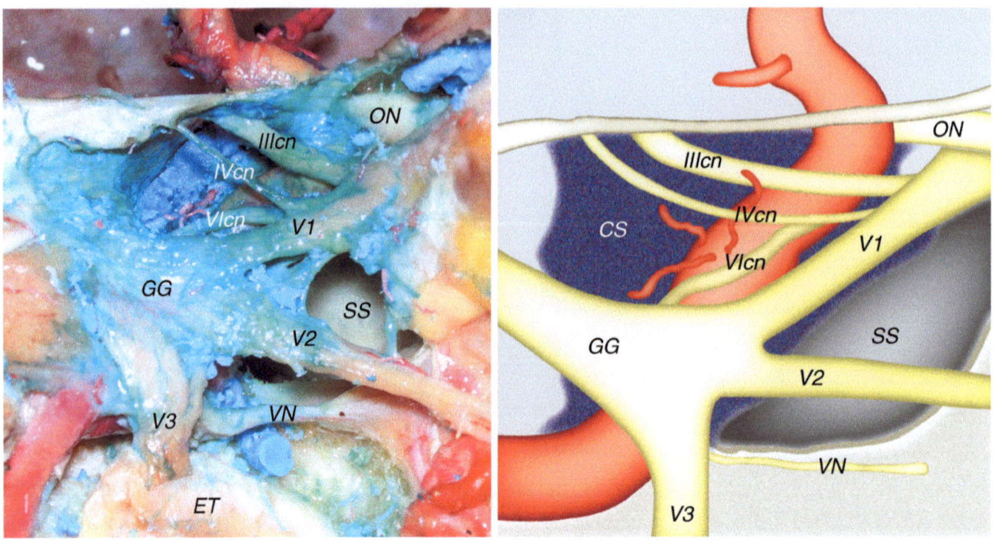

Fig. 3.41 Lateral vision of the right cavernous sinus

CS **cavernous sinus,** ***ET*** **eustachian tube,** ***GG*** **gasserian ganglion,** ***ON*** **optic nerve,** ***SS*** **sphenoid sinus,** ***VN*** **vidian nerve,** ***V1*** **first branch of the trigeminal nerve,** ***V2*** **second branch of the trigeminal nerve,** ***V3*** **third branch of the trigeminal nerve,** ***IIIcn*** **oculomotor nerve,** ***IVcn*** **trochlear nerve,** ***VI*** **abducens nerve**

In the posterior part of the CS the trochlear nerve is below the oculomotor nerve, while anteriorly it turns upward and becomes the most superior structure of the CS (at the level of the optic strut) (Iaconetta et al. 2012).

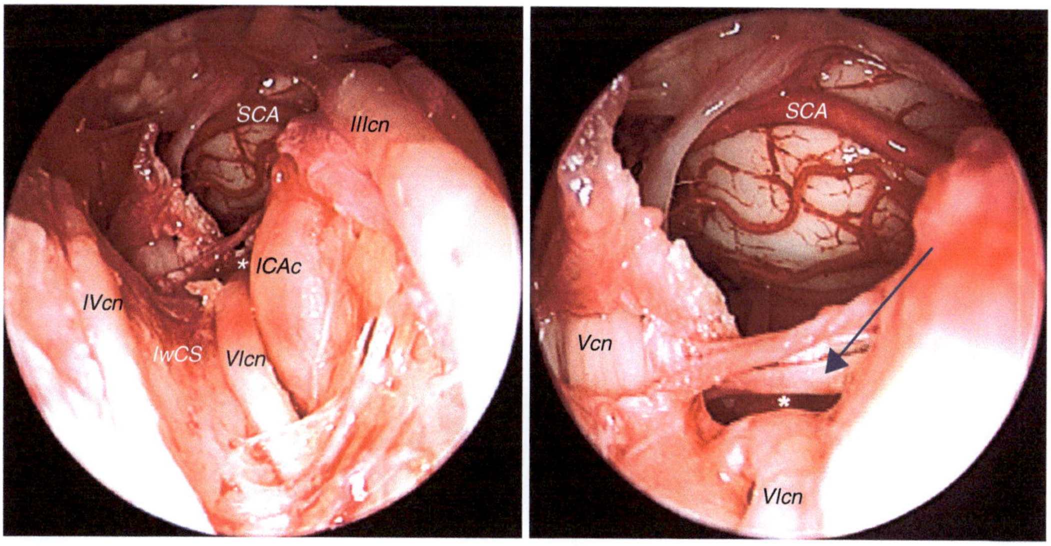

Fig. 3.42 Endoscopic vision of the cavernous sinus. Vision obtained through a right supraorbital approach with a 30° down-facing lens focusing on the cavernous sinus

ICAc **cavernous portion of the internal carotid artery,** ***lwCS*** **lateral wall of the cavernous sinus,** ***SCA*** **superior cerebellar artery,** ***IIIcn*** **oculomotor nerve,** ***IVcn*** **trochlear nerve,** ***Vcn*** **root of the trigeminal nerve,** ***VIcn*** **abducens nerve,** ***blue arrow*** **Gruber's ligament,** ***white asterisk*** **Dorello's canal**

The abducens nerve in most case is a single trunk throughout its entire course (Zhang et al. 2012). There are some variants, and one should be aware that the nerve can fuse with the oculomotor nerve for all its course (Zhang et al. 2012). The surgeon must be prepared to face other rare variations, such as different fasciculi within the CS. Globally, the incidence of a duplicated abducens nerve has been reported, ranging from 8 % to 18 % (Nathan et al. 1974; Iaconetta et al. 2001; Ozveren et al. 2003). In the prepontine cistern, when the duplication is present, AICA passes through the bundles. Furthermore, the incidence of a bilaterally duplicated nerve has been reported as frequently as 8 % of the time (Nathan et al. 1974; Ozveren et al. 2003). The abducens nerve can pass above the Gruber's ligament in 12 % of cases (Lang 1995).

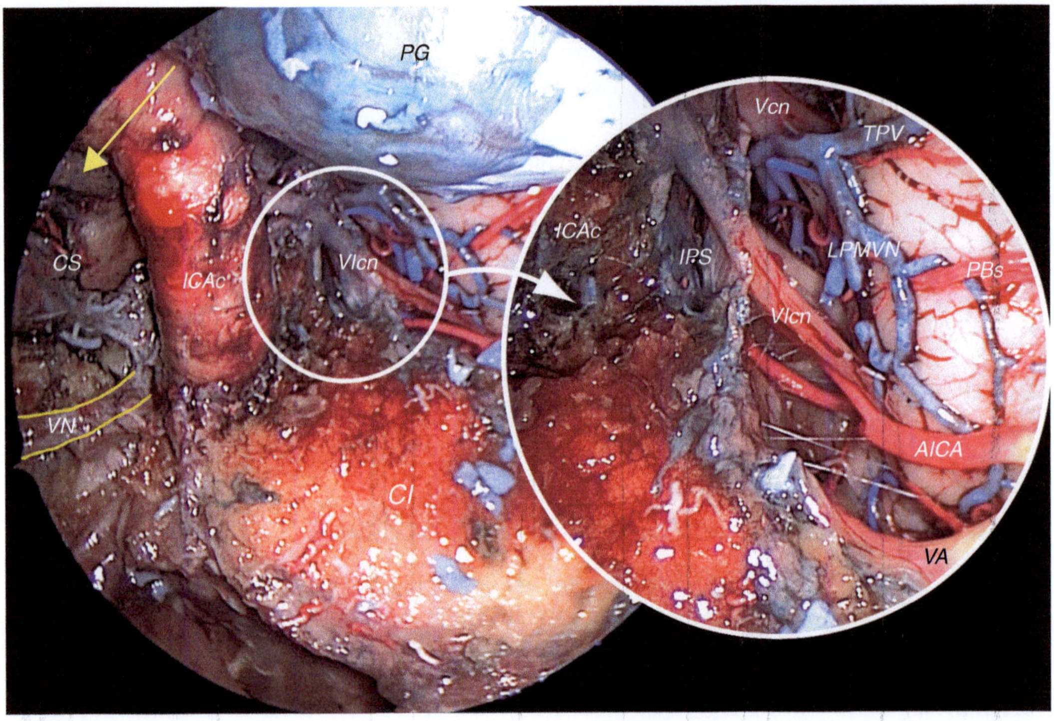

Fig. 3.43 Clival and cavernous region with a focus on the pathway of the abducens nerve

AICA **anterior-inferior cerebellar artery,** ***Cl*** **clivus,** ***CS*** **cavernous sinus,** ***ICAc*** **cavernous portion of the internal carotid artery,** ***IPS*** **inferior petrosal sinus,** ***LPMVN*** **lateropontomesencephalic venous network,** ***PBs*** **pontine branches,** ***PG*** **pituitary gland,** ***TPV*** **transverse pontine vein,** ***VA*** **vertebral artery,** ***VN*** **vidian nerve (bordered in** ***yellow*****),** ***Vcn*** **trigeminal nerve,** ***VIcn*** **abducens nerve,** ***yellow arrow*** **cavernous portion of the abducens nerve**

The abducens nerve enters through the lower part of the posterior wall of the CS. The inferior limit of the posterior wall of the cavernous sinus is situated at the upper margin of the petro-clival fessure.

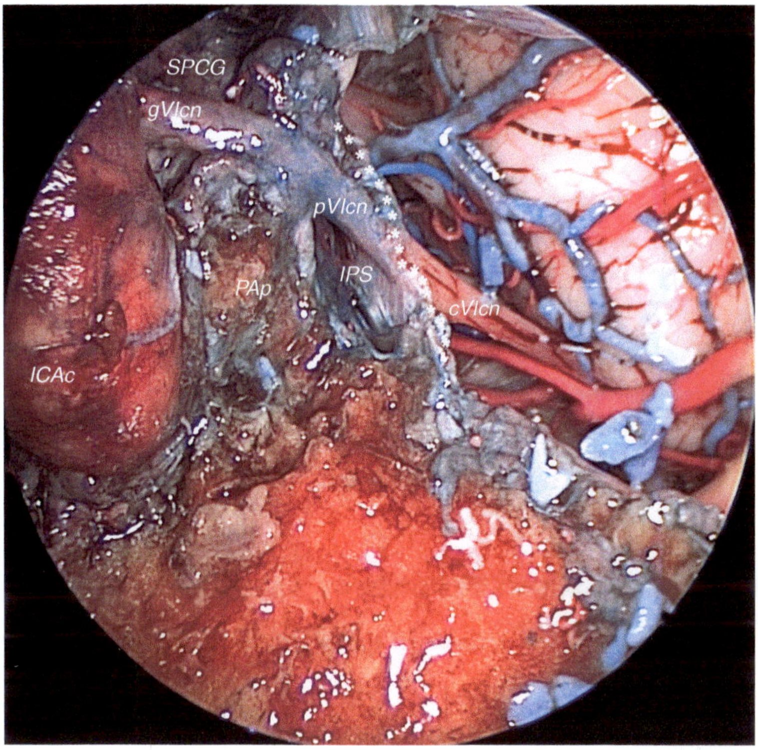

Fig. 3.44 Abducens nerve: posterior segments

ICAc **cavernous portion of the internal carotid artery,** ***IPS*** **inferior petrosal sinus,** ***PAp*** **petrous apex,** ***SPCG*** **sphenopetroclival gulf,** ***cVIcn*** **cisternal segment of the abducens nerve,** ***gVIcn*** **gulfar segment of the abducens nerve,** ***pVIcn*** **petrosal segment of the abducens nerve,** ***white asterisks*** **dura of the posterior cranial fossa**

At the transition between the inferior petrosal and the gulfar segment, the abducens nerve changes its trajectory drastically from approximately 45° to 5–10° flat and almost parallel to the sellar floor. The gulfar segment can be identified at the intersection of the sellar floor and the proximal parasellar internal carotid artery (ICA) (Barges-Coll et al. 2010).

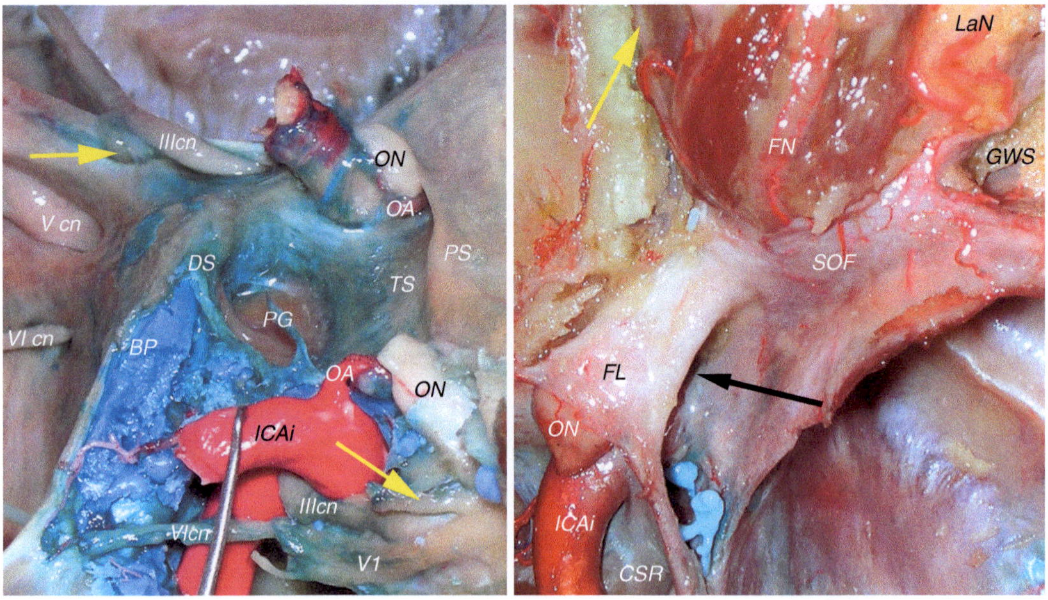

Fig. 3.45 Superolateral and superior vision of the cavernous sinus, superior orbital fissure, and orbital apex

BP **basilar plexus,** ***CSR*** **cavernous sinus roof,** ***DS*** **dorsum sellae,** ***FL*** **falciform ligament,** ***FN*** **frontal nerve,** ***GWS*** **greater wing of the sphenoid,** ***ICAi*** **intracranial portion of the internal carotid artery,** ***LaN*** **lacrimal nerve,** ***OA*** **ophthalmic artery,** ***ON*** **optic nerve,** ***PG*** **pituitary gland,** ***PS*** **planum sphenoidale,** ***SOF*** **superior orbital fissure,** ***TS*** **tuberculum sellae,** ***Vcn*** **trigeminal nerve,** ***V1*** **first branch of the trigeminal nerve,** ***IIIcn*** **oculomotor nerve,** ***VIcn*** **abducens nerve,** ***yellow arrow*** **trochlear nerve,** ***black arrow*** **optic strut (partially removed)**

The term *cavernous sinus* addresses only the venous aspect, neglecting the neural and soft tissue components. A more comprehensive and rational term is lateral sellar compartment (Parkinson 1990). This space is in continuation with the contents of the superior orbital fissure and the orbit (Froelich et al. 2009). The superior orbital fissure is a 3D space that contains connecting structures (lateral sellar orbital junction) between the lateral sellar compartment and the orbit (Froelich et al. 2009). This space can be further divided into an anterior lateral sellar compartment and the orbital apex. The anterior lateral sellar compartment is located anterior to the anterior loop of the cavernous portion of the internal carotid artery.

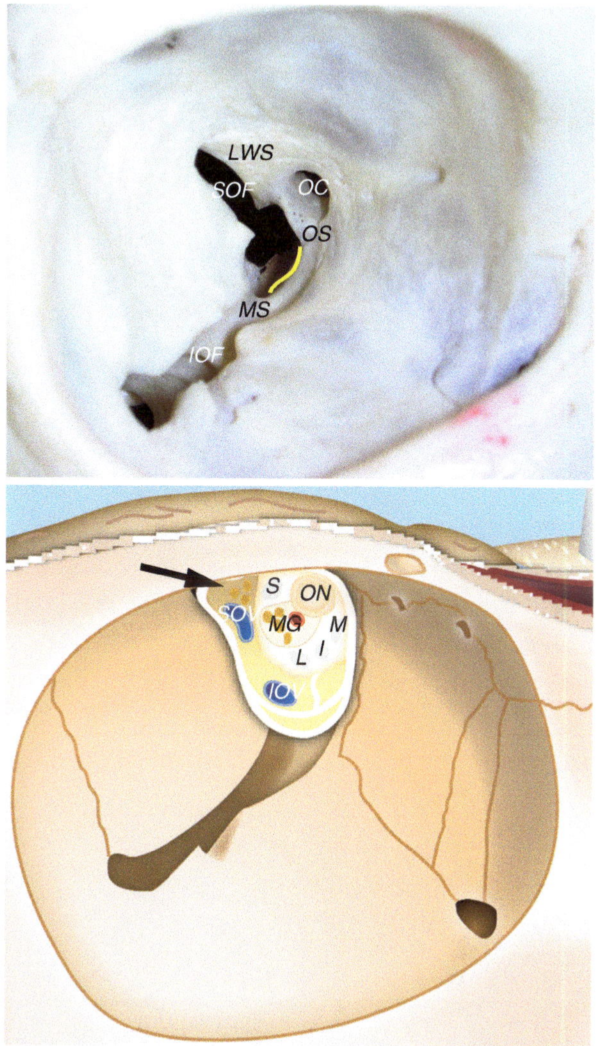

Fig. 3.46 Superior orbital fissure

I **inferior rectus muscle tendon,** ***IOF*** **inferior orbital fissure,** ***IOV*** **inferior ophthalmic vein,** ***L*** **lateral rectus muscle tendon,** ***LWS*** **lesser wing of the sphenoid,** ***M*** **medial rectus muscle tendon,** ***MG*** **medial group of nerve (oculomotor, nasociliary, abducens),** ***MS*** **maxillary strut,** ***OC*** **optic canal,** ***ON*** **optic nerve,** ***OS*** **optic strut,** ***S*** **superior rectus muscle tendon,** ***SOF*** **superior orbital fissure,** ***SOV*** **superior ophthalmic vein,** ***yellow line*** **indicates the "nasal" part of the superior orbital fissure,** ***black arrow*** **lateral group of nerves (frontal, lacrimal, trochlear)**

Only the medial portion of the SOF is a connection between the lateral sellar compartment and the orbit. The medial portion of the SOF contains the lateral sellar orbital junction above the IOF and the posterior extension of the PPF below the level of the IOF (Froelich et al. 2009). The lateral portion is not crossed by any neural structures, and it is covered by temporal fossa dura. The four rectus muscles insert posteriorly, through the common tendon, on the infraoptic tubercle, a small depression below the optic strut. This tendon forms a tendinous cone with two openings: the superomedial and superolateral foramina. More anteriorly, the common tendon splits into a superior and inferior tendon. From the inferior tendon originate the medial, inferior, and lateral rectus muscles, and from the superior originates the superior rectus muscle.

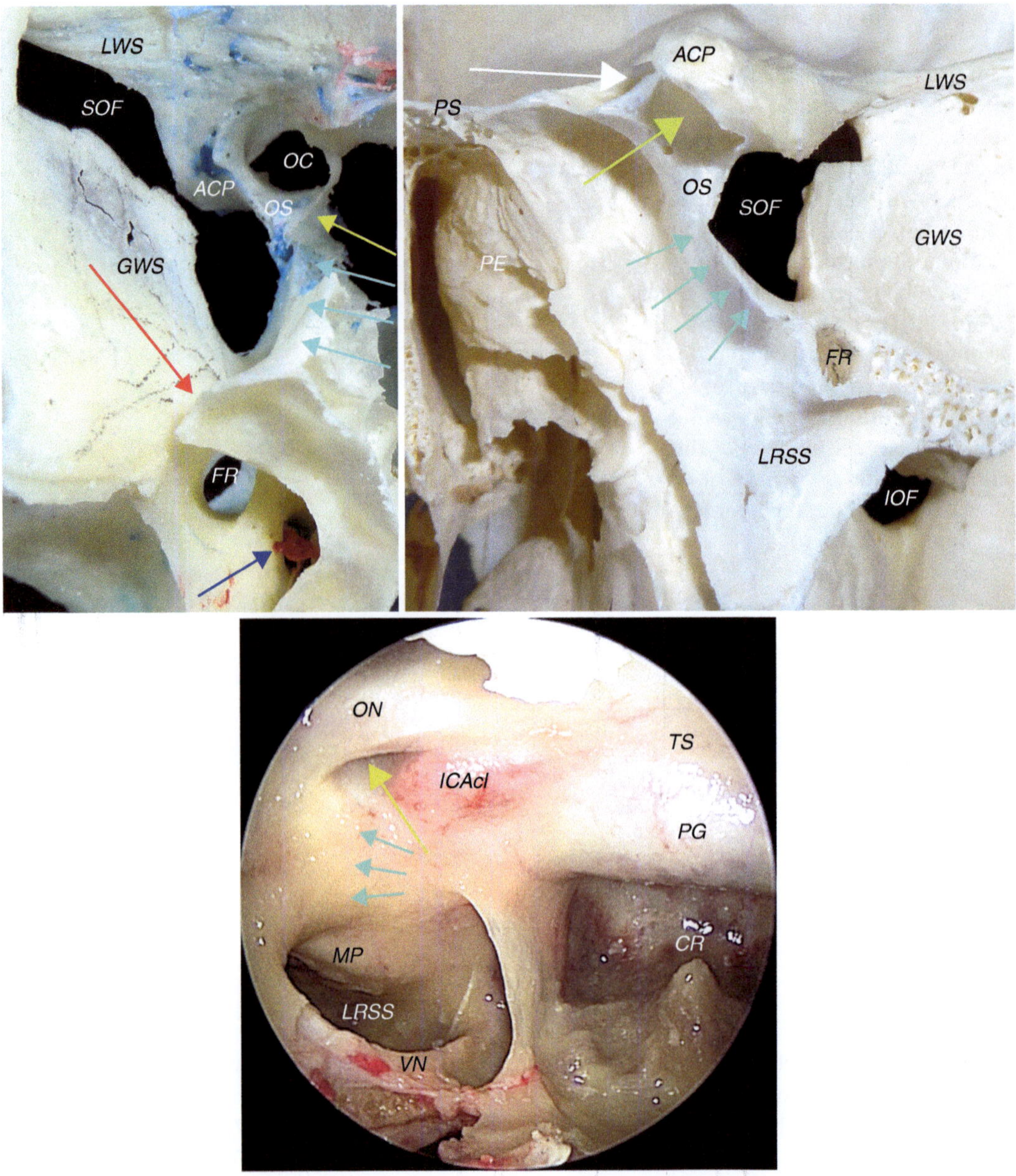

Fig. 3.47 Superior orbital fissure, osteology (anterior and posterior views) and endoscopic perspective

ACP **anterior clinoid process,** ***CR*** **clival recess,** ***FR*** **foramen rotundum,** ***GWS*** **greater wing of sphenoid,** ***ICAcl*** **clinoidal portion of the internal carotid artery,** ***IOF*** **inferior orbital fissure,** ***LRSS*** **lateral recess of the sphenoid sinus,** ***LWS*** **lesser wing of the sphenoid,** ***MP*** **maxillary prominence,** ***OC*** **optic canal,** ***ON*** **optic nerve,** ***OS*** **optic strut,** ***PE*** **posterior ethmoid,** ***PG*** **pituitary gland,** ***PS*** **planum sphenoidale,** ***SOF*** **superior orbital fissure,** ***TS*** **tuberculum sellae,** ***VN*** **vidian nerve,** ***red arrow*** **inferior orbital fissure,** ***white arrow*** **optic canal,** ***blue arrow*** **vidian canal and vidian artery,** ***yellow arrow*** **lateral opticocarotid recess,** ***blue-sky arrows*** **medial aspect of the superior orbital fissure**

The lateral opticocarotid recess corresponds to the pneumatisation of the optic strut. The clinoidal segment of the internal carotid artery faces the posterior aspect of the optic strut.

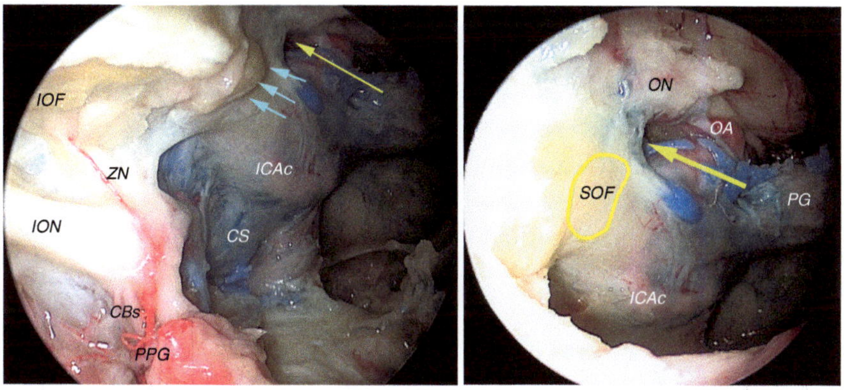

Fig. 3.48 Superior orbital fissure

***CBs* connecting branches between *V2* and *PPG*, *CS* cavernous sinus, *ICAc* cavernous portion of the internal carotid artery, *IOF* inferior orbital fissure, *ION* infraorbital nerve, *OA* ophthalmic artery, *ON* optic nerve, *PG* pituitary gland, *PPG* pterygopalatine ganglion, *SOF* superior orbital fissure, *ZN* zygomatic nerve, *yellow arrow* optic strut removed, *blue-sky arrows* superior orbital fissure**

V2 presented a safe landmark to reach the lower part of the CS and the vertical segment of the ICAc. Average distance from the FR at PPF and the vertical segment of ICAc is 35 mm (Amin et al. 2010). The CS apex can be exposed endoscopically by removing a bony triangle given by V1 superiorly, V2 inferiorly, and a line connecting FR and SOF anteriorly. Clinically, the SOF and CS apex represents a continuum. An important vein travelling the SOF is quite constant. It is immediately under the periorbit, outside the muscular cone, and reaches the cavernous venous compartment. This vein can be a limiting factor for drilling the SOF area (Dallan et al. 2013).

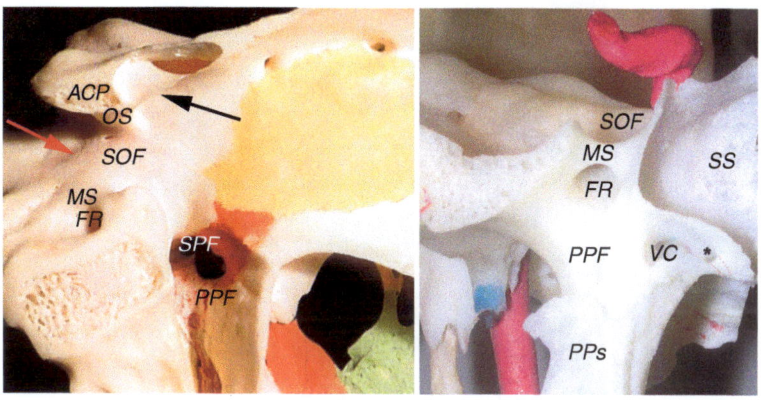

Fig. 3.49 Superior orbital fissure and pterygopalatine fossa relationship

***ACP* anterior clinoid process, *FR* foramen rotundum, *MS* maxillary strut, *OS* optic strut, *PPF* pterygopalatine fossa, *PPs* pterygoid plates, *SOF* superior orbital fissure, *SPF* sphenopalatine foramen, *SS* sphenoid sinus, *VC* vidian canal, *black arrow* optic canal, *red arrow* carotid sulcus, *black asterisk* palatovaginal canal**

At the level of the PPF, the FR lies about 7 mm superolateral to the SPF (Isaacs and Goyal 2007). Note the 3-dimensionality of the superior orbital fissure in the coronal, axial, and sagittal plane. Superior orbital fissure (SOF) is bordered by the optic strut (superiorly) and the maxillary strut (inferiorly). So, from an endoscopic endonasal viewpoint the nasal window to SOF is above V2, and below the lateral optico-carotid recess.

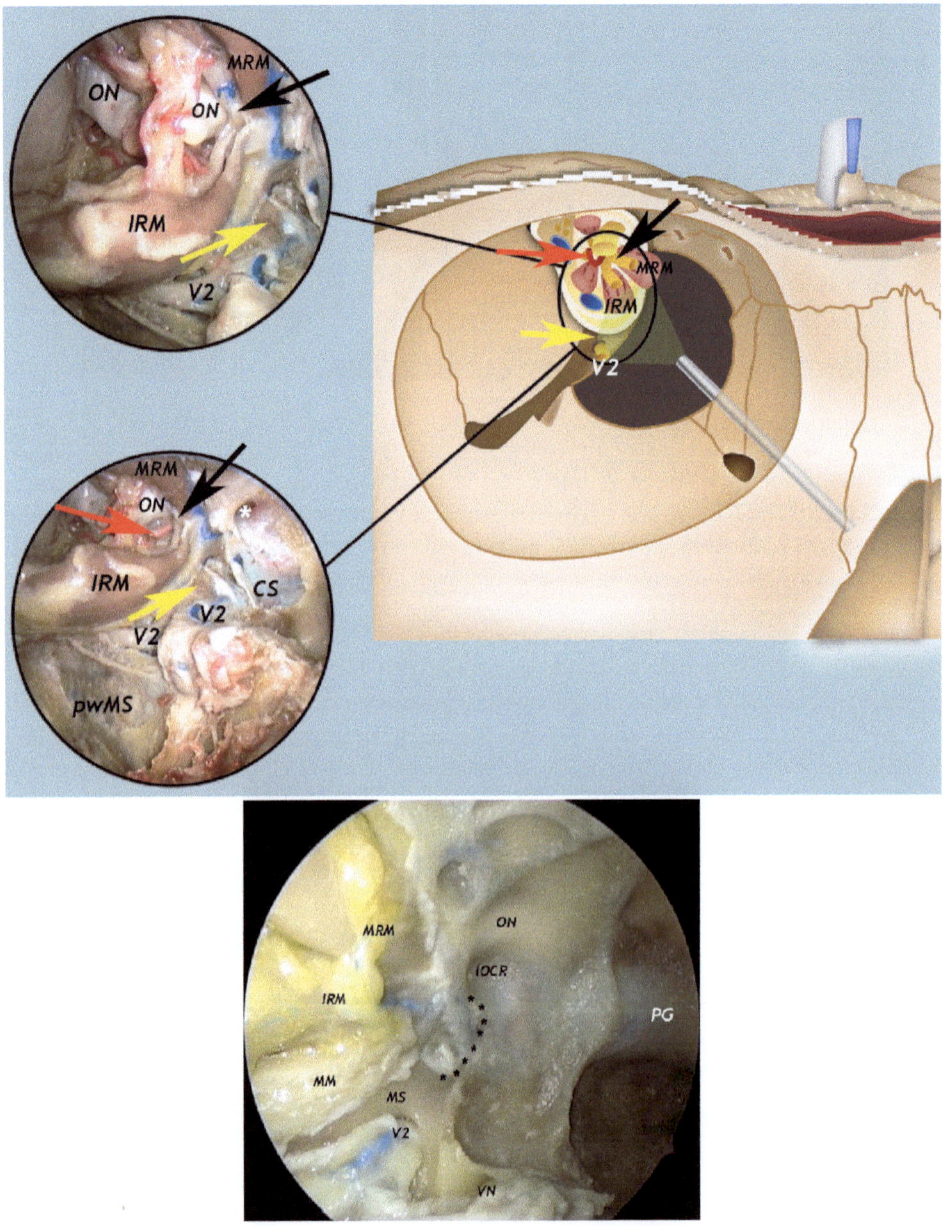

Fig. 3.50 Superior orbital fissure: endoscopic endonasal views

CS* cavernous sinus, *IRM* inferior rectus muscle, *lOCR* lateral optico-carotid recess, *MM **Muller's muscle, *MRM* medial rectus muscle, *ON* optic nerve, *pwMS* posterior wall of the maxillary sinus, *VN* vidian nerve, *V2* second branch of the trigeminal nerve, *white asterisk* indicates lateral optico-carotid recess, *black asterisks* indicate the nasal part of the superior orbital fissure, *black arrow* indicates the division of the oculomotor nerve, *red arrow* indicates ophthalmic artery, *yellow arrow* indicates maxillary strut**

The muller's muscle extends for the whole length of the inferior orbital fissure, passes above the maxillary strut and enters the superior orbital fissure. The maxillary strut is identified as a really constant bony landmark useful for indicating the superior orbital fissure and the "front door" to the cavernous sinus. At the level of the superior orbital fissure, once the fascial layer has been removed, the tendon of the IRM and MRM is evident. By dividing this tendon is possible to identify the 2 main branches of the oculomotor nerve, and laterally to it, the first segment of the ophthalmic artery (Dallan et al. 2013).

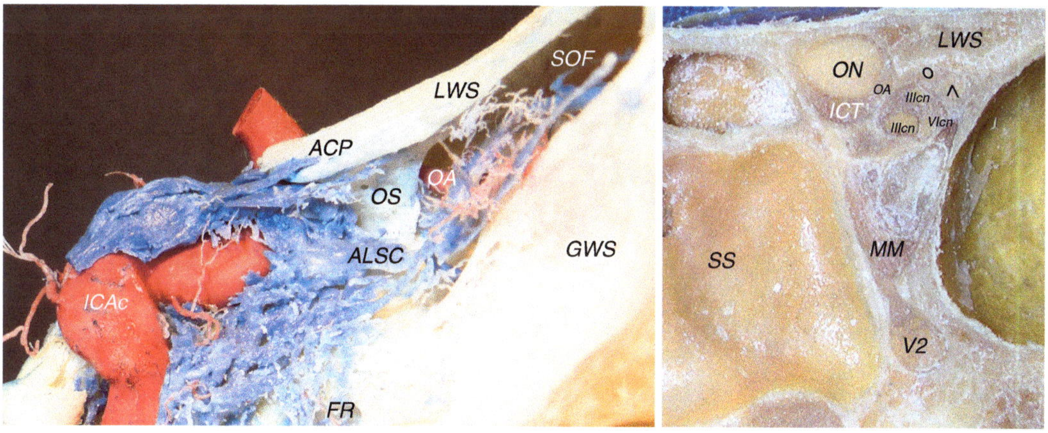

Fig. 3.51 Anterior sellar compartment region, coronal *view*, posterior perspective

ACP **anterior clinoid process,** ***ALSC*** **anterior lateral sellar compartment,** ***FR*** **foramen rotundum,** ***GWS*** **greater wing of the sphenoid,** ***ICAc*** **cavernous portion of the internal carotid artery,** ***ICT*** **inferior common tendon,** ***LWS*** **lesser wing of the sphenoid,** ***MM*** **muscle of Muller,** ***OA*** **ophthalmic artery,** ***ON*** **optic nerve,** ***OS*** **optic strut,** ***SOF*** **superior orbital fissure,** ***SS*** **sphenoid sinus,** ***V2*** **second branch of the trigeminal nerve,** ***IIIcn*** **oculomotor nerve,** ***VIcn*** **abducens nerve,** ***black circle*** **frontal nerve,** ***black arrowhead*** **nasociliary nerve**

The anterior sellar compartment is anterior to the anterior bend of the ICAc. Its floor is given by Muller's muscle. It presents a superior nervous compartment and an inferior venous compartment. The superior compartment of the anterior lateral sellar compartment can be divided into medial and a lateral groups of nerves. The medial includes the superior and inferior division of the oculomotor nerve and nasociliary and abducens nerves. The lateral group is composed of the trochlear, frontal, and lacrimal nerves. The inferior venous compartment is given by the confluence of the superior ophthalmic vein (*SOV*) and inferior ophthalmic vein (*IOV*), which drain into the cavernous sinus (Froelich et al. 2009). In the annulus, the nasociliary nerve passes medially, and it is located between the two divisions of the oculomotor nerve; the abducens nerve runs superiorly and laterally to reach the lateral rectus muscle.

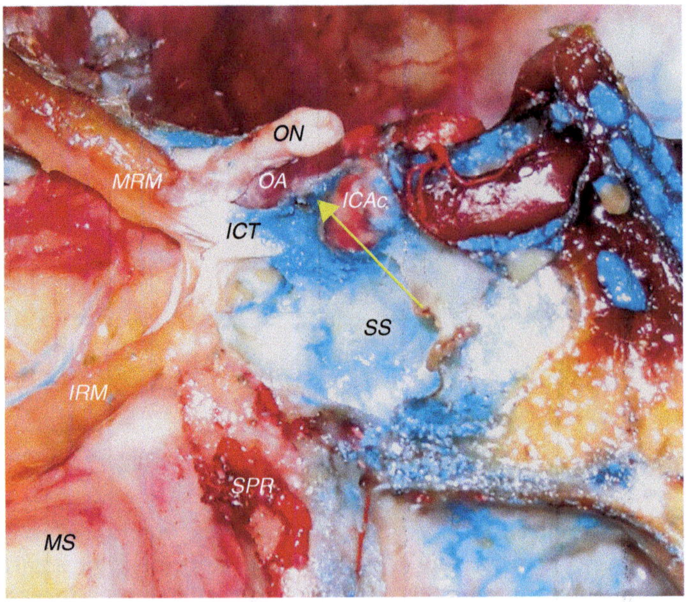

Fig. 3.52 Anterior sellar compartment region

ICAc **cavernous portion of the internal carotid artery,** ***ICT*** **inferior common tendon,** ***IRM*** **inferior rectus muscle,** ***MRM*** **medial rectus muscle,** ***MS*** **maxillary sinus,** ***OA*** **ophthalmic artery,** ***ON*** **optic nerve,** ***SPR*** **sphenopalatine region,** ***SS*** **sphenoid sinus,** ***yellow arrow*** **lateral opticocarotid recess**

Usually, the ophthalmic veins enter the anteroinferior part of the cavernous sinus (*CS*) below cranial nerves III and IV (Reisch et al. 2002). Just before entering the superior orbital fissure, the ophthalmic nerve splits in three branches: nasociliary, lacrimal, and frontal.

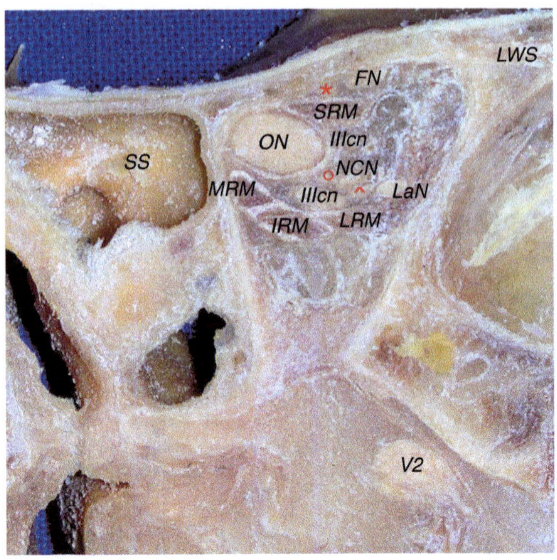

Fig. 3.53 Orbital apex, right side, posterior view

FN **frontal nerve,** ***IRM*** **inferior rectus muscle,** ***LaN*** **lacrimal nerve,** ***LRM*** **lateral rectus muscle,** ***LWS*** **lesser wing of the sphenoid,** ***MRM*** **medial rectus muscle,** ***NCN*** **nasociliary nerve,** ***ON*** **optic nerve,** ***SRM*** **superior rectus muscle,** ***SS*** **sphenoid sinus,** ***V2*** **second branch of the trigeminal nerve,** ***IIIcn*** **oculomotor nerve,** ***red asterisk*** **trochlear nerve,** ***red arrowhead*** **abducens nerve,** ***red circle*** **ophthalmic artery**

The orbital apex is divided into the intra- and extraconal compartments. Within the intraconal space, the superomedial and superolateral foramens are observed. Through the superomedial annular foramen, the optic nerve and the ophthalmic artery pass. Through the superolateral foramen, the oculomotor, nasociliary, and abducens nerves pass. The extraconal compartment is passed by the trochlear, lacrimal, and frontal nerves. The frontal and trochlear nerves ascend above the superior rectus muscle. The pterygopalatine fossa presents an extension within the superior orbital fissure (*SOF*), inferior to the lateral sellar compartment and Muller's muscle. It is composed of fat, small veins, and nerve fibres associated with the pterygopalatine ganglion (PPG) (Weninger and Prahmas 2000).

Supracavernous Segment

3.3 Anatomic Layout

3.3.1 Clinoidal Segment

The clinoidal segment is bordered by the inferior and superior dural ring. The roof of the CS is given by the extension of the dura just beneath the anterior clinoid process. This dura forms the *caroticoclinoid ligament*, lying between the anterior and middle clinoid process. This ligament fixes the vessel to the carotid sulcus. So, the middle clinoid process can be considered as marking the inferior border of the paraclinoid segment on its medial wall. As a whole, the medial and anteroinferior venous compartment of the CS are separated from the paraclinoid compartment. Just underneath the proximal dural ring, III, IV and V1 can be found running toward the superior orbital fissure. The superior dural ring is given by the extension of the dura covering the superior surface of the anterior clinoid process. This ring is not closely attached to the ICA, and a small cuff of arachnoid can surround the artery (Reisch et al. 2002).

3.3.2 Cisternal or Supraclinoid Segment

Personally, we prefer the term *cisternal segment* instead of supraclinoid segment. This segment extends between the distal dural ring and the carotid bifurcation, where the artery divides into the anterior and middle cerebral arteries (MCA). It presents a posterosuperior direction and passes laterally to the optic chiasm until it reaches the anterior perforate substance, where it bifurcates. In the cisternal segment, the intracranial portion of the ICA (ICAi) usually gives some branches/arteries: *ophthalmic*, *anterior choroidal* (AchA), *posterior communicating* (PcomA), *perforating*, and *SHA*. The ophthalmic artery presents a short intradural course, and it is located under the optic nerve. The AchA passes laterally around the cerebral peduncle and into the temporal horn, while the PcomA presents a posteromedial course parallel to the oculomotor nerve. During its intracranial pathway, the ICAi gives off a series of perforating branches. The first of these, in close proximity to the ophthalmic segment, arises from the posterior and medial aspect of the artery and supplies the pituitary stalk (SHAs), the optic chiasm, and less frequently the optic nerve and optic tract. The branches from the PcomA address the optic tract, floor of the third ventricle, and the area around the mammillary bodies. From the prebifurcation area, branches supplying the anterior perforated substance, the optic tract, and the uncus arise from the posterior aspect of the vessel.

3.3.3 Vascular Branches

The Superior Hypophyseal and the Infundibular Arteries

The *SHAs* usually arise from the first part of the cisternal segment of the ICA and terminate on the pituitary stalk and gland, but that can also send branches to the optic nerves and chiasm and the floor of the third ventricle. The *infundibular arteries* originate from the PcomA and are mainly directed to the infundibulum. Both the infundibular and the SHAs pass medially, below the chiasm, to reach the tuber cinereum. They form several anastomoses around the pituitary stalk, creating the *circuminfundibular plexus* (Rhoton 2003). Secondary braches from this plexus are directed to the anterior lobe of the pituitary gland, the tuber cinereum, the optic chiasm, and nerves.

Ophthalmic Artery

Usually, the ophthalmic artery arises below the optic nerve, above the dural roof of the CS. Rarely, it arises from the intracavernous segment (8 %) (Rhoton 2003), clinoidal segment, or middle meningeal artery. It can branch meningeal rami, which, if present, go to the ventral aspect of the optic nerve and chiasm. The cisternal segment of the ophthalmic artery is usually very short and covered laterally by the anterior clinoid process.

Posterior Communicating Artery

The PcomA arises from the posterior surface of the cisternal segment of the ICA. It runs backward and medially below the tuber cinereum, above the sella turcica, and parallel and medial to cranial nerve III to connect with the posterior cerebral artery. It gives rise to several branches, mostly from the superior and lateral surfaces, that reach the tuber cinereum, the premammillary part of the floor of the third ventricle, the posterior perforated substances, and the interpeduncolar fossa. The largest branch to the premammillary region is called the *premammillary artery* and belongs to the group of the *anterior thalamoperforating arteries*.

Anterior Choroidal Artery

Usually, the AchA arises from the ICA as a single artery, in most cases close to the PcomA. In rare cases (2 %), it arises from the PcomA or the MCA (Lang 1995; Rhoton 2003). In the great majority of cases, it arises from the cisternal segment of the ICA lateral to the optic tract and passes below or along the optic tract (usually medially to it) to get the lateral surface of the cerebral peduncle. It gives rise to different perforating arteries, reaching the optic tract, uncus, cerebral peduncle, and so on. The extreme variability of this network makes any attempt at description of limited significance.

Anterior Cerebral Artery

The anterior cerebral artery (ACA) is the smaller of the two terminal branches of the ICA. It arises lateral to the optic chiasm and below the anterior perforated substance. The artery courses anteromedially above the optic chiasm and nerve to enter the interhemispheric fissure. In front of the lamina terminalis, before entering the fissure, the ACA is connected by means of the anterior communicating artery (AcomA) to the ACA of the contralateral side. The AcomA complex is usually above the optic chiasm (70 % of cases) (Rhoton 2003). The AcomA is similar to the textbook description in three-fourths of cases. In about 10 % of cases, it can be hypoplastic or even duplicated and triplicated (Lang 1995). Other authors reported a higher percentage of duplicated (30 %) and triplicated (10 %) arteries (Perlmutter and Rhoton 1976). It usually sends several perforating branches for the anterior part of the diencephalon-lamina terminalis and surrounding regions (superior surface of the optic chiasm) (Lang 1995; Rhoton 2003). Also, the ACA, usually in proximity of the AcomA, sends a variable number of branches to the anterior part of the diencephalon, the lateral regions of the lamina terminalis, and the optic chiasm. Usually, the precommunicating segment (A1) courses above the optic chiasm, while the postcommunicating segment (A2) enters the pericallosal cistern and courses around the genu of the corpus callosum. If A1 is long, it can present a tortuous course and may be in close proximity of the planum sphenoidale. A1 sends a mean of five branches to the lower hypothalamic region. The *recurrent artery of Heubner (RAH)* is a branch of the ACA (in most cases from proximal A2) (Perlmutter and Rhoton 1976) that doubles back to the major artery and passes above the carotid bifurcation and MCA to feed the anterior perforated substance. In two-thirds of the cases, given its long course, the RAH participates in supplying the olfactory bulbs and tracts and the orbital parts of the frontal lobes (Lang 1995). Usually, the RAH presents a strict relationship with A1. According to Lang, in 30 % of cases the vessel is double (Lang 1995), while Perlmutter and Rhoton reported in more than 70 % of cases the presence of 2–4 arteries (Perlmutter and Rhoton 1976). Accessory MCAs have been described as arising from the ACA (Lang 1995). The frontopolar and the frontoorbital arteries are almost always present and usually arise from A2. The frontopolar artery usually courses on the basal surface of the anterior cranial fossa supplying the gyrus rectus and the medial part of the orbital gyri (Rhoton 2003).

Middle Cerebral Artery

The MCA is considered the continuation of the ICA and is rarely absent and duplicated (McCormick 1969). Its origin is at the medial end of the sylvian fissure, lateral to the optic chiasm and below the anterior perforated substance. At the level of the anterior perforated substance, it offers several branches, the *lenticulostriate arteries*.

3.4 Anatomic Pictures

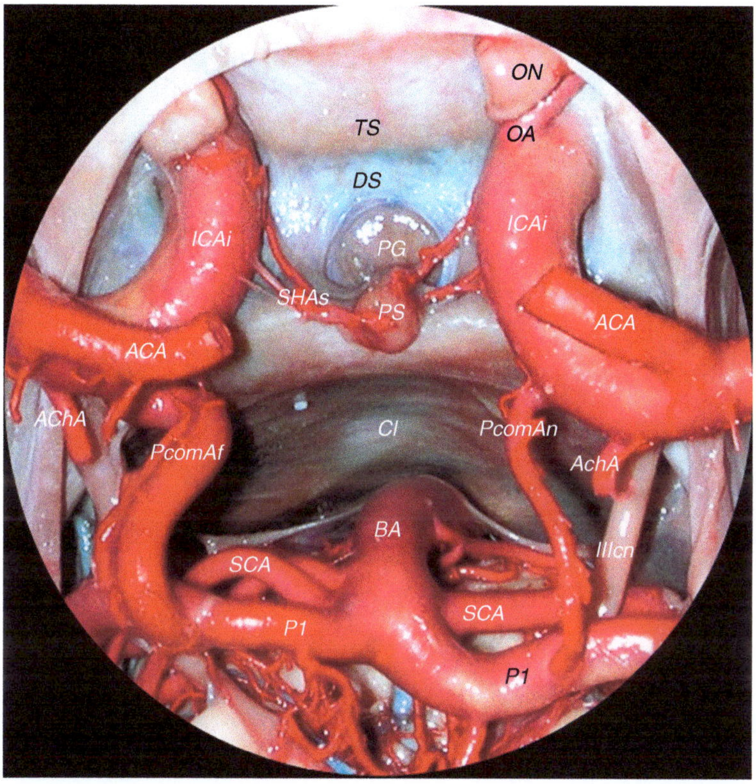

Fig. 3.54 Supracavernous segment, Willis's circle from above

***ACA* anterior cerebral artery, *AchA* anterior choroidal artery, *BA* basilar artery, *Cl* clivus, *DS* diaphragma sellae, *ICAi* intracranial portion of the internal carotid artery, *OA* ophthalmic artery, *ON* optic nerve, *PcomAf* posterior communicating artery (fetal configuration), *PcomAn* posterior communicating artery (normal configuration), *PG* pituitary gland, *PS* pituitary stalk, *P1* first segment of the posterior cerebral artery, *SCA* superior cerebellar artery, *SHAs* superior hypophyseal arteries, *TS* tuberculum sellae, *IIIcn* oculomotor nerve**

The *PcomA* is the most variable vessel of Willis's circle. If PcomA is wider than P1, it is said to be of the fetal type. This happens in about 20 % of cases. In 1 % of cases, it is absent (Lang 1995). The diaphragma sellae extends from the TS to the upper rim of the dorsum sellae and the posterior clinoid processes. Usually the DS originates some millimeters below the TS. The diaphragmatic foramen can be passed by the hypophyseal cistern (especially in adults) (Lang 1995). The size of the diaphragmatic foramen depends on the age and it is usually larger in older people.

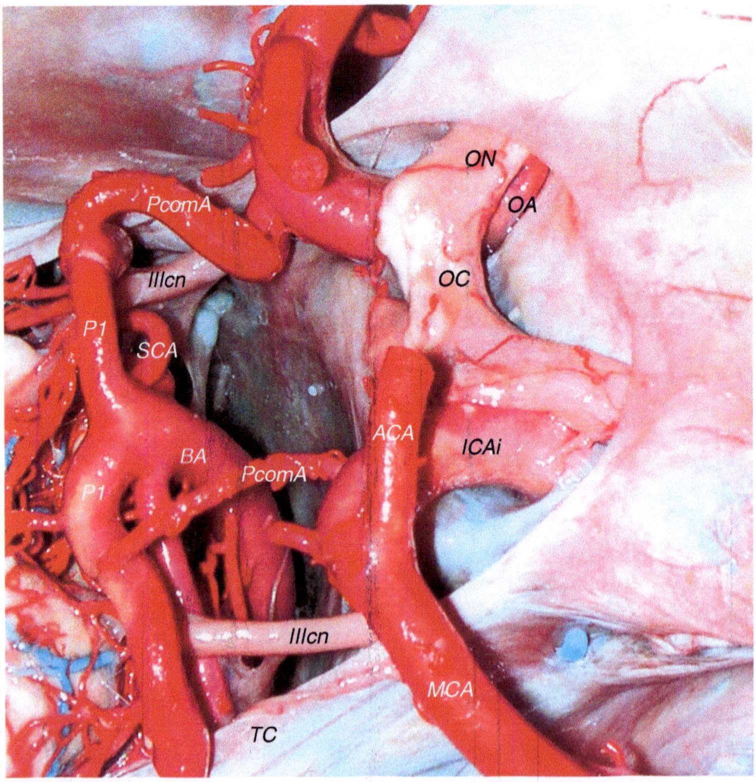

Fig. 3.55 Superolateral vision of the circle of Willis

***ACA* anterior cerebral artery, *BA* basilar artery, *ICAi* intracranial portion of the internal carotid artery, *MCA* middle cerebral artery, *OA* ophthalmic artery, *OC* optic chiasm, *ON* optic nerve, *PcomA* posterior communicating artery, *P1* first segment of the posterior cerebral artery, *SCA* superior cerebellar artery, *TC* tentorium cerebelli, *IIIcn* oculomotor nerve**

The optic nerve in the cranial cavity may be of variable length, resulting in a variable position of the optic chiasm. In most cases, the OC lies directly over the pituitary gland (>90 %), while in about 5 % of cases is located anteriorly (prefixed-above the tuberculum sellae); in less than 5 % of cases, it is located posteriorly (postfixed-above the dorsum sellae) (Janfaza and Nadol 2001).

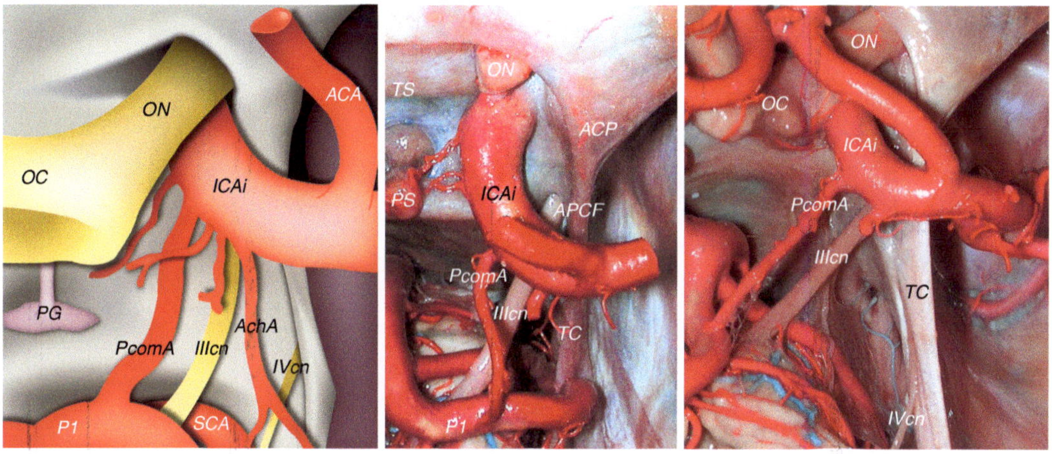

Fig. 3.56 Reconstruction and pictures of the roof of the cavernous sinus and suprasellar region from above

ACA **anterior cerebral artery,** ***AchA*** **anterior choroidal artery,** ***ACP*** **anterior clinoid process,** ***APCF*** **anterior petroclinoid fold,** ***ICAi*** **intracranial portion of the internal carotid artery,** ***OC*** **optic chiasm,** ***ON*** **optic nerve,** ***PcomA*** **posterior communicating artery,** ***PG*** **pituitary gland,** ***PS*** **pituitary stalk,** ***P1*** **first segment of the posterior cerebral artery,** ***SCA*** **superior cerebellar artery,** ***TC*** **tentorium cerebelli,** ***TS*** **tuberculum sellae,** ***IIIcn*** **oculomotor nerve,** ***IVcn*** **trochlear nerve**

The trochlear nerve in 80 % of cases enters at the posterior end of the roof of the cavernous sinus (*CS*) and in 20 % at the lower surface of the TC (Lang 1995).

The trochlear nerve is divided into 5 segments: cisternal, tentorial, cavernous, fissural and orbital. The cisternal segment exits the midbrain and courses through the quadrigeminal and ambiens cisterns towards the TC. The tentorial segment starts when the nerve pierces the TC, usually posterior to the postero-lateral margin of the oculomotor triangle. This segment ends at the level of the anterior petro-clinoid fold. This portion is in close relationship with the spheno-petro-clival venous gulf and the petrous apex (Iaconetta et al. 2012). And it can be fed at this level by: 1_terminal branches of the accessory middle meningeal artery, 2_tentorial branch from the inferolateral trunk, and 3_the Bernasconi-Cassinari artery.

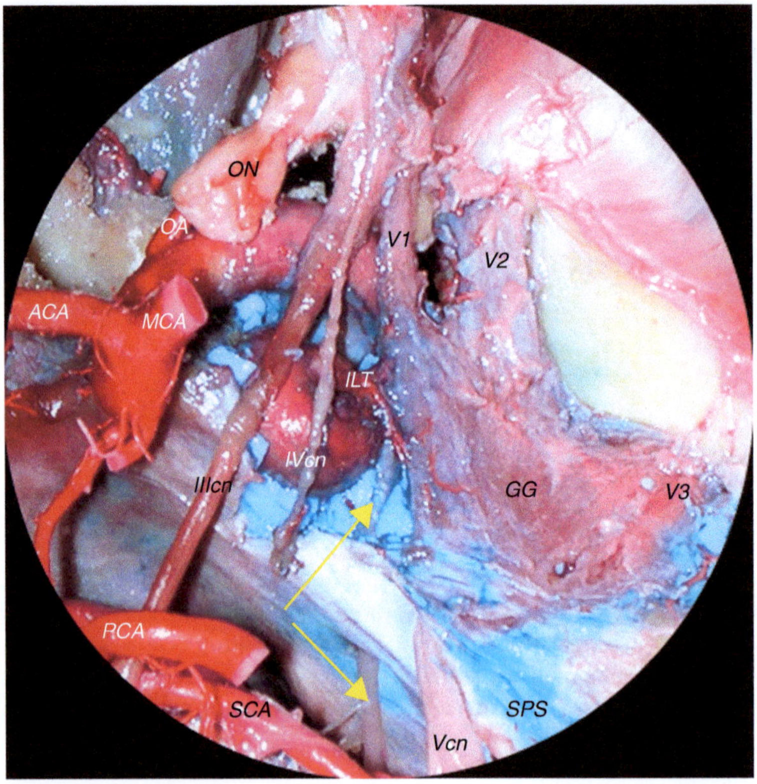

Fig. 3.57 Cavernous sinus, trigeminal ganglion, and Meckel's cave regions from above

***ACA* anterior cerebral artery, *GG* Gasserian ganglion, *ICAc* cavernous portion of the internal carotid artery, *ILT* inferolateral trunk, *OA* ophthalmic artery, *ON* optic nerve, *MCA* middle cerebral artery, *PCA* posterior cerebral artery, *SCA* superior cerebellar artery, *SPS* superior petrosal sinus, *Vcn* trigeminal nerve, *V1* first branch of the trigeminal nerve, *V2* second branch of the trigeminal nerve, *V3* third branch of the trigeminal nerve, *IIIcn* oculomotor nerve, *IVcn* trochlear nerve, *yellow arrows* abducens nerve**

The Meckel's cave (*MC*) is a dural recess extending from the posterior cranial fossa into the middle cranial fossa. The subarachnoid space extends around the roots of the trigeminal nerve above the petrous ridge and forms an arachnoid pocket that terminates at the ganglion. The dural layer of the MC can be followed until the foramina (Sabanci et al. 2011). The porus trigeminus, through which the trigeminal roots (sensory and motor) pass, corresponds to the mouth of the MC. The MC's mouth is placed, at the petrous apex, just below the SPS (Sabanci et al. 2011).

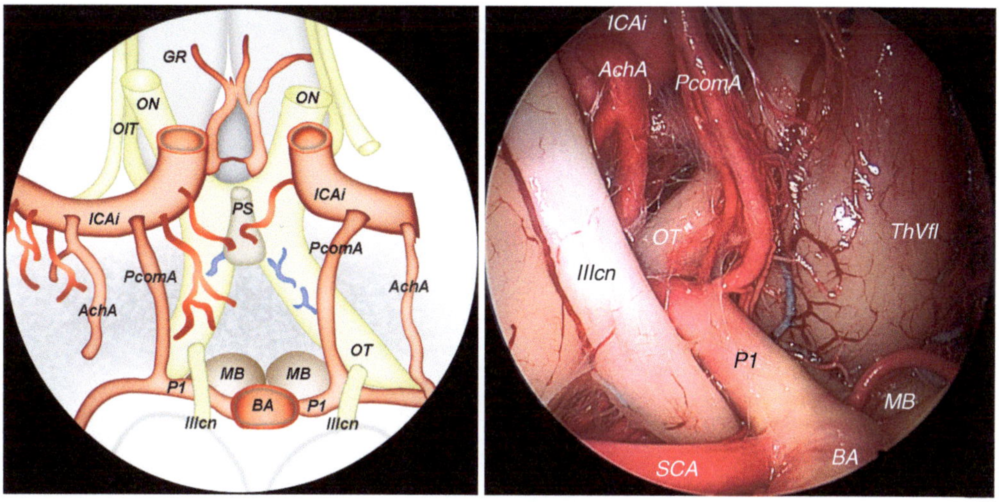

Fig. 3.58 Willis's circle from below (posterior part)

AchA **anterior choroidal artery,** ***BA*** **basilar artery,** ***GR*** **gyrus rectus,** ***ICAi*** **intracranial segment of the internal carotid artery,** ***MB*** **mammillary body,** ***OlT*** **olfactory tract,** ***ON*** **optic nerve,** ***OT*** **optic tract,** ***PcomA*** **posterior communicating artery,** ***PS*** **pituitary stalk,** ***P1*** **first segment of the posterior cerebral artery,** ***SCA*** **superior cerebellar artery,** ***ThVfl*** **floor of the third ventricle,** ***IIIcn*** **oculomotor nerve**

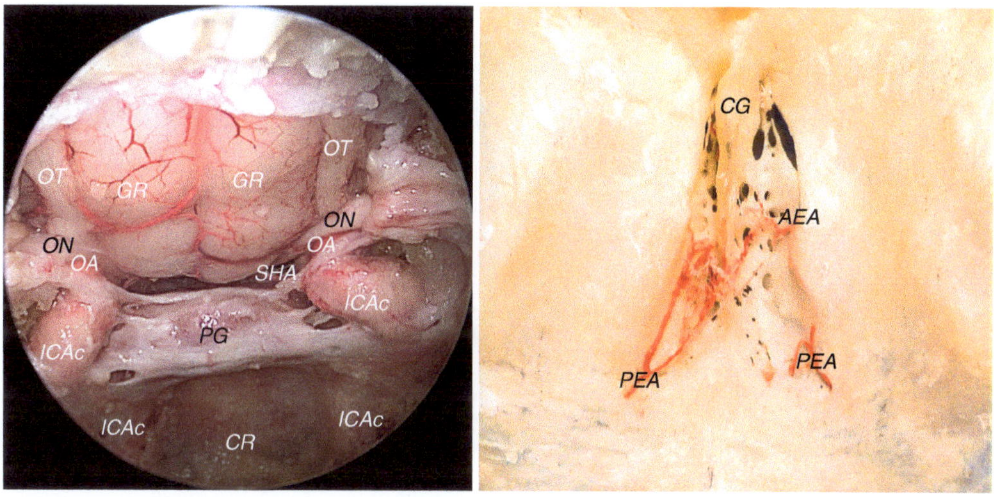

Fig. 3.59 Endoscopic view of the sellar region and anterior cranial fossa structures and view from above of the cribriform plate region

AEA **anterior ethmoidal artery,** ***CG*** **crista galli,** ***CR*** **clival recess,** ***GR*** **gyrus rectus,** ***ICAc*** **cavernous portion of the internal carotid artery,** ***OA*** **ophthalmic artery,** ***ON*** **optic nerve,** ***OT*** **olfactory tract,** ***PEA*** **posterior ethmoidal artery,** ***PG*** **pituitary gland,** ***SHA*** **superior hypophyseal artery**

The crista galli is the superior extension of the nasal septum, and the anterior end of the cerebral falx attaches to it. The ethmoidal arteries supply the dura of the anterior cranial fossa. They run in the dura along the lateral border of the cribriform plate. A branch of the AEA may be large enough to be named the anterior meningeal artery (Janfaza and Nadol 2001).

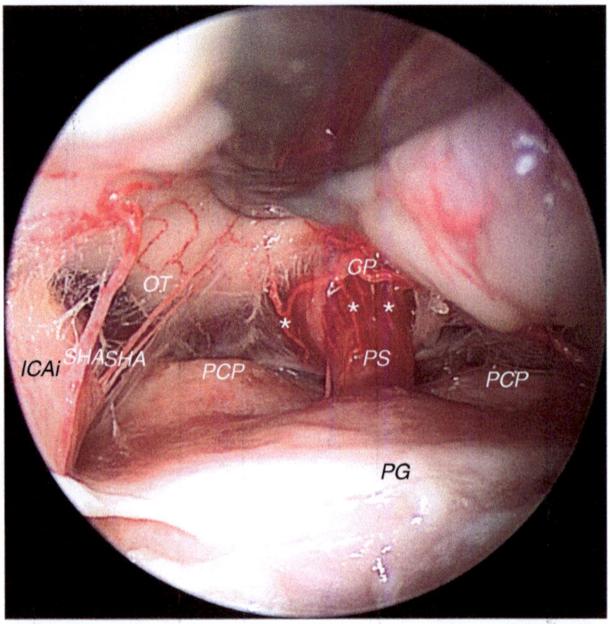

Fig. 3.60 Endoscopic view of the pituitary stalk. The complex vascular network around it, coming from the superior hypophyseal arteries, is clearly evident

CP **circuminfundibular plexus,** ***ICAi*** **intracranial portion of the internal carotid artery,** ***OT*** **optic tract,** ***PCP*** **posterior clinoid process,** ***PG*** **pituitary gland,** ***PS*** **pituitary stalk,** ***SHA*** **superior hypophyseal artery,** ***white asterisks*** **coaxial branches**

The SHAs usually arise from the intracranial portion of the internal carotid artery (or from the carotid cave). They mainly supply the optic chiasm and the infundibular region of the hypothalamus.

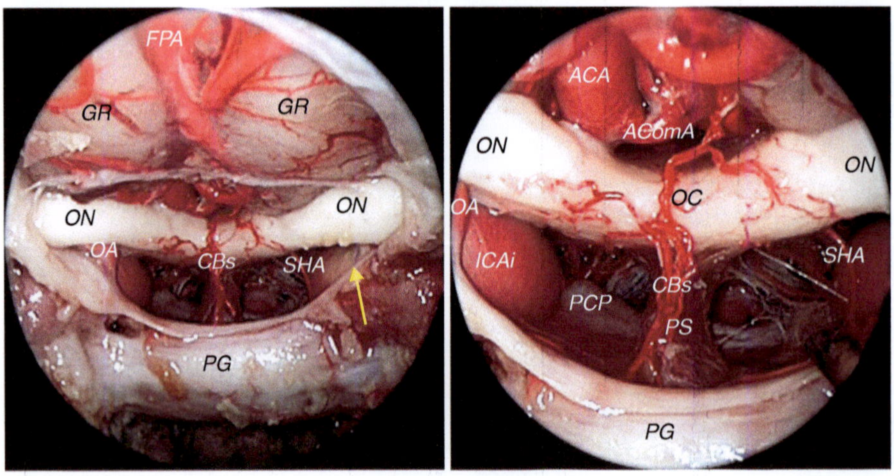

Fig. 3.61 Endoscopic view of the sellar region and anterior cranial fossa structures

ACA **anterior cerebral artery,** ***AcomA*** **anterior communicating artery,** ***CBs*** **chiasmatic branches,** ***FPA*** **frontopolar artery,** ***GR*** **gyrus rectus,** ***ICAi*** **intracranial portion of the internal carotid artery,** ***OA*** **ophthalmic artery,** ***OC*** **optic chiasm,** ***ON*** **optic nerve,** ***PCP*** **posterior clinoid process,** ***PG*** **pituitary gland,** ***PS*** **pituitary stalk,** ***SHA*** **superior hypophyseal artery,** ***yellow arrow*** **upper dural ring**

The optic chiasm receives its blood supply from the superior hypophyseal artery, the anterior cerebral arteries, and the carotid arteries (Janfaza et al. 2001). The chiasmatic cistern is located in front of the optic chiasm and above the sella turcica. In the lateral border of the chiasmatic cistern the first part of the ICAi is visible.

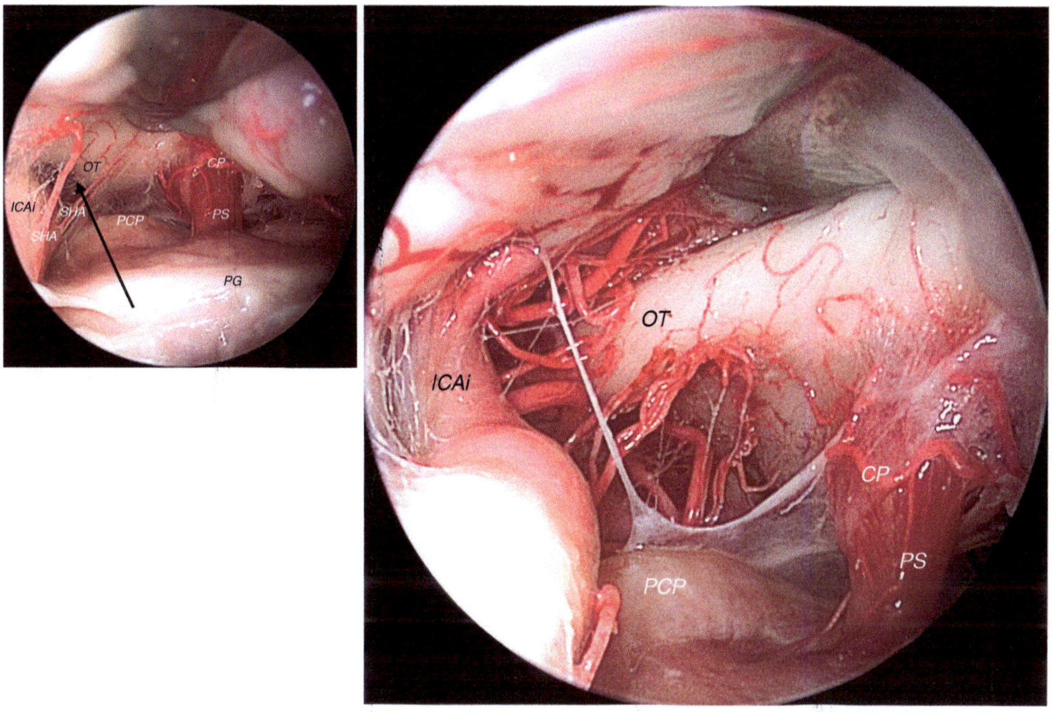

Fig. 3.62 Endoscopic view of the intracranial segment of the internal carotid artery. The smaller picture shows a general overview

CP **circuminfundibular plexus,** ***ICAi*** **intracranial portion of the internal carotid artery,** ***OT*** **optic tract,** ***PCP*** **posterior clinoid process,** ***PG*** **pituitary gland,** ***PS*** **pituitary stalk,** ***SHA*** **superior hypophyseal artery,** ***black arrow*** **indicates the direction of the view (as seen in the bigger picture)**

Within the medial part of the carotid cistern a tremendous arterial network given by the superior hypophyseal arteries, the infundibular arteries and perforating branches from the internal carotid artery is visible.

The superior hypophyseal arteries and infundibular arteries (from the posterior communicating artery) form a complex network around the pituitary stalk, named circuminfundibular plexus (Rhoton 2003). This plexus gives rise to descending (for the anterior lobe of PG) and ascending (for tuber cinereum, median eminence and inferior surface of optic chiasm) branches (Rhoton 2003).

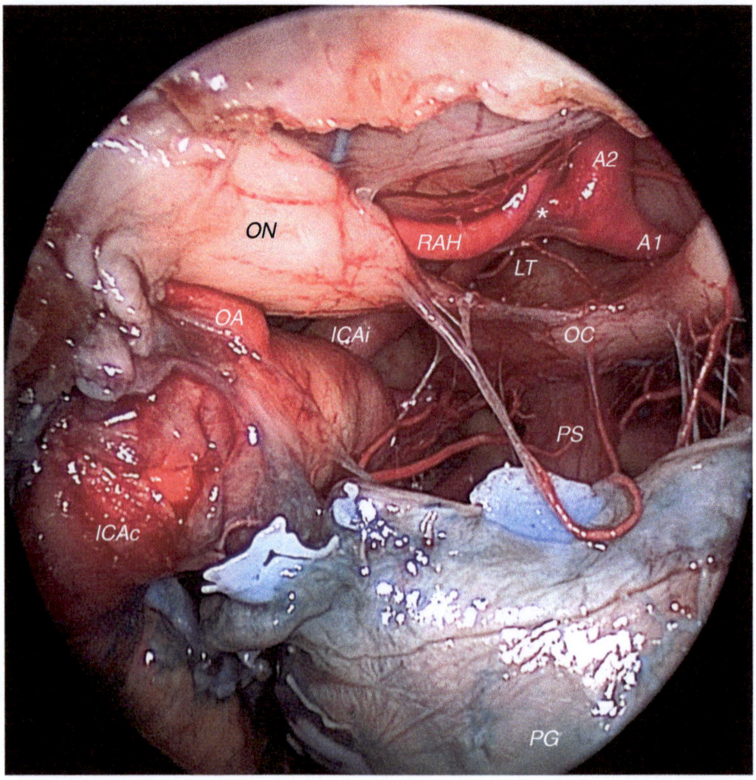

Fig. 3.63 Endoscopic view of the pituitary stalk, right supraclinoid internal carotid artery, and optic pathways

***A1* first segment of the anterior cerebral artery, *A2* second (postcommunicating) segment of the anterior cerebral artery, *ICAc* cavernous portion of the internal carotid artery, *ICAi* intracranial portion of the internal carotid artery, *LT* lamina terminalis, *OA* ophthalmic artery, *OC* optic chiasm, *ON* optic nerve, *PG* pituitary gland, *PS* pituitary stalk, *RAH* recurrent artery of Heubner, *white asterisk* anterior communicating artery**

The lamina terminalis cistern is situated above the optic chiasm (Martins et al. 2011). Within this cistern, A1 and A2, as well as the anterior communicating artery and the first part of the recurrent artery of Heubner, are evident.

The recurrent artery of Heubner usually origins from the post-communicating segment of the anterior cerebral artery (ACA). It doubles back the ACA to reach the medial part of the Sylvian fissure, below the anterior perforated substance. Sometimes its path is so long that the artery loops below the basal surface of the frontal lobes. Not frequently more than one recurrent arteries can be present (Rhoton 2003). According to Lang the artery is double in about 30% of cases (Lang 1995).

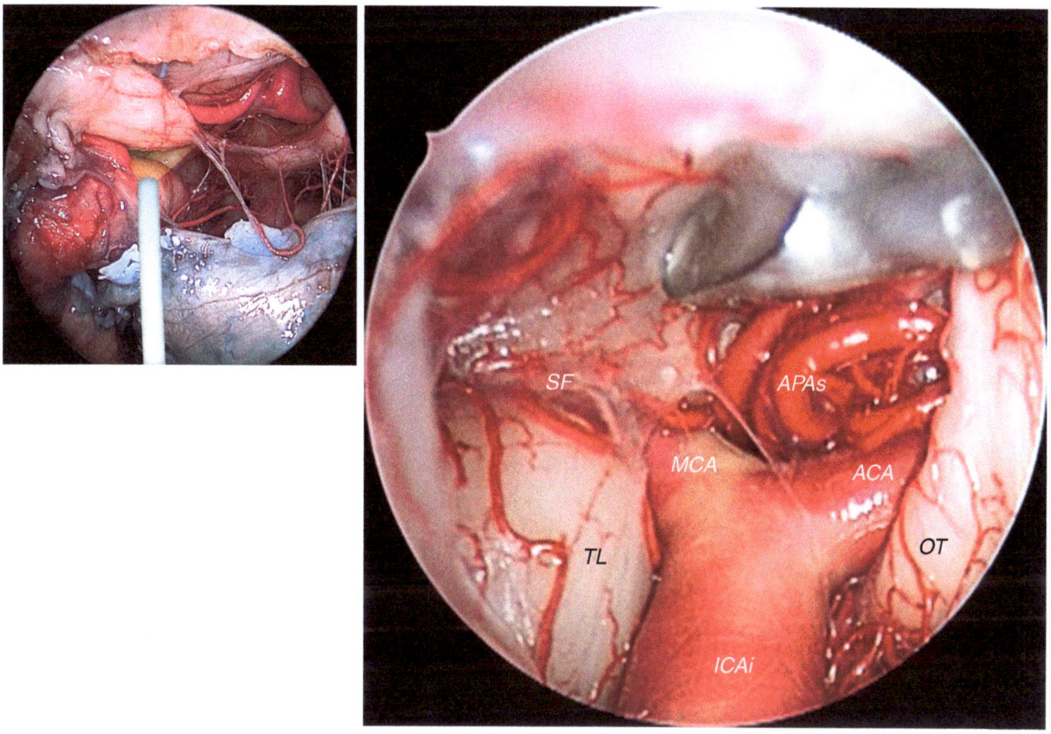

Fig. 3.64 Endoscopic vision of the anterior perforated substance region. Vision obtained with a 0° lens passing inferiorly and then laterally to the optic nerve and tract

***ACA* anterior cerebral artery, *APAs* anterior perforating arteries, *ICAi* intracranial portion of the internal carotid artery, *MCA* middle cerebral artery, *OT* optic tract, *SF* Sylvian fissure, *TL* temporal lobe**

The initial part of M1 segment and the posterior part of medial orbital gyri are evident in the anterior compartment of the Sylvian cistern.

MCA origins at the medial end of the sylvian fissure, lateral to the optic chiasm and below to the anterior perforate substance (Rhoton 2003). Passing below the anterior perforated substance it gives rise to perforating branches (named lenticulostriate arteries). Rarely MCA can be absent (unilaterally) or doubled (Lang 1995). In about 10% of cases the recurrent artery of Heubner originates in the precommunicating part of the ACA (Lang 1995).

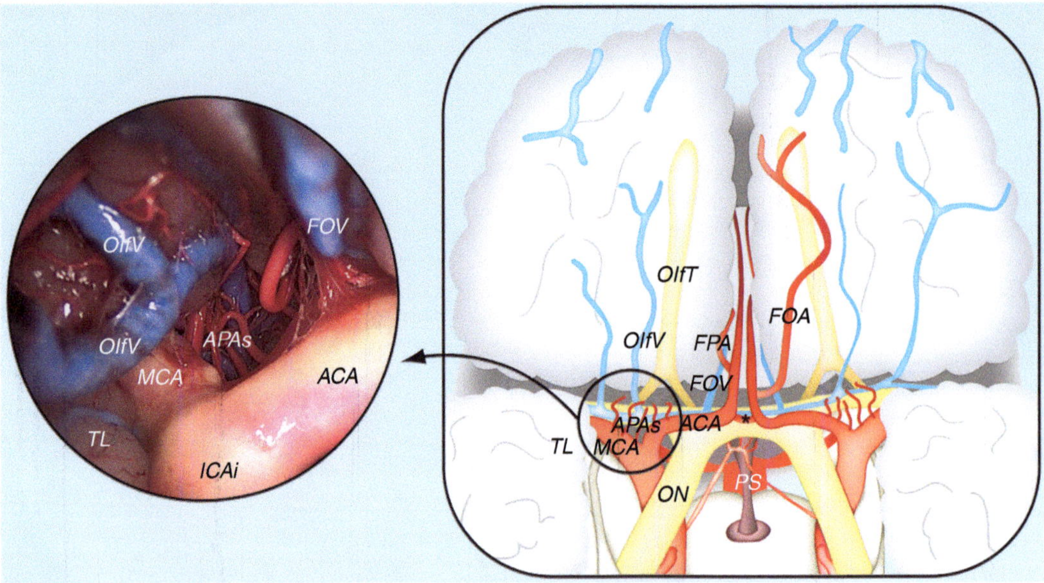

Fig. 3.65 Endoscopic vision of the anterior perforated substance region. In the drawing the frontal lobes have been pushed upward

ACA **anterior cerebral artery,** ***APAs*** **anterior perforating arteries,** ***FOA*** **fronto-orbital artery,** ***FOV*** **fronto-orbital vein,** ***FPA*** **fronto-polar artery,** ***ICAi*** **intracranial segment of the internal carotid artery,** ***MCA*** **middle cerebral artery,** ***OlfT*** **olfactory tract,** ***OlfV*** **olfactory vein,** ***ON*** **optic nerve,** ***PS*** **pituitary stalk,** ***TL*** **temporal lobe,** ***black asterisk*** **anterior communicating artery**

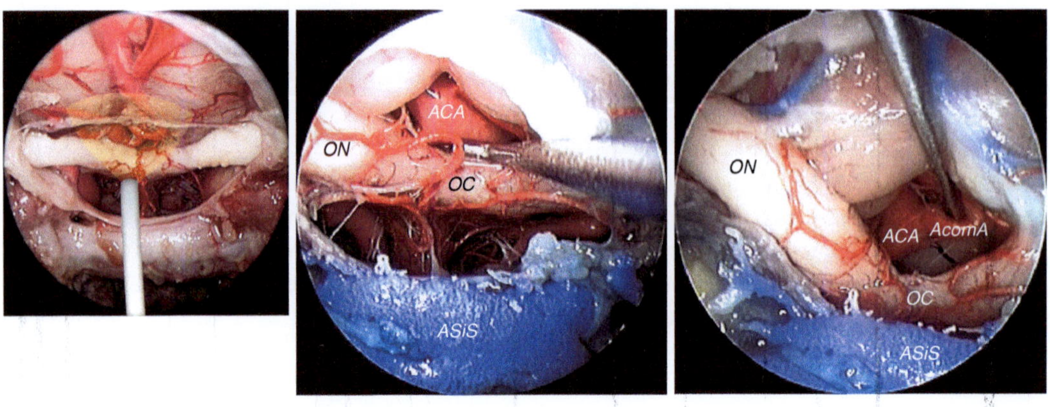

Fig. 3.66 Endoscopic view of the suprasellar region

ACA **anterior cerebral artery,** ***AcomA*** **anterior communicating artery,** ***ASiS*** **anterior superior intercavernous sinus,** ***OC*** **optic chiasm,** ***ON*** **optic nerve**

The anterior cerebral artery arises at the medial end of the Sylvian fissure, below the anterior perforated substance and lateral to the optic chiasm. And it runs anteromedially, lying above the optic chiam and/or optic nerve, to get the interemispheric fissure. Close to the fissure, it is conneted to the opposite ACA by the AcomA, giving rise to the ACA-AcomA complex.

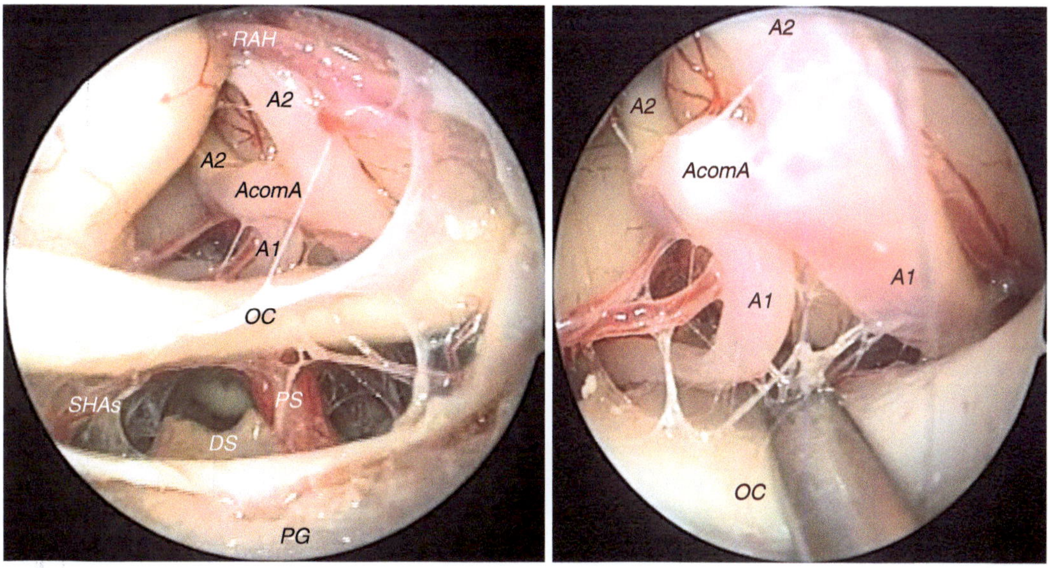

Fig. 3.67 Endoscopic view of the suprachiasmatic region. The vascular network given by anterior cerebral arteries is evident

***AcomA* anterior communicating artery, *A1* first segment of the anterior cerebral artery, *A2* second segment of the anterior cerebral artery, *DS* dorsum sellae, *OC* optic chiasm, *PG* pituitary gland, *PS* pituitary stalk, *RAH* recurrent artery of Heubner, *SHAs* superior hypophyseal arteries**

A normal ACA-AcomA complex is one in which an AcomA connects A1s of nearly equal size, and in these cases the diameter of AcomA is about 1mm less than A1's one (Rhoton 2003). But AcomA shows a great variability, both in terms of size, shape and numbers. In about 10 % of cases, AcomA is duplicated, or it can also be present as a plexus. In the same percentage, it can be hypoplastic (Lang 1995).

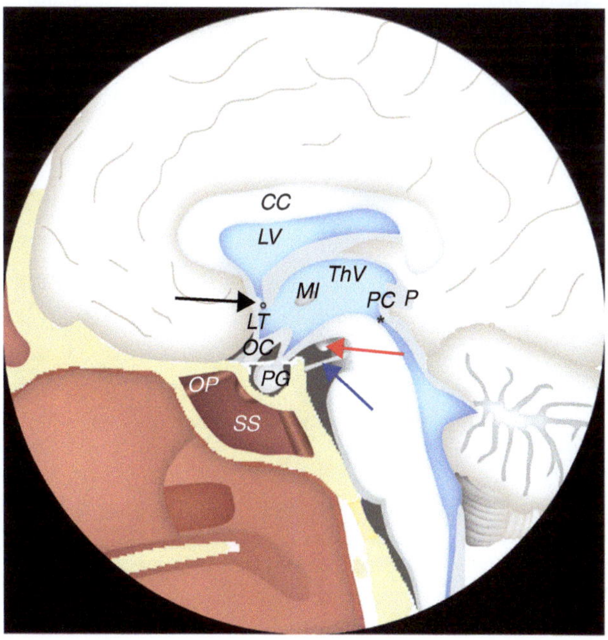

Fig. 3.68 Midsagittal reconstruction of the ventricular system

***CC* corpus callosum, *LT* lamina terminalis, *LV* lateral ventricle, *MI* massa intermedia, *OC* optic chiasm, *OP* optic prominence, *P* pineal gland, *PC* posterior commissure, *PG* pituitary gland, *SS* sphenoid sinus, *ThV* third ventricle, *black arrow* anterior commissure, *blue arrow* oculomotor nerve, *red arrow* mammillary body, *black asterisk* opening of the Sylvius' aqueduct, *black circle* foramen of Monro**

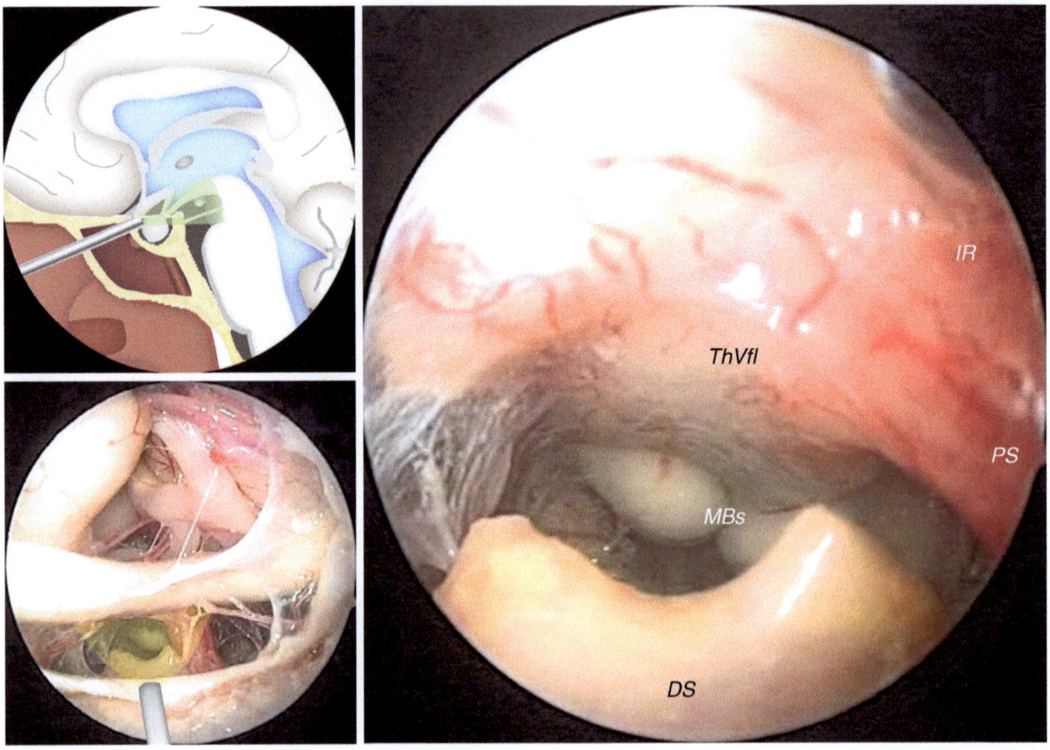

Fig. 3.69 Endoscopic view of the floor of the third ventricle. The dorsum sellae and the upper premesencephalic (mammillary bodies) region are evident

DS **dorsum sellae,** ***IR*** **infundibular region (infundibulum),** ***MBs*** **mammillary bodies,** ***PS*** **pituitary stalk,** ***ThVfl*** **floor of the third ventricle**

The interpeduncular cistern is located between the cerebral peduncles. It is posterior to the chiasmatic cistern and in continuation with it (Janfaza and Nadol 2001). The pontine cistern is caudal to the interpeduncular cistern. Inferiorly, there are the medullary cisterns, at the level of the cerebellomedullary angle. The infundibulum is the inferior projection of the hypothalamus. It lies immediately behind the optic chiasm and gives origin to the pituitary stalk. It is the connection between the hypothalamus and the posterior lobe of the pituitary gland.

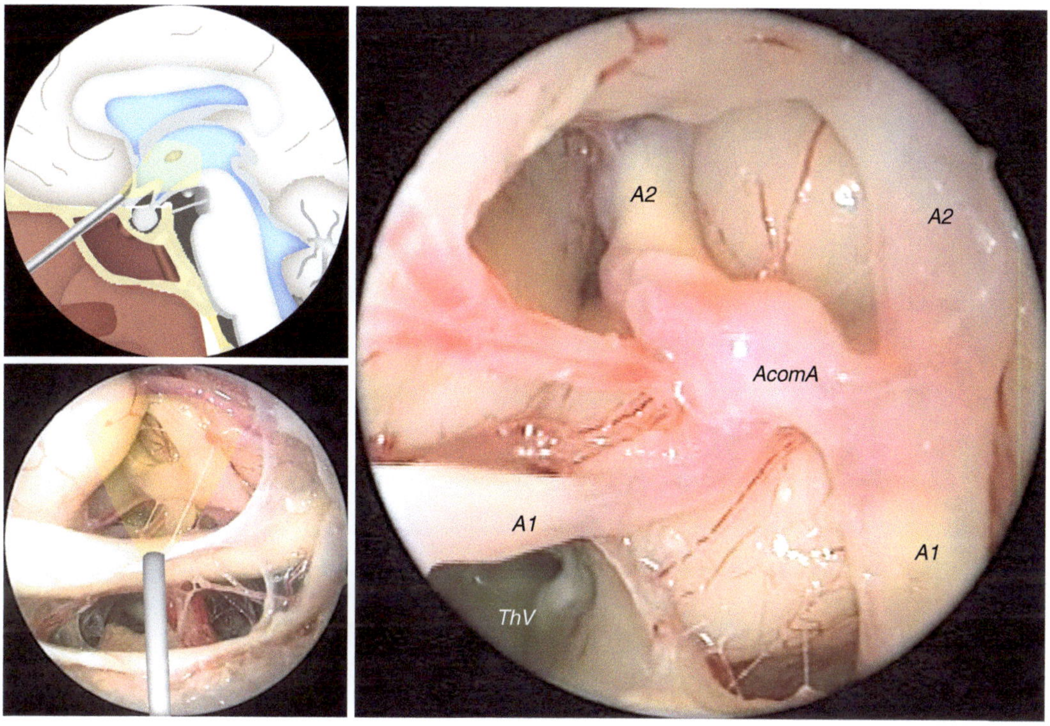

Fig. 3.70 Endoscopic view of the suprachiasmatic region. The anterior communicating artery complex is evident

***AcomA* anterior communicating artery, *A1* first segment of the anterior cerebral artery, *A2* second segment of the anterior cerebral artery, *ThV* third ventricle**

The lamina terminalis cistern is located above the anterior aspect of the lamina terminalis, and it is in continuation with the chiasmatic cistern and the pericallosal cistern. This last one is reached when the interhemispheric fissure is opened (Abuzayed et al. 2010). At this level, the origin of the fronto-orbital and frontopolar artery can be seen. Opening the lamina terminalis below the AcomA allows entrance into the anterior part of the third ventricle. A2 usually ascends, in front of the lamina terminalis, to pass into the longitudinal fissure between the cerebral hemispheres. A2s are typically not side by side in the way to the pericallosal cistern (Rhoton 2003).

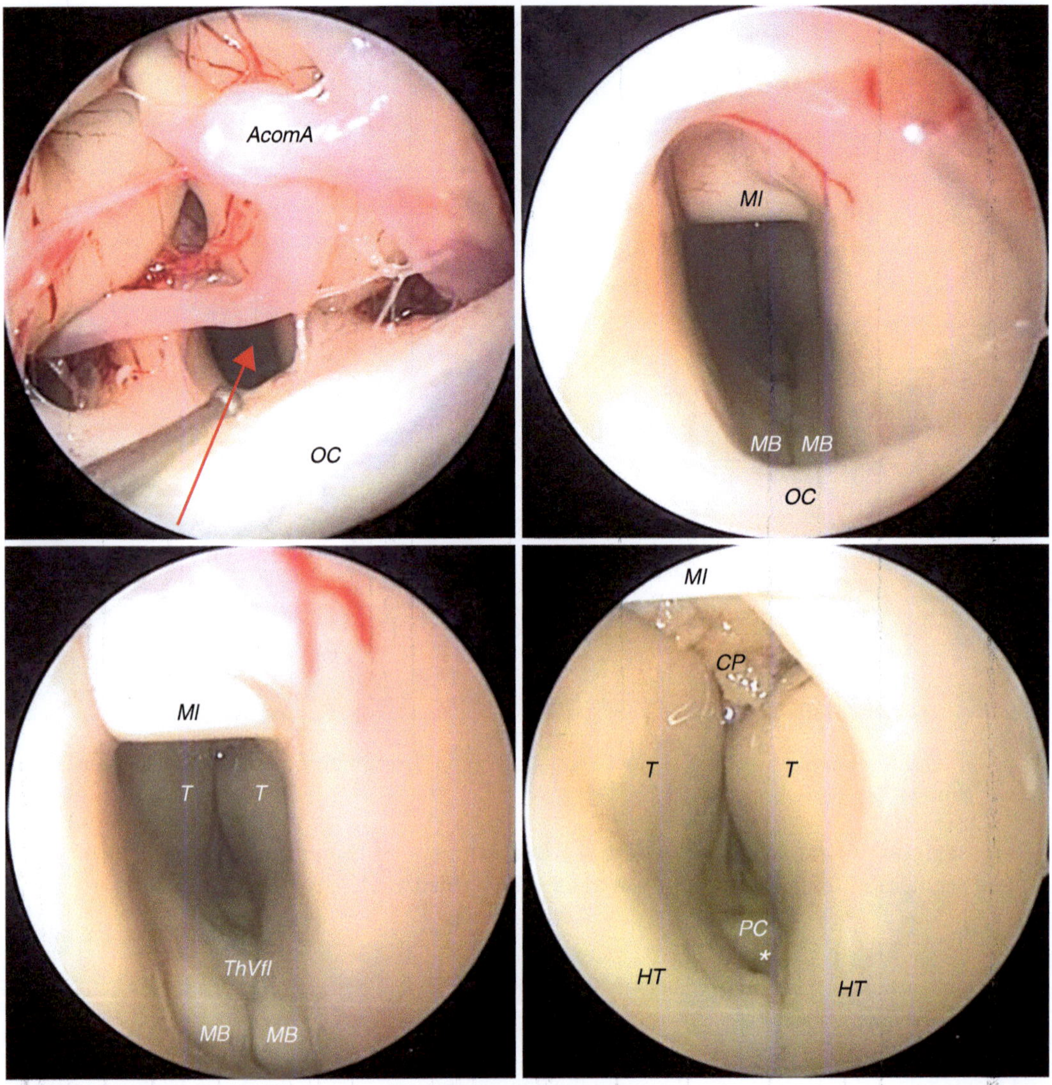

Fig. 3.71 Endoscopic transnasal view of the third ventricle

***AcomA* anterior communicating artery, *CP* choroid plexus, HT hypothalamus, *MB* mammillary bodies, *MI* massa intermedia, *OC* optic chiasm, *PC* posterior commissure, *T* thalamus, *ThVfl* floor of the third ventricle, *white asterisk* opening of the Sylvius aqueduct, *red arrow* front door to the third ventricle**

The anterior wall of the third ventricle is given by the lamina terminalis. The roof of this ventricle is given by the tela choroidea, which presents paired choroid plexuses.

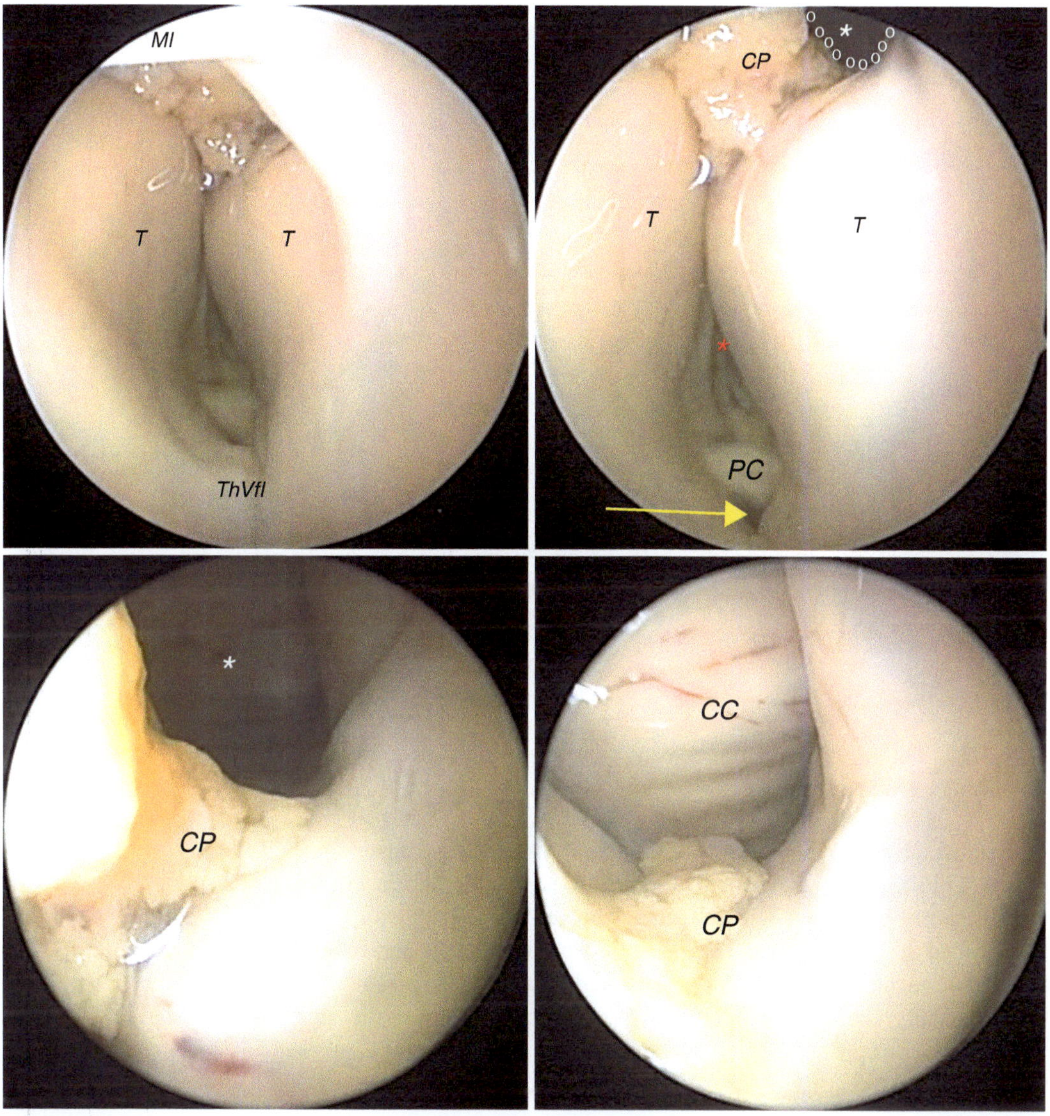

Fig. 3.72 Endoscopic transnasal view of the third ventricle and the lateral ventricles (*left side*)

CC **corpus callosum,** ***CP*** **choroid plexus,** ***MI*** **massa intermedia,** ***PC*** **posterior commissure,** ***T*** **thalamus,** ***ThVfl*** **floor of the third ventricle,** ***yellow arrow*** **opening of the Silvius aqueduct,** ***red asterisk*** **suprapineal recess,** ***white asterisk*** **(*left*) lateral ventricle,** ***white circles*** **foramen of Monro**

Lateral ventricles are located in the cerebral hemispheres. They communicate with the third ventricle by the foramen of Monro.

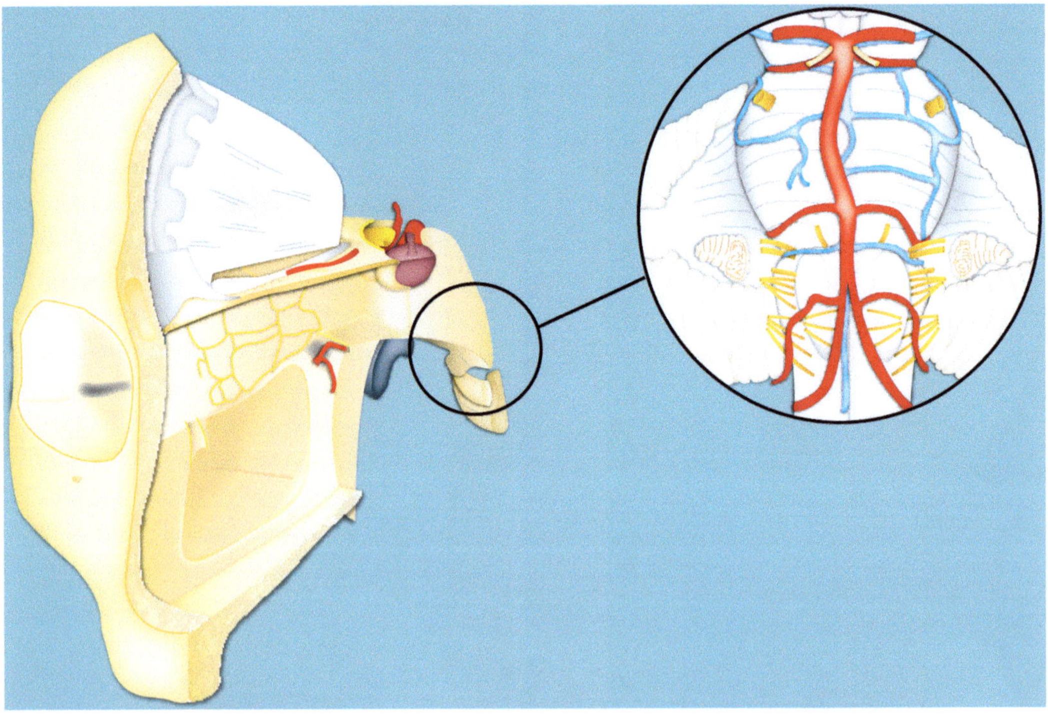

Fig. 3.73 Three-dimensional reconstruction showing the operative window to the posterior cranial fossa and upper spine

Through a clival window, the posterior cranial fossa and the upper spine can be exposed. The lateral limits of this approach are given by the vertical segment of the cavernous internal carotid artery (*ICA*) and inferiorly by the hypoglossal canal. The vertical segments of the cavernous portion of the ICA (also called the paraclival ICA) are separated by a distance of approximately 17 mm (Lang 1995). The "lacerum" segments of the ICA are separated by an average distance of 21 mm (Morera et al. 2010); more caudally, the anterior intercondylar distance (19 mm) represents the limit for the endonasal approach to the upper spine.

The clivus is separated laterally from the petrous part of the temporal bone by the petro-occipital fissure, that is usually filled in adults with cartilaginous tissue (to give a synchondrosis). With age the synchondrosis may ossify and small ossicles may be found (Riolan's ossicles).

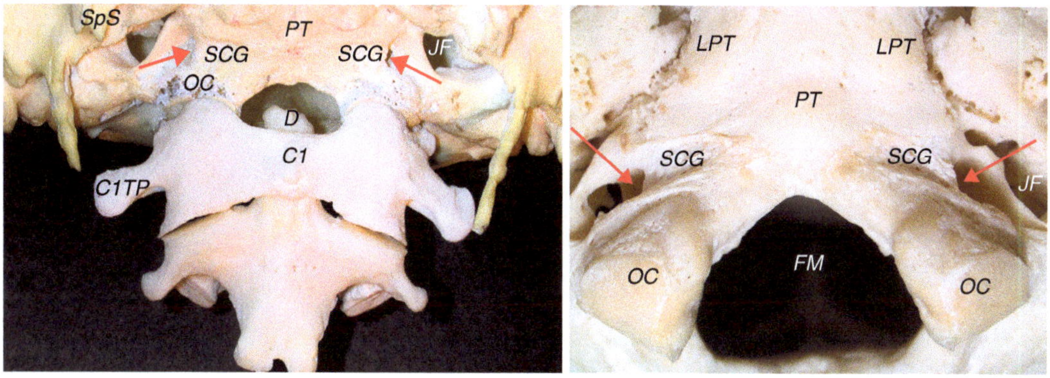

Fig. 3.74 Osteology of the inferior clival and foramen magnum region

C1 **atlas,** ***C1TP*** **transverse process of C1,** ***D*** **dens,** ***FM*** **foramen magnum,** ***JF*** **jugular foramen,** ***LPT*** **lateral pharyngeal tubercle,** ***OC*** **occipital condyle,** ***PT*** **pharyngeal tubercle,** ***SCG*** **supracondylar groove,** ***SpS*** **spine of the sphenoid,** ***red arrows*** **extracranial orifice of the hypoglossal canal**

The SCG represents a reliable landmark for hypoglossal canal (HC) identification (Morera et al. 2010). The HC divides the condylar region into the tubercular compartment (superior) and the condylar compartment (inferior). The tubercular compartment corresponds to the jugular tubercle, and its lateral limit is the medial edge of the JF. It presents a close relationship with cranial nerves IX, X, and XI. The condylar compartment is caudally located with respect to the HC. Anatomically speaking, the OC is in close relationship with the vertebral artery. The HC is about 9 mm above the intradural entry of the vertebral artery (Lang 1995). Rarely, a persistent hypoglossal artery may be present and connect through the HC extracranial segment of the internal carotid artery (*ICA*) with the basilar artery. Arterial branches from the external carotid system (usually from the ascending pharyngeal artery) can be seen passing through the HC.

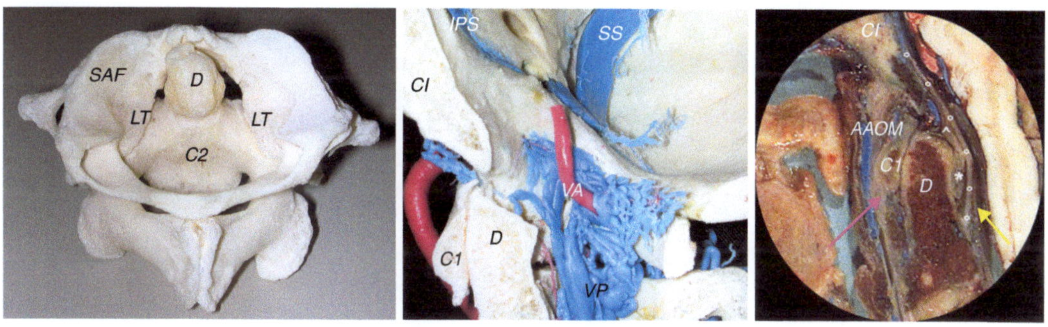

Fig. 3.75 Craniocervical junction: superior and sagittal views

AAOM **anterior atlanto-occipital membrane,** ***Cl*** **clivus,** ***C1*** **atlas,** ***C2*** **axis,** ***D*** **dens,** ***IPS*** **inferior petrosal sinus,** ***LT*** **lateral tubercle,** ***SAF*** **superior articular facet,** ***SS*** **sigmoid sinus,** ***VA*** **vertebral artery,** ***yellow arrow*** **dura,** ***pink arrow*** **anterior atlanto-axial membrane,** ***white asterisk*** **transverse ligament,** ***white arrowhead*** **superior extension of the cruciform ligament,** ***white circles*** **tectorial membrane**

At the level of the craniovertebral junction, the dura is covered by the tectorial membrane, which represents the superior extension of the posterior longitudinal ligament of the spinal canal (Cavallo et al. 2011). The AAOM attaches the anterior aspect of the atlas to the anterior rim of the foramen magnum. It is the anterior wall of the supraodontoid space, which houses alar and apical ligaments as well as fat and veins (Haffajee et al. 2008).

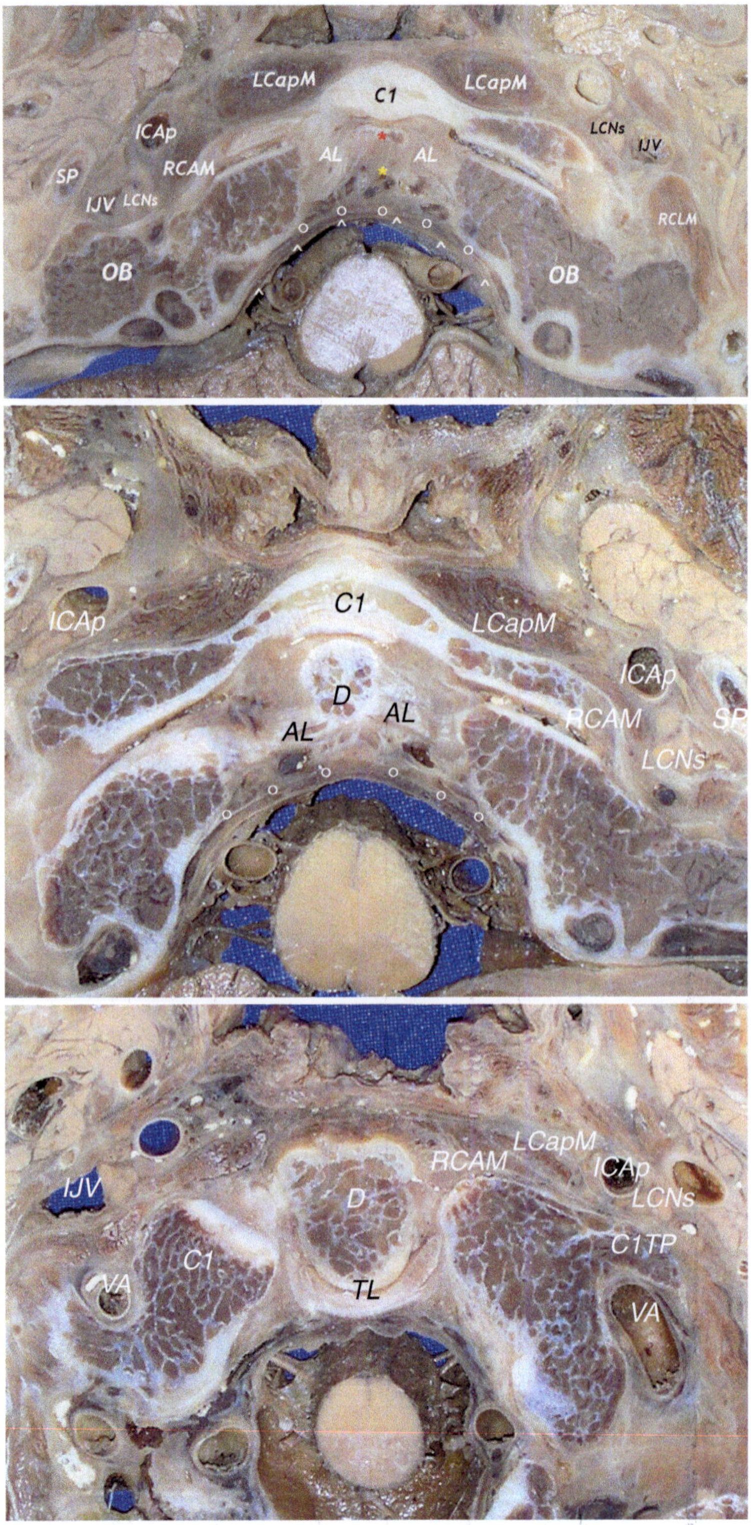

Fig. 3.76 Craniocervical junction: axial views

AL **alar ligament,** ***C1*** **atlas,** ***C1TP*** **transverse process of the atlas,** ***D*** **dens,** ***ICAp*** **parapharyngeal portion of the internal carotid artery,** ***IJV*** **internal jugular vein,** ***LCapM*** **longus capitis muscle,** ***LCNs*** **lower cranial nerves,** ***OB*** **occipital bone,** ***RCAM*** **rectus capitis anterior muscle,** ***RCLM*** **rectus capitis lateralis muscle,** ***SP*** **styloid process,** ***TL*** **transverse ligament,** ***VA*** **vertebral artery,** ***red asterisk*** **cranial portion of the dens,** ***yellow asterisk*** **superior extension of the cruciform ligament,** ***white circles*** **tectorial membrane,** ***white arrow-heads*** **dura mater**

The alar ligaments attach the axis to the base of the skull. The transverse ligament is the most important part of the cruciform ligament. It locks the odontoid process (dens) anteriorly against the posterior aspect of the anterior arch of C1. It attaches to the lateral tubercles of the atlas. The tectorial membrane, epidural fat, and dura are located dorsal to the transverse ligament.

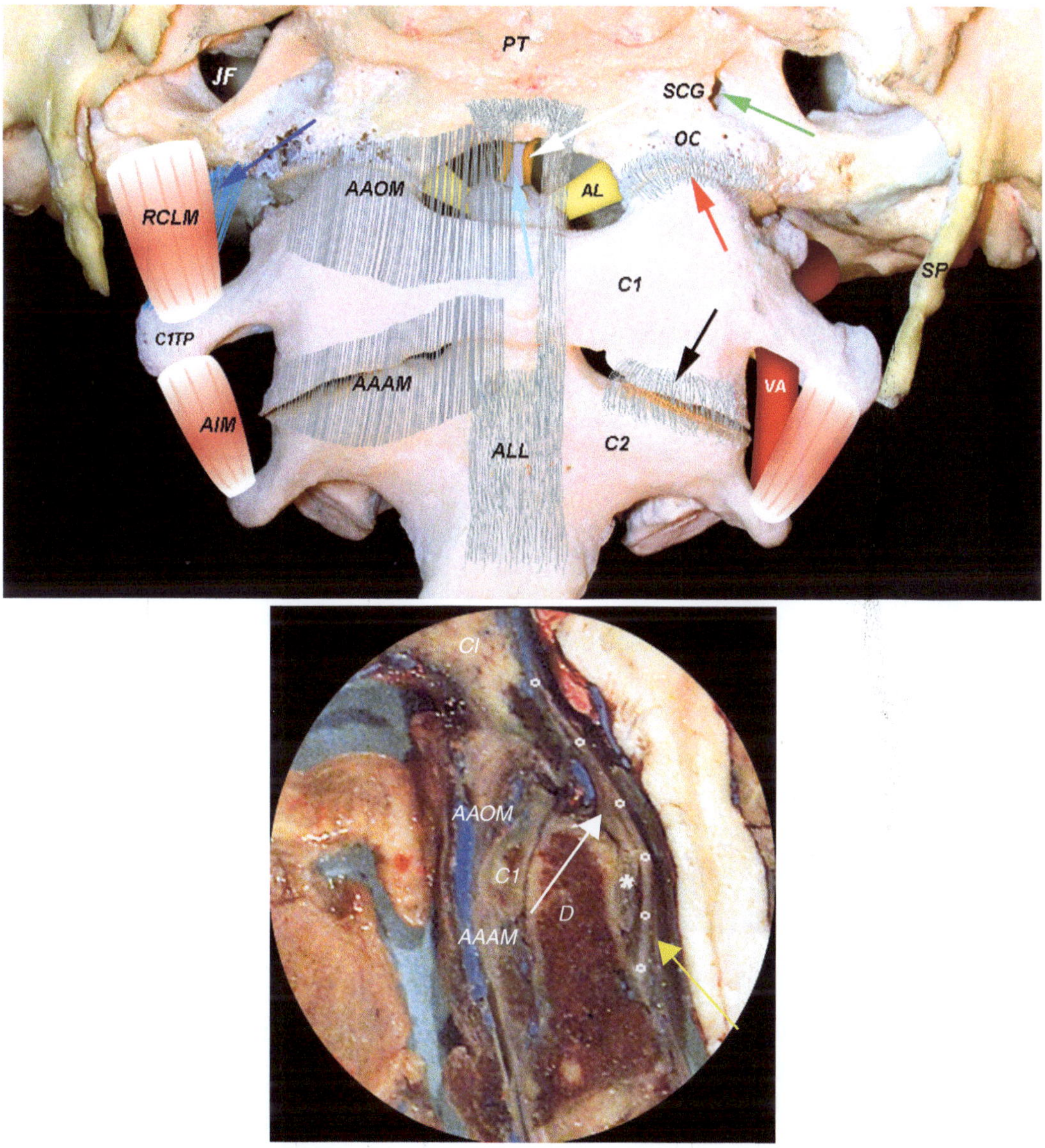

Fig. 3.77 Craniocervical junction

AAAM **anterior atlanto-axial membrane,** ***AAOM*** **anterior atlanto-occipital membrane,** ***AIM*** **anterior intertransversarius muscle,** ***AL*** **alar ligament,** ***ALL*** **anterior longitudinal ligament,** ***Cl*** **clivus,** ***C1*** **atlas,** ***C1TP*** **transverse process of C1,** ***C2*** **axis,** ***D*** **dens,** ***JF*** **jugular foramen,** ***OC*** **occipital condyle,** ***PT*** **pharyngeal tubercle,** ***RCLM*** **rectus capitis lateralis muscle,** ***SCG*** **supracondylar groove,** ***SP*** **styloid process,** ***VA*** **vertebral artery,** ***blue-sky arrow*** **apical ligament,** ***white arrow*** **superior part of the cruciform ligament,** ***green arrow*** **external orifice of hypoglossal canal,** ***black arrow*** **atlantoaxial joint,** ***red arrow*** **atlanto-occipital joint,** ***blue arrow*** **lateral atlanto-occipital ligament,** ***yellow arrow*** **dura of the posterior cranial fossa and upper spine,** ***white asterisk*** **transverse ligament,** ***white circles*** **tectorial membrane**

The tectorial membrane (TM) is a thin structure acting as the posterior border of the supraodontoid space. It presents an intimate relationship with the dura mater (posteriorly) and with the accessory atlanto-axial and cruciform ligaments (anteriorly). TM firmly adheres to the cranial base and body of the axis but not to the posterior aspect of the dens (Tubbs et al. 2011).

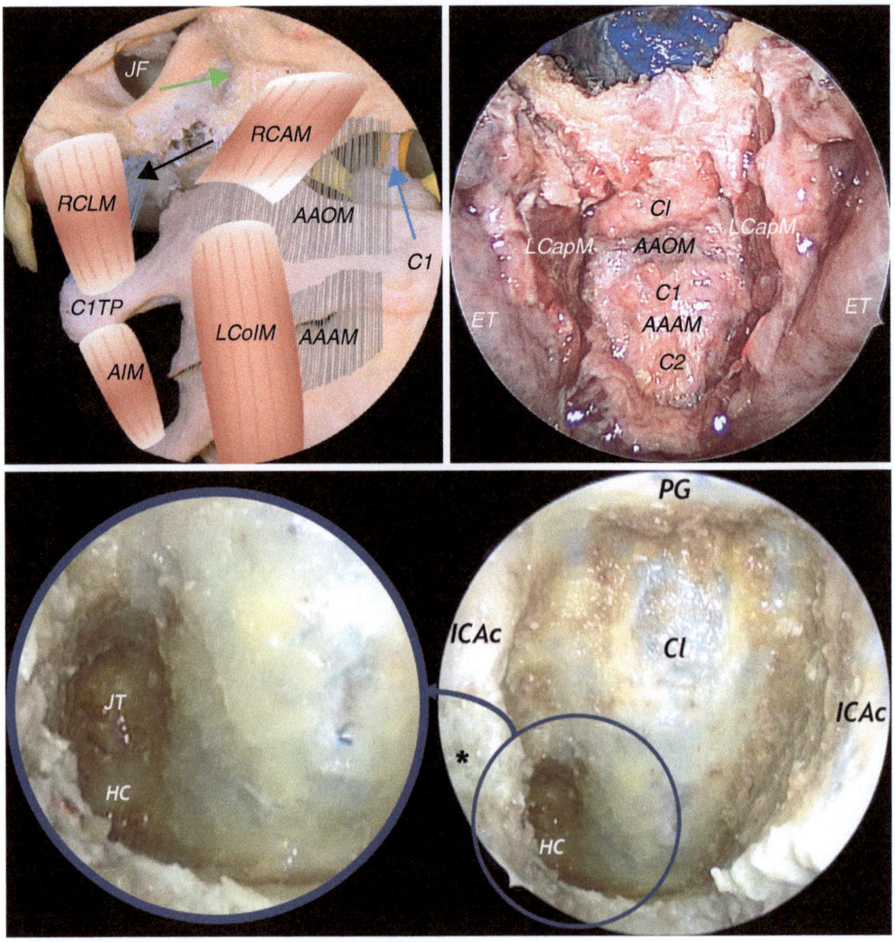

Fig. 3.78 Craniocervical junction

AAAM **anterior atlanto-axial membrane,** ***AAOM*** **anterior atlanto-occipital membrane,** ***AIM*** **anterior intertrasversarius muscle,** ***Cl*** **clivus,** ***C1*** **atlas,** ***C1TP*** **transverse process of C1,** ***C2*** **axis,** ***ET*** **eustachian tube,** ***JF*** **jugular foramen,** ***JT*** **jugular tubercle,** ***HC*** **hypoglossal canal,** ***ICAc*** **cavernous portion of the internal carotid artery,** ***LCapM*** **longus capitis muscle,** ***LColM*** **longus colli muscle,** ***PG*** **pituitary gland,** ***RCAM*** **rectus capitis anterior muscle,** ***RCLM*** **rectus capitis lateralis muscle,** ***blue-sky arrow*** **apical ligament,** ***green arrow*** **external orifice of the hypoglossal canal,** ***black arrow*** **lateral atlanto-occipital ligament,** ***black asterisk*** **foramen lacerum**

The foramen lacerum (FL) is located lateral to the floor of the sphenoid sinus at the level of the spheno-petro-clival confuence. In respect to the FL, the JT is postero-medially located. Therefore to access the jugular tubercle from anteriorly a complete exposure of the foramen lacerum is needed. The hypoglossal canal forms the inferior limit of the jugular tubercle, while the inferior petrosal sinus forms the supero-lateral limit (Fernandez-Miranda et al. 2012).

The longus capitis and rectus capitis anterior muscle attach on the inferior surface of the clivus. Below the RCAM the occipito-cervical joint capsule lies. The area of attachement of the RCAM has been named inferior clival line (Fernandez-Miranda et al. 2012) and correspond to the supracondylar groove (that is a landmark for the hypoglossal canal).

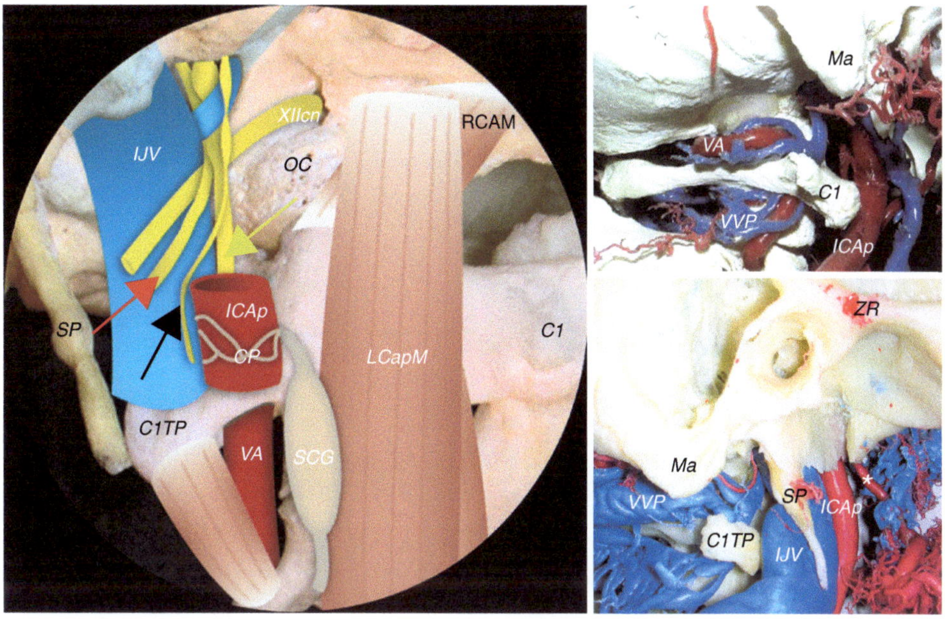

Fig. 3.79 Craniocervical junction

CP **sympathetic carotid plexus,** ***C1*** **atlas,** ***C1TP*** **transverse process of C1,** ***ICAp*** **parapharyngeal portion of the internal carotid artery,** ***IJV*** **internal jugular vein,** ***LCapM*** **longus capitis muscle,** ***Ma*** **mastoid (tip),** ***OC*** **occipital condyle,** ***RCAM*** **rectus capitis anterior muscle,** ***SCG*** **superior cervical ganglion,** ***SP*** **styloid process,** ***VA*** **vertebral artery,** ***VVP*** **vertebral venous plexus,** ***ZR*** **zygomatic root,** ***XIIcn*** **hypoglossal nerve,** ***yellow arrow*** **vagus nerve,** ***red arrow*** **accessory nerve,** ***black arrow*** **glossopharyngeal nerve,** ***white asterisk*** **middle meningeal artery**

The VAs pass through the transverse foramina of the first six vertebrae and exit from the transverse foramen of C1, running backward and medially over the posterior arch of C1, and pierce the posterior atlanto-occipital membrane and the spinal dura. They are surrounded extracranially by a venous plexus that does not enter the intradural space.

The VA, at the level of the transverse process of the atlas, is located on the medial side of the rectus capitis lateralis muscle. The extradural segment of VA gives rise to posterior meningeal and posterior spinal arteries and branches to the deep cervical muscles.

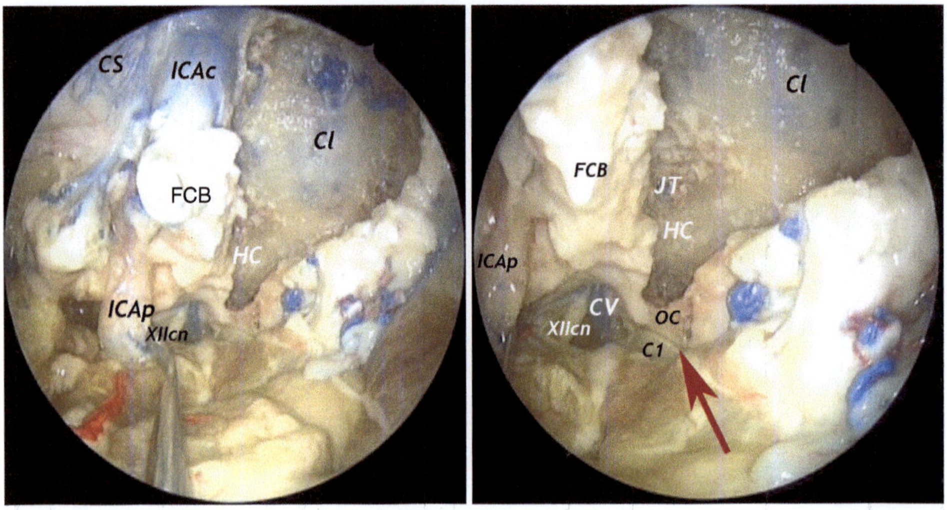

Fig. 3.80 Endoscopic endonasal views of the hypoglossal canal and nerve (extracranial segment)

***C1* atlas, *Cl* clivus, *CS* cavernous sinus, *CV* condylar vein, *FCB* fibrocartilago basalis, *HC* hypoglossal canal, *ICAc* cavernous portion of the internal carotid artery, *ICAp* parapharyngeal portion of the internal carotid artery, *JT* jugular tubercle, *OC* occipital condyle, *XIIcn* hypoglossal nerve, *violet arrow* atlanto-occipital joint**

The JT is bordered supero-laterally by the inferior petrosal sinus and inferiorly by the hypoglossal canal. From an anterior perspective the medial aspect of the JT is placed postero-medially to the lower portion of the foramen lacerum, filled by the FCB (Fernandez-Miranda et al. 2012). The hypoglossal nerve exits from the hypoglossal canal medial to the ICAp. It lies posteriorly to the vagus nerve and passes laterally between the internal jugular vein and ICAp. The hypoglossal nerve is usually accompained, within the hypoglossal canal, by an emissary vein and arterial branches from ascending pharyngeal artery and occipital artery.

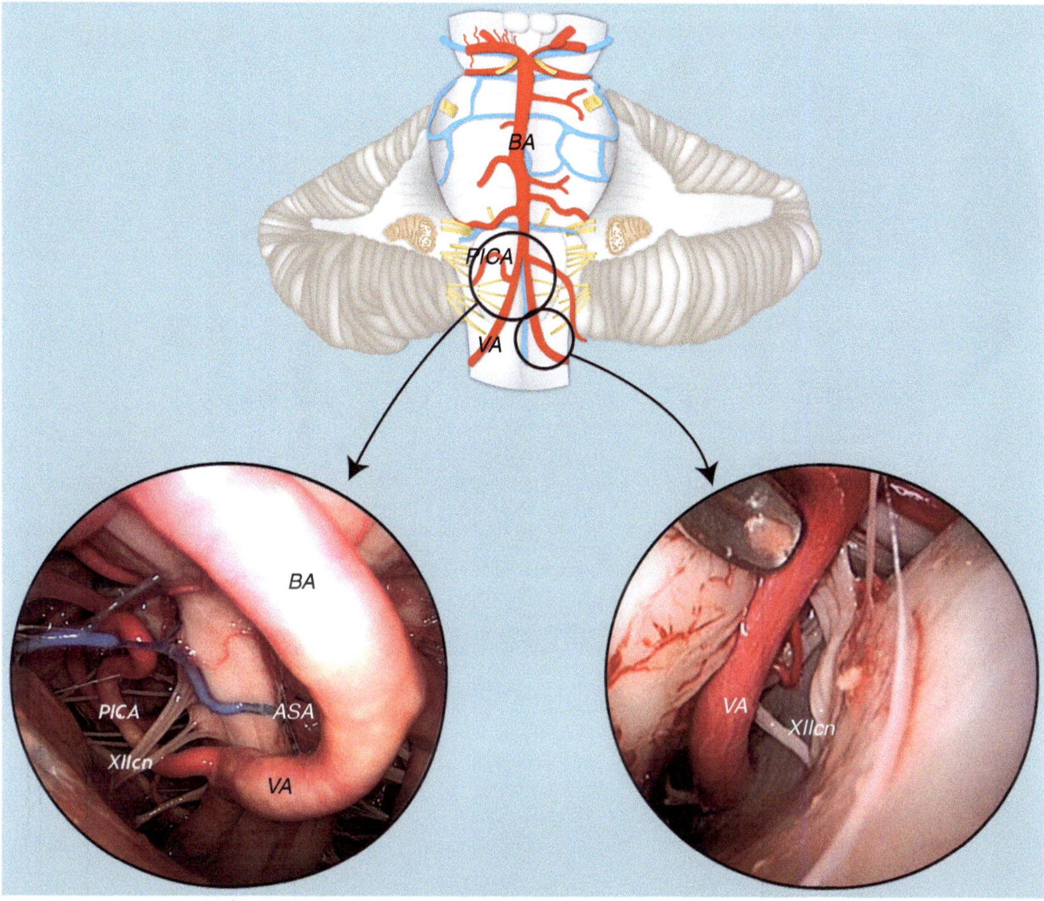

Fig. 3.81 Endoscopic view of the medulla oblongata and upper spine regions

***ASA* anterior spinal artery, *BA* basilar artery, *PICA* posteroinferior cerebellar artery, *VA* vertebral artery, *XIIcn* hypoglossal nerve**

The most important arteries in relationship with the craniocervical junction are the vertebral artery, the posteroinferior cerebellar artery, and the anterior spinal artery. In about 4 % of cases, PICA presents an extradural origin, at the level of the pars atlantis of the VA (Lang 1995). The intradural segment of the VA is crossed by the XIIcn.

The paired anterior spinal arteries arise from VAs and join to form a single trunk (in front of spinal cord). In most cases the junction of the spinal arteries is above the level of the foramen magnum (Rhoton 2003).

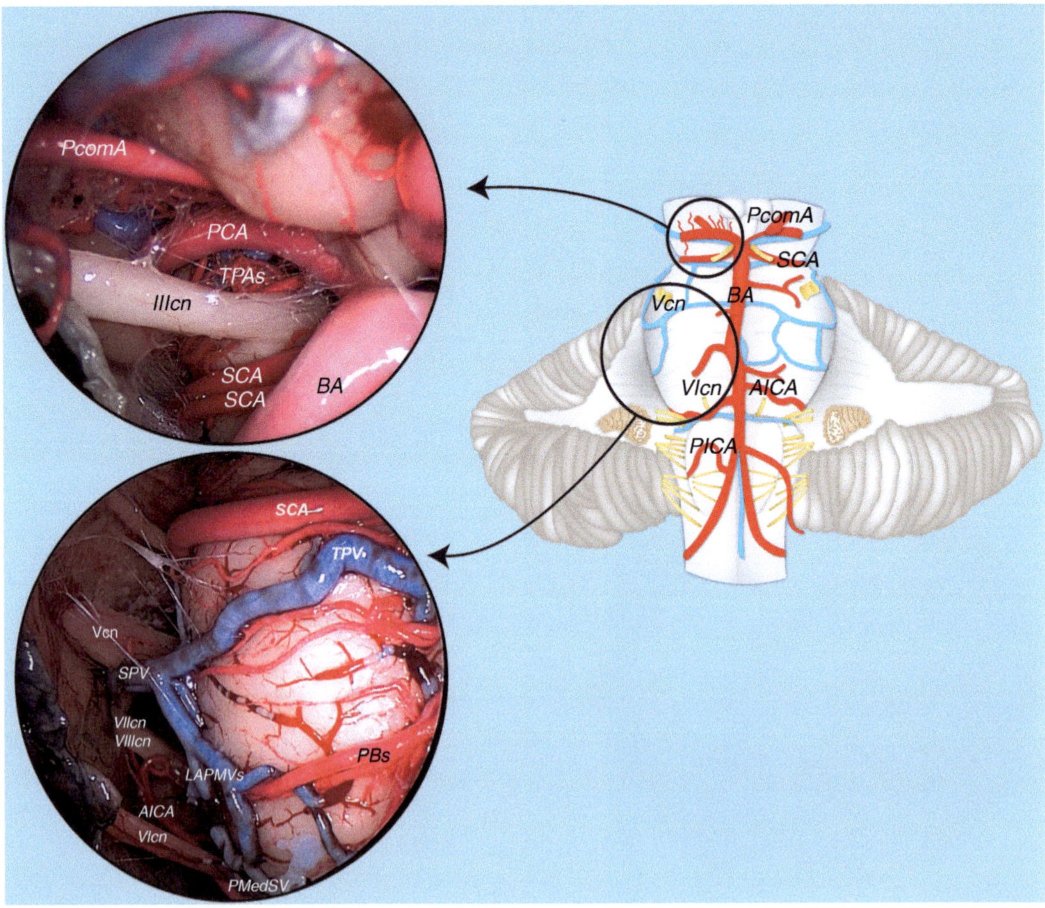

Fig. 3.82 Posterior cranial fossa (pontomesencephalic region); vision obtained with a 45° endoscope through a clival window

AICA **anteroinferior cerebellar artery,** ***BA*** **basilar artery,** ***LPMVN*** **lateropontomesencephalic venous network,** ***PBs*** **pontine branches,** ***PcomA*** **posterior communicating artery,** ***PICA*** **postero-inferior cerebellar artery,** ***PMedSV*** **pontomedullary sulcus vein,** ***SCA*** **superior cerebellar artery,** ***SPV*** **superior petrosal vein,** ***TPAs*** **talamoperforating arteries,** ***TPV*** **transverse pontine vein,** ***IIIcn*** **oculomotor nerve,** ***Vcn*** **trigeminal nerve,** ***VIcn*** **abducens nerve,** ***VIIcn*** **facial nerve,** ***VIIIcn*** **vestibulo-cochlear (statoacoustic) nerve**

The SCA courses posteriorly around the cerebral peduncles or the upper border of the pons.

The BA, PcomA, first segment of PCA and the oculomotor nerve are evident in the interpeduncolar cistern. This cistern is bordered by the cerebral peduncles and the leaves of the Liliequist's membrane (LM). The posterior wall of the cistern is given by the posterior perforated substance and the upper border at the level of the posterior edge of the mammillary bodies. The lower border is the junction of the midbrain and pons.

Below the interpeduncolar cistern stays the prepontine cistern, that is bordered anteriorly by the clivus and posteriorly by the pons. It is separated from the interpeduncolar cistern by the mesencephalic leaf of LM.

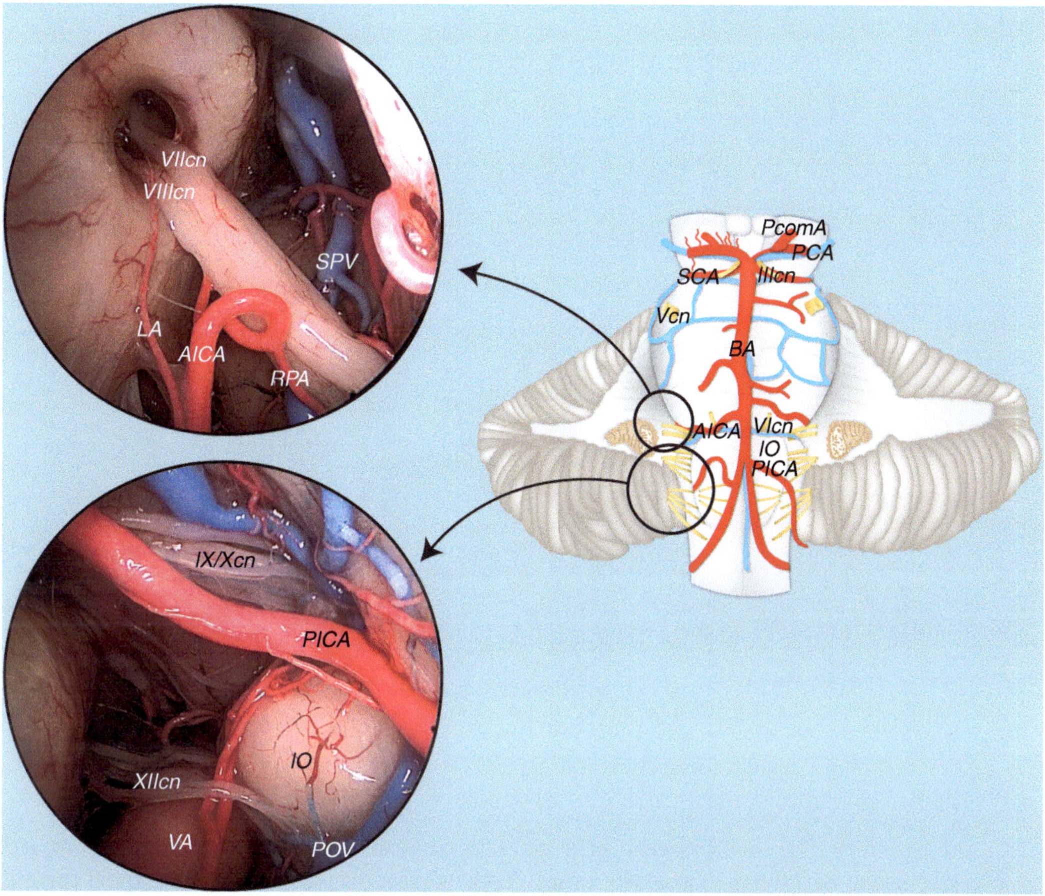

Fig. 3.83 Posterior cranial fossa (jugular and hypoglossal areas); vision obtained with a 45° endoscope through a clival window

***AICA* anteroinferior cerebellar artery, *BA* basilar artery, *IO* inferior olive, *LA* labyrinthine artery, *PCA* posterior cerebral artery, *PcomA* posterior communicating artery, *PICA* posteroinferior cerebellar artery, *POV* preolivary vein, *RPA* recurrent perforating artery, *SCA* superior cerebellar artery, *SPV* superior petrosal vein, *VA* vertebral artery, *IIIcn* oculomotor nerve, *Vcn* trigeminal nerve, *VIcn* abducens nerve, *VIIcn* facial nerve, *VIIIcn* vestiboloacoustic (statoacoustic) nerve, *IXcn* glossopharyngeal nerve, *Xcn* vagus nerve, *XIIcn* hypoglossal nerve**

The LA usually originates from the AICA, rarely directly from the BA. It feeds the inner ear.

AICA and SCA course through the cerebellopontine cistern. AICA enters the lower part of cerebellopontine cistern and it usually bifurcates into its rostral and caudal trunks within the cistern. PICA origins from the VA, near the inferior olive, and passes posteriorly around the medulla. It could pass rostral, caudal or even between the rootlets of the hypoglossal nerve.

RPA(s) are arteries that present a recurrent course and reach the root entry zone of the VII and VIII cns. They send branches to these nerves and to the brainsterm around the root entry zone.

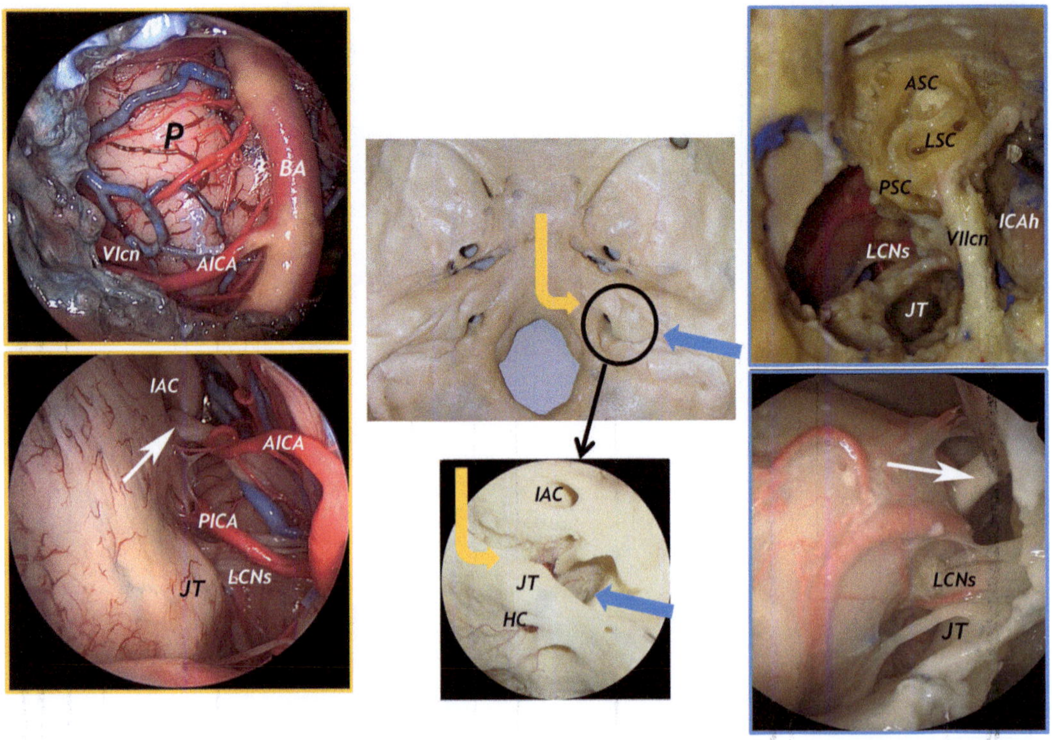

Fig. 3.84 Intracranial jugular foramen region

AICA **antero-inferior cerebellar artery,** ***ASC*** **anterior semicircular canal,** ***BA*** **basilar artery,** ***HC*** **hypoglossal canal,** ***IAC*** **internal acoustic canal,** ***ICAh*** **horizontal portion of the internal carotid artery,** ***JT*** **jugular tubercle,** ***LCNs*** **lower cranial nerves,** ***LSC*** **lateral semicircular canal,** ***P*** **pons,** ***PICA*** **postero-inferior cerebellar artery,** ***PSC*** **posterior semicircular canal,** ***VIcn*** **abducens nerve,** ***VIIcn*** **facial nerve,** ***white arrow*** **vestibolocochlear nerve**

The upper surface of the jugular process of the occipital bone presents an oval prominence named jugular tubercle. It is placed superomedially to the JF and above the hypoglossal canal (Rhoton 2003). The glossopharyngeal, vagus and accessory nerves (LCNs) penetrate the dura on the medial side of the intrajugular process of the temporal bone. In the cerebello-medullary cistern the LCNs cross the posterior surface of the JT on their way to JF (Fernandez-Miranda et al. 2012).

Arterial branches from the ascending pharyngeal and occipital arteries pass through the JF and HC.

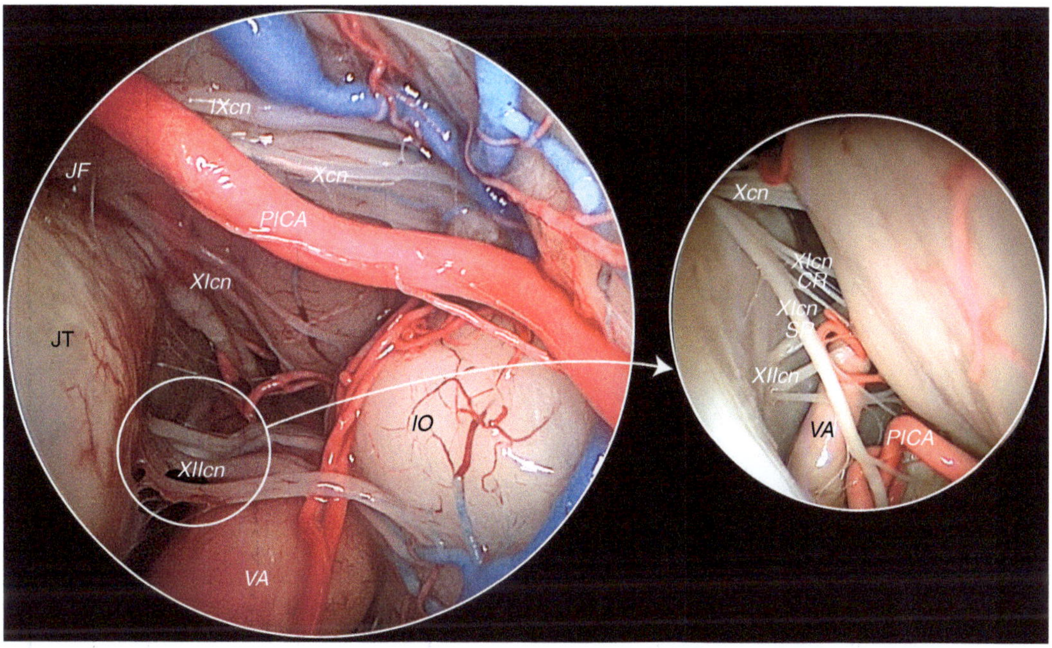

Fig. 3.85 Intracranial hypoglossal region. Anterior endoscopic transnasal-transclival vision is compared with a posterior retrosigmoid endoscopic one

***JF* jugular foramen, *JT* jugular tubercle, *IO* inferior olive, *PICA* posteroinferior cerebellar artery, *VA* vertebral artery, *IXcn* glossopharygeal nerve, *Xcn* vagus nerve, *XIcnCR* cervical roots of accessory nerve, *XIcnSR* spinal roots of accessory nerve, *XIIcn* hypoglossal nerve**

Cranial nerves IX and X present a close relationship with the first portion of the PICA. They are protected by the arachnoid membrane (Roche et al. 2008). The roots of cranial nerve XIcn from the spine pass through the foramen magnum posterior to the vertebral artery. Within the hypoglossal canal, XIIcn is surrounded by a venous plexus and dural and arachnoid sheets. Branches of the ascending pharyngeal artery coursing through the hypoglossal canal are seen in about 50 % of cases (Lang 1995). Also branches from the posterior meningeal artery have been described (Janfaza and Nadol 2001). The transcisternal vein to the area of the JF can be seen. Also, veins to the hypoglossal canal can be present. The hypoglossal nerve do not exit with VA. It can have maximum 3 outlets. On the contrary, C1 roots exit with the VA.

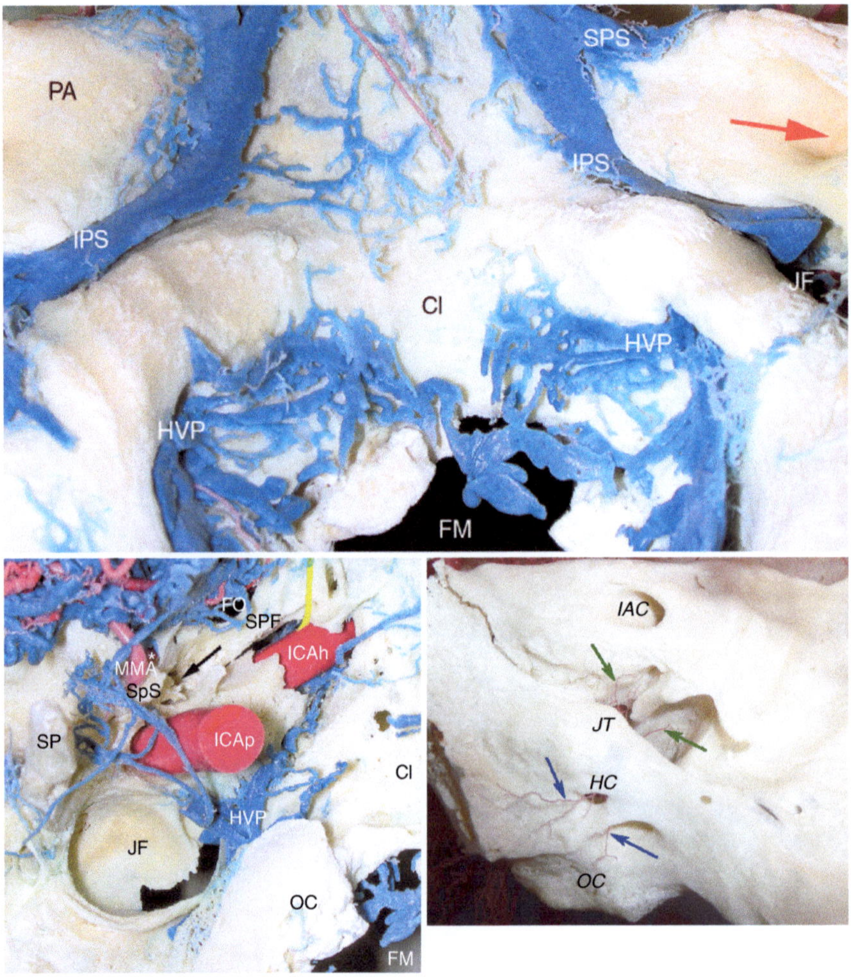

Fig. 3.86 Endocranial and esocranial views of dry skull: jugular foramen and hypoglossal regions

Cl **clivus,** ***FM*** **foramen magnum,** ***FO*** **foramen ovale,** ***HC*** **hypoglossal canal,** ***HVP*** **hypoglossal venous plexus,** ***JF*** **jugular foramen,** ***JT*** **jugular tubercle,** ***IAC*** **internal acoustic canal,** ***ICAh*** **horizontal portion of the internal carotid artery,** ***ICAp*** **parapharyngeal portion of the internal carotid artery,** ***IPS*** **inferior petrosal sinus,** ***MMA*** **middle meningeal artery,** ***OC*** **occipital condyle,** ***PA*** **petrous apex,** ***SP*** **styloid process,** ***SPF*** **sphenopetrosal fissure,** ***SPS*** **superior petrosal sinus,** ***SpS*** **spine of the sphenoid,** ***black arrow*** **position of the bony tube,** ***red arrow*** **internal acoustic meatus,** ***blue arrows*** **arteries passing through the hypoglossal canal,** ***dark green arrows*** **arteries passing through the jugular foramen,** ***white asterisk*** **foramen spinosum**

The IPS usually connects the cavernous sinus (CS) to the bulb of the internal jugular vein (IJV). Rarely (10 %), it drains in the IJV below the cranial base and not in the jugular bulb. In these cases IPS passes usually through a foramen present in the petro-occipital fissure. Passing through the JF, it is usually between cranial nerves IX and X. Usually, the IPS passes beneath the superior petro-sphenoidal ligament (l. of Gruber) with the abducens nerve. The SPS connects the CS to the sigmoid sinus. Most commonly, it passes superiorly to the opening of the Meckel's cave, but sometimes can be inferior to it, or it can even split and surround it. The basilar plexus is located between periosteum and dura at the level of the clivus. The HVP communicates with the JF venous channel in the JF area. Through the posterior condylar canal passes an emissary vein joining the sigmoid sinus and the suboccipital venous plexus.

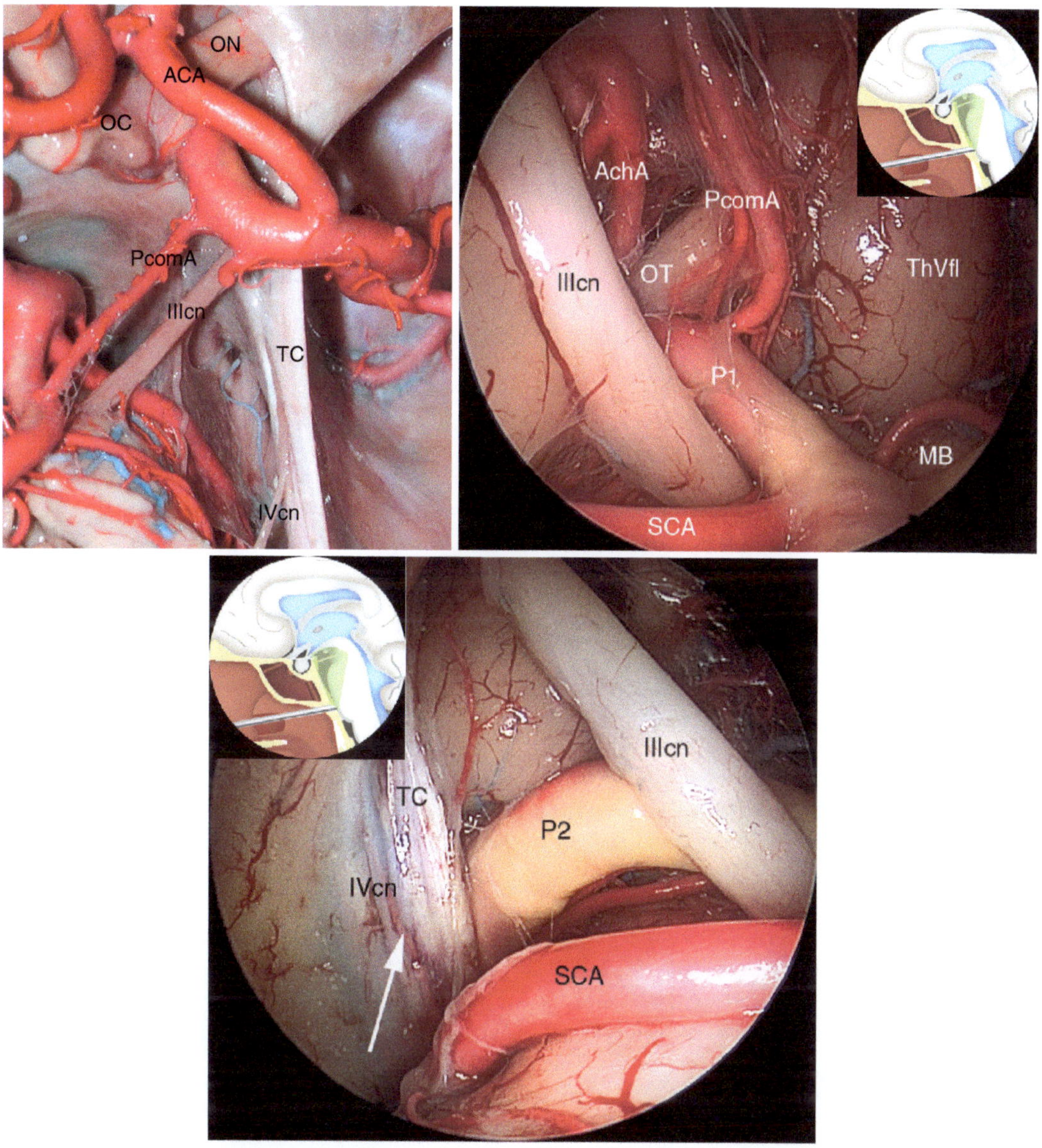

Fig. 3.87 Tentorial region: superior view and endoscopic transclival views obtained with a 45° up-facing scope

ACA **anterior cerebral artery,** ***AchA*** **anterior choroidal artery,** ***MB*** **mammillary body,** ***OC*** **optic chiasm,** ***ON*** **optic nerve,** ***OT*** **optic tract,** ***PcomA*** **posterior communicating artery,** ***P1*** **first segment of the posterior cerebral artery,** ***P2*** **second segment of the posterior cerebral artery,** ***SCA*** **superior cerebellar artery,** ***TC*** **tentorium cerebelli,** ***ThVfl*** **floor of the third ventricle,** ***IIIcn*** **oculomotor nerve,** ***IVcn*** **trochlear nerve,** ***white arrow*** **a tentorial artery**

The TC separates the convex upper surface of the cerebellum from the posterior portions of both the cerebral hemispheres. It attaches to the posterior clinoid process, the superior border of the petrous ridge, and the sulci for the lateral sinuses. The PcomA courses posteromedially below the floor of the third ventricle. From its superior and lateral surface, several perforators penetrate the floor of the third ventricle between the optic chiasm and the cerebral peduncle. The TC, with the trochlear nerve inside, can be visualized passing inferiorly to the IIIcn.

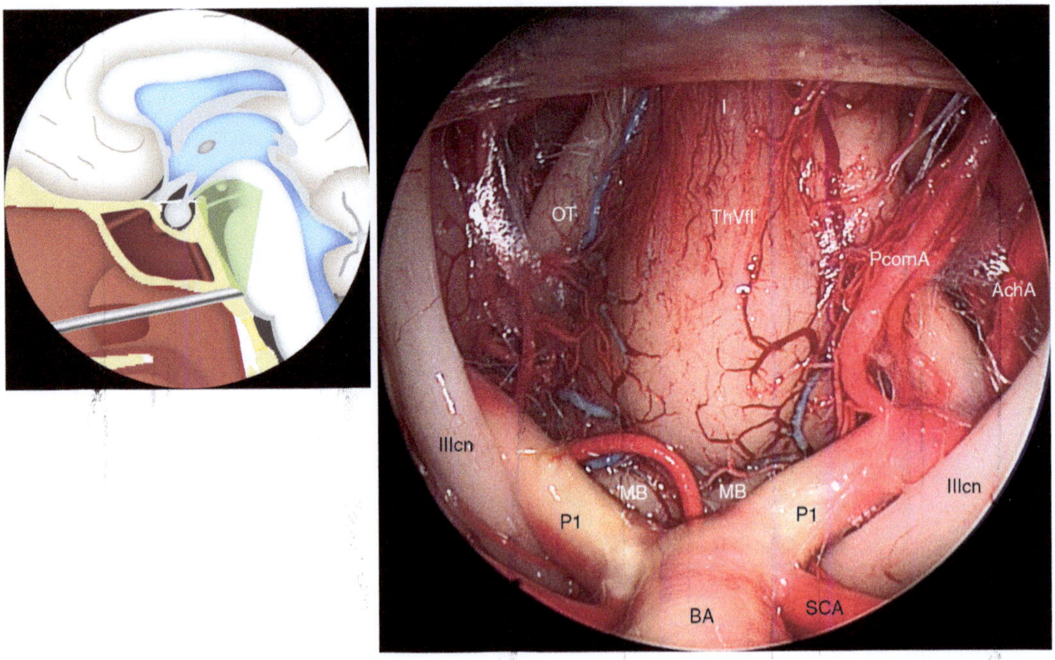

Fig. 3.88 Endoscopic view of the floor of the third ventricle. The dorsum sellae and the upper brain stem region are evident. Vision obtained through a clival window using a 45° up-facing scope

AchA **anterior choroidal artery,** ***BA*** **basilar artery,** ***MB*** **mammillary body,** ***OT*** **optic tract,** ***PcomA*** **posterior communicating artery,** ***P1*** **first segment of the posterior cerebral artery,** ***SCA*** **superior cerebellar artery,** ***ThVfl*** **floor of the third ventricle,** ***IIIcn*** **oculomotor nerve**

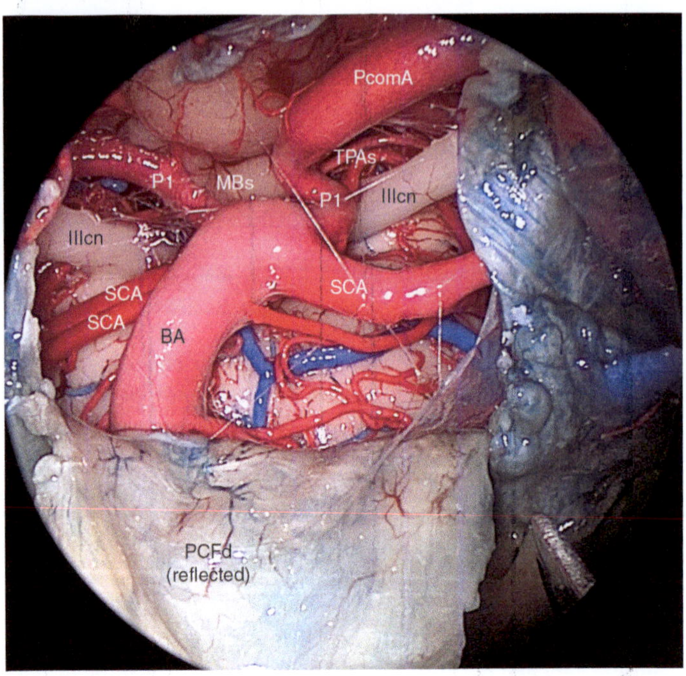

Fig. 3.89 Basilar apex region. Vision obtained after pituitary transposition

BA **basilar artery,** ***MBs*** **mammillary bodies,** ***PCFd*** **posterior cranial fossa dura,** ***PcomA*** **posterior communicating artery,** ***P1*** **first segment of the posterior cerebral artery,** ***SCA*** **superior cerebellar artery,** ***TPAs*** **talamoperforating arteries,** ***IIIcn*** **oculomotor nerve**

References

Abuzayed B, Tanriover N, Akar Z et al (2010) Extended endoscopic endonasal approach to the suprasellar parachiasmatic cisterns: anatomic study. Childs Nerv Syst 26:1161–1170

Amin SM, Nasr AY, Saleh HA et al (2010) Endoscopic orientation of the parasellar region in sphenoid sinus with ill-defined bony landmarks: an anatomic study. Skull Base 20:421–428

Barges-Coll J, Fernandez-Miranda JC, Prevedello DM et al (2010) Avoiding injury to the abducens nerve during expanded endonasal endoscopic surgery: anatomic and clinical case studies. Neurosurgery 67:144–154

Cavallo LM, Esposito I, De Notaris M et al (2011) Endoscopic anatomy of the clivus and posterior fossa. In: Stamm AC (ed) Transnasal endoscopic skull base and brain surgery. Tips and pearls. Thieme, New York

Conti M, Prevedello DM, Madhok R et al (2008) The antero-medial triangle: the risk for cranial nerve ischemia at the cavernous sinus lateral wall. Anatomic cadaveric study. Clin Neurol Neurosurg 110:682–686

Dallan I, Castelnuovo P, De Notaris M et al (2013) Endoscopic endonasal anatomy of the superior orbital fissure and orbital apex regions: critical considerations for clinical applications. Eur Arch Otorhinolaryngol 270:1643–1649

D'Avella E, Tschabitscher M, Santoro A et al (2008) Blood supply to the intracavernous cranial nerves: comparison of the endoscopic and microsurgical perspectives. Neurosurgery 62(Suppl 2):305–311

Dolenc VV (1989) Anatomy and surgery of the cavernous sinus. Springer, New York

Fernandez-Miranda JC, MoreraVA, Snyderman CH et al (2012) Endoscopic endonasal transclival approach to the jugular tubercle. neurosurgery 71(Suppl 1):146–159

Fields WS (1968) The significance of persistent trigeminal artery. Carotid-basilar anastomosis. Radiology 91: 1095–1101

Froelich S, Abdel Aziz KM, van Loveren HR et al (2009) The transition between the cavernous sinus and orbit. In: Dolenc V, Rogers L (eds) Cavernous sinus. Springer, Vienna

Haffajee MR, Thomson C, Govender S (2008) The supraodontoid space or "apical cave" at the craniocervical junction: a microdissection study. Clin Anat 21:404–415

Herzallah IR, Casiano RR (2007) Endoscopic endonasal study of the internal carotid artery and variations. Am J Rhinol 21:262–270

Iaconetta G, Tessitore E, Samii M (2001) Duplicated abducens nerve and its course: microanatomical study and surgery-related considerations. J Neurosurg 95:853–858

Iaconetta G, de Notaris M, Benet A et al (2012) The trochlear nerve: microanatomic and endoscopic study. Neurosurg Rev PMID 23065103

Inoue T, Rhoton AL Jr, Theele D et al (1990) Surgical approaches to the cavernous sinus: a microsurgical study. Neurosurgery 26:903–932

Isaacs SJ, Goyal P (2007) Endoscopic anatomy of the pterygopalatine fossa. Am J Rhinol 21:644–647

Isolan G, de Oliveira E, Mattos LP (2005) Microsurgical anatomy of the arterial compartment of the cavernous sinus. Arq Neuropsiquiatr 63:259–264

Janfaza P, Montgomery WW (2001) Pterygomaxillary (pterygopalatine) fossa and the autonomic nervous system. In: Janfaza P, Nadol JB Jr, Galla R, Fabian RL, Montgomery WW (eds) Surgical anatomy of the head and neck. Lippincott Williams & Wilkins, Philadelphia

Janfaza P, Nadol JB Jr (2001) Scalp, cranium, and brain. In: Janfaza P, Nadol JB Jr, Galla R, Fabian RL, Montgomery WW (eds) Surgical anatomy of the head and neck. Lippincott Williams & Wilkins, Philadelphia

Janfaza P, Rubin PAD, Azar N (2001) Orbit. In: Janfaza P, Nadol JB Jr, Galla R, Fabian RL, Montgomery WW (eds) Surgical anatomy of the head and neck. Lippincott Williams & Wilkins, Philadelphia

Jinkins JR (2000) Atlas of neuroradiologic embryology, anatomy, and variants. Lippincott Williams & Wilkins, Philadelphia

Jittapiromsak P, Sabuncuoglu H, Deshmukh P et al (2010) Anatomical relationship of intracavernous internal carotid artery to intracavernous neural structures. Skull Base 20:327–336

Krisht A, Barnett DW, Barrow DL et al (1994) The blood supply of the intracavernous cranial nerves: an anatomic study. Neurosurgery 34:275–279

Labib MA, Prevedello DM, Fernandez-Miranda JC et al (2013) The medial opticocarotid recess: an anatomical study of an endoscopic "key landmark" to ventral cranial base. Neurosurgery 72(1 Suppl Operative):66–76

Lang J (1995) Skull base and related structures: atlas of clinical anatomy. Schattauer, Stuttgart

Lasjaunias PL (1981) Craniofacial and upper cervical arteries: functional, clinical and angiographic aspects. Lippincott Williams & Wilkins, Baltimore

Lasjaunias P, Moret J, Mik J (1977) The anatomy of the inferolateral trunk (ILT) of the internal carotid artery. Neuroradiology 13:215–220

Martins C, de Alencastro LF, Cardoso ACC et al (2011) Anatomy of the nasal cavity and paranasal sinuses. In: Stamm AC (ed) Transnasal endoscopic skull base and brain surgery. Tips and pearls. Thieme, New York

Martins C, Yasuda A, Campero A et al (2011) Microsurgical and endoscopic anatomy of the parasellar region. In: Stamm AC (ed) Transnasal endoscopic skull base and brain surgery. Tips and pearls. Thieme. New York

McCormick WF (1969) Vascular disorder of nervous tissue: anomalies, malformations and aneurisms. The structure and function of nervous tissue. In: Bourne GH (ed) Biochemistry and disease. Academic Press, New York

Morera VA, Fernandez-Miranda JC, Prevedello DM et al (2010) "Far-medial" expanded endonasal approach to the inferior third of the clivus: the transcondylar and transjugular tubercle approaches. Neurosurgery 66(6 Suppl Operative):211–219

Nathan H, Ouaknine G, Kosary IZ (1974) The abducens nerve: anatomical variations in its course. J Neurosurg 41:561–566

Ozveren MF, Sam B, Akdemir I et al (2003) Duplication of the abducens nerve at the petroclival region: an anatomic study. Neurosurgery 52:645–652

Parkinson D (1964) Collateral circulation of cavernous carotid artery: anatomy. Can J Surg 7:251–268

Parkinson D (1990) Surgical anatomy of the lateral sellar compartment (cavernous sinus). Clin Neurosurg 36:219–239

Perlmutter D, Rhoton AL Jr (1976) Microsurgical anatomy of the anterior cerebral-anterior communicating-recurrent artery complex. J Neurosurg 45:259–272

Reisch R, Vutskits FR et al (2002) Topographic microsurgical anatomy of the paraclinoid carotid artery. Neurosurg Rev 25:177–183

Rhoton AL Jr (2002) The cavernous sinus, the cavernous venous plexus and carotid collar. Neurosurgery 51(Suppl 1):375–410

Rhoton AL Jr (2003) Cranial anatomy and surgical approaches. Lippincott Williams & Wilkins, Philadelphia

Roche PH, Mercier P, Sameshima T et al (2008) Surgical anatomy of the jugular foramen. Adv Tech Stand Neurosurg 33:233–263

Sabanci PA, Batay F, Civelek E et al (2011) Meckel's cave. World Neurosurg 76(3–4):335–341

Salas E, Ziyal IM, Sekhar LN et al (1998) Persistent trigeminal artery: an anatomic study. Neurosurgery 43:557–561

Silver JM, Wilkins RH (1991) Persistent embryonic intracranial and extracranial vessels. In: Wilkins RH, Rengachary SS (eds) Neurosurgery update II vascular, spinal, pediatric, and functional neurosurgery. McGraw-Hill, New York

Suttner N, Mura J, Tedeschi H et al (2000) Persistent trigeminal artery: a unique anatomic specimen-analysis and therapeutic implications. Neurosurgery 47: 428–433

Tekdemir I, Tuccar E, Cubuk HE et al (1998) Branches of the intracavernous internal carotid artery and the blood supply of the intracavernous cranial nerves. Anat Anz 180:343–348

Tran-Dinh H (1987) Cavernous branches of the internal carotid artery: anatomy and nomenclature. Neurosurgery 20:205–210

Tubbs RS, Hansasuta A, Loukas M et al (2007) Branches of the petrous and cavernous segments of the internal carotid artery. Clin Anat 20:596–601

Tubbs RS, Hallock JD, Radcliff V et al (2011) Ligaments of the craniocervical junction. J Neurosurg Spine 14: 697–709

Weninger WJ, Prahmas D (2000) Compartments of the adult parasellar region. J Anat 197:681–686

Willinsky R, Lasjaunias P, Bernstein A (1987) Intracavernous branches of the internal carotid artery (ICA). Comprehensive review of their variations. Surg Radiol Anat 9:201–215

Yasargil MG (1984) Intracranial arteries. In: Microneurosurgery. Georg Thieme, Stuttgart

Yasuda A, Campero A, Martins C et al (2005) Microsurgical anatomy and approaches to the cavernous sinus. Neurosurgery 56(ONS Suppl 1):4–27

Zhang Y, Yu H, Shen BY et al (2012) Microsurgical anatomy of the abducens nerve. Surg Radiol Anat 34(1): 3–14

Index

P. Castelnuovo et al., *Surgical Anatomy of the Internal Carotid Artery*,
DOI 10.1007/978-3-642-29664-2, © Springer-Verlag Berlin Heidelberg 2013

F

G

H

I

J

L

MIX
Papier aus verantwortungsvollen Quellen
Paper from responsible sources
FSC® C105338

If you have any concerns about our products,
you can contact us on
ProductSafety@springernature.com

In case Publisher is established outside the EU,
the EU authorized representative is:
Springer Nature Customer Service Center GmbH
Europaplatz 3, 69115 Heidelberg, Germany

Printed by Libri Plureos GmbH
in Hamburg, Germany